PEDIATRIC
CARE PLANNING

Third Edition

Kathleen Morgan Speer, RN, PhD, CPNP
Pediatric Nurse Practitioner–Case Manager
Children's Medical Center of Dallas

D1354077

Springhouse Corporation
Springhouse, Pennsylvania

Staff

Vice President
Matthew Cahill

Clinical Director
Judith Schilling McCann, RN, MSN

Art Director
John Hubbard

Managing Editor
David Moreau

Clinical Project Manager
Patricia Kardish Fischer, RN, BSN

Editors
Karen Diamond, Margaret MacKay Eckman

Copy Editors
Cynthia C. Breuninger (manager), Priscilla DeWitt, Barbara Long, Brenna H. Mayer, Pamela Wingrod

Designers
Arlene Putterman (associate art director), Mary Ludwicki

Manufacturing
Deborah Meiris (director), Patricia K. Dorshaw (manager), Otto Mezei (book production manager)

Editorial Assistants
Beverly Lane, Liz Schaeffer

Indexer
Manjit K. Sahai

Printed in the United States of America.
PCP3-011198

℞ A member of the Reed Elsevier plc group

Library of Congress Cataloging-in-Publication Data

Speer, Kathleen Morgan
Pediatric care planning/Kathleen Morgan Speer. – 3rd ed.
        p.   cm.
    Includes bibliographical references and index.
    1. Pediatric nursing. 2. Nursing care plans. I. Title
    [DNLM: 1. Pediatric Nursing — methods. 2. Patient Care Planning. 3. Home Care Services. WY 159 S7415p 1999]
RJ245.S63 1999
610.73'62—DC21
DNLM/DLC   98-37811
ISBN 0-87434-943-5 (alk. paper)   CIP

Contents

Contributors and reviewers

Consultants

Marilyn Borgerson,
RN, MASN, CPE
Advanced Nurse Practitioner
Children's Medical Center of Dallas

Mary Breen,
RN, MSN
Advanced Nurse Practitioner
Children's Medical Center of Dallas

Carolanne Capron,
RN, BSN, MEd
Department Director
Wesley Medical Center
Wichita, Kans.

Linda Dillon,
RN, MSN, PhD
Instructor
Baylor University
Dallas

Paula Dimmitt,
RN, MS, CPNP
Advanced Nurse Practitioner
Children's Medical Center of Dallas

Michelle Faxel,
RN, MS
Director of Nursing Education
The Children's Hospital Medical Center of
Northern California
Oakland

Sally Finical,
RN, BSN
Staff Nurse
University of Arizona Medical Center
Tucson

Carol Gaggini,
RN, MN
Advanced Nurse Practitioner
Children's Medical Center of Dallas

Chris Geyer,
RN, MSN
Educator
Baylor University Medical Center
Dallas

Becky Johnston,
RN, BSN, MS
Instructor
El Centro Community College
Dallas

Lynn Kiewel,
RN, BSN
Former Staff Nurse
Children's Medical Center of Dallas

Diane Lesh,
RN, MSN
Nurse Practitioner
Dallas City Health Department

Kathy Morin,
RN, MSN
Clinical Nurse Specialist
Winnipeg (Canada) Children's Hospital

Claudia Odgers,
RN, MSN
Formerly, Quality Assurance Auditor
Blue Cross/Blue Shield
Topeka, Kans.

Nancy Quay,
RN, MSN
Former Clinical Nurse Specialist
Children's Medical Center of Dallas

Deborah Salsbury,
RN, BSN
Neonatal Intensive Care Unit Nurse
Stormont-Vail Regional Medical Center
Topeka, Kans.

Martha Sanford,
RN, PhD
Assistant Professor
Baylor University
Dallas

Bonnie Saucier,
RN, PhD
Formerly, Division Director of Health Sciences
Midwestern State University
Wichita Falls, Tex.

Suzanne Schuyler,
RN, MSN
Missionary and Former Clinical Nurse Specialist
Children's Medical Center of Dallas

Maureen Smith,
RN, BSN
Assistant Director
Children's Medical Center of Dallas

Kathy Soltis,
RN, BSN
Staff Nurse
Children's Medical Center of Dallas

Carolyn Swann,
RN, MSN
Director of Operations
Developmental Specialist and Neonatologist
Dallas

Lillian Waring,
RN, EdD
Former Associate Professor
Midwestern State University
Wichita Falls, Tex.

Penny Williams,
RN, MSN
Educator
Children's Medical Center of Dallas

Kelly Yager,
RN, BSN
Case Manager
Cigna
Dallas

Donna N. Roddy,
RN, BSN, MSN
Director, Practical Nursing and Surgical Technology
Chattanooga (Tenn.) State Technical Community
College

Reviewers

Sandra Faux,
RN, PhD
Associate Professor
Rush University College of Nursing
Chicago

Joanne M. Resnic,
RN, BSN, MBA
Implementation Manager
Paidos Health Management Services, Inc.
Paoli, Pa.

Virginia Richardson,
RN, DNS, CPNP
Assistant Dean for Student Affairs
Indiana University School of Nursing
Indianapolis

Acknowledgments

I give my many thanks to all the contributors of this book. They worked tirelessly from deadline to deadline.

To the physicians that I am privileged to be associated with—Drs. Shaw, Coble, Stenton, Blair, Rose, and Kalil—thank you for your support and collegiality.

To the staff of Children's, as always you encourage me to do my best.

To Gary, Shannon, Barbara, and Missy — I love you always.

Preface

Children are very different from adults. This is most evident to nurses when treating children diagnosed with illnesses similar to those of adults. Invariably, children respond quite differently. For this reason, nurses need special guidelines when planning the care of pediatric patients.

The third edition of this care planning book addresses many of the major illnesses affecting pediatric patients. However, it also includes important information on subjects not included or difficult to find in most pediatric care planning books — information on home health care, perioperative care, and care of children undergoing diagnostic procedures.

Given mounting interest in cost containment, home health care will become an increasingly important aspect of nursing. Providing care in the home requires that nurses work independently and without the immediate support of a hospital setting. Therefore, nurses caring for pediatric patients in the home need special knowledge and skills.

Likewise, nurses working with pediatric patients in surgical and postanesthesia care units also require special knowledge and skills concerning thermoregulation, fluid and electrolyte maintenance, anesthesia induction, and shock. And nurses dealing with children undergoing diagnostic studies must understand the specific procedures and know how to provide proper care throughout the procedure.

In this book, general plans of care are listed alphabetically by medical diagnosis within each body system section. Under each diagnostic head, a description of the illness appears followed by assessment guidelines, which are listed according to body system. A nursing diagnosis, which appears beneath the assessment information, includes a specific expected outcome and a listing of interventions and corresponding rationales. When more than one nursing diagnosis is given for a particular illness, the diagnoses are prioritized according to level of importance. Most plans of care also include information on home health teaching to share with the entire family. Several plans also include sample critical pathways, useful for guiding patient care.

Although this book is not meant to be exhaustive, it includes a wealth of information on pediatric care. Nurses at all academic and professional levels will find this a useful tool when working with children.

Kathleen Morgan Speer, RN, PhD, CPNP
Pediatric Nurse Practitioner–Case Manager
Children's Medical Center of Dallas

Introduction

Because children differ greatly from adults—both physiologically and psychologically — pediatric care is considered a specialty. To better respond to children's special needs, many of today's health care facilities are equipped with separate pediatric units in which nurses and other health care professionals can provide treatment based on their patients' individual needs. However, many other health care facilities do not have such highly specialized units. Consequently, in such settings, acutely ill children sometimes do not receive the special attention and care they require—and deserve.

Regardless of the clinical setting, nurses need practical, hands-on information to provide the best possible care for their pediatric patients. One of the best tools available to practicing nurses as well as to students and instructors is a set of concise, clinically relevant plans of care—such as those presented in this book.

Using this book

Pediatric Care Planning, Third Edition, includes individual plans of care that focus on various aspects of pediatric nursing, including acute illness in the hospital setting, perioperative care, diagnostic studies, and home care. These plans, newly updated and revised, provide essential information on specific disorders, treatments, procedures, and problems commonly encountered by nurses working with pediatric patients.

Parts 1 to 10 contain a series of plans alphabetized within separate body system categories, including a new plan on tuberculosis. Each plan of care begins with an introduction describing a medical disorder or treatment commonly encountered in pediatric patients. Also included in each plan is a list of assessment findings categorized according to body system and a series of NANDA-approved nursing diagnoses (the current list of NANDA-approved diagnoses appears in appendix D). After each nursing diagnosis come expected outcomes for that diagnosis and related interventions and rationales. A documentation checklist specific to the information covered completes each plan.

Part 11, "Perioperative care," consists of a series of plans dealing with various pediatric problems encountered during the preoperative and postoperative periods. Each plan of care includes an introduction describing the problem, assessment findings, nursing diagnoses with expected outcomes and related interventions and rationales, and a documentation checklist.

Part 12, "Diagnostic studies," focuses on plans for specific procedures used in diagnosing illnesses common to pediatric patients. Each plan begins with an introduction describing the procedure, followed by a list of possible indications for testing. Also included in each plan are nursing diagnoses with expected outcomes and related interventions and rationales as well as a documentation checklist.

Part 13, "Home health care," contains a series of plans for treating pediatric patients in the home setting. Similar to the plans of care in other sections, each plan includes an introduction describing the treatment, a list of assessment findings, nursing diagnoses with expected outcomes and related interventions and rationales, and a documentation checklist.

The appendices offer several useful, quick-reference charts and graphs essential to nurses working with pediatric patients in any clinical setting.

When using this book, nurses as well as students and instructors are urged to keep in mind that each patient is unique and that these plans are intended only as a general guide to pediatric care. Individual plans of care should be adapted to meet the special needs of each patient.

Part 1

Respiratory system

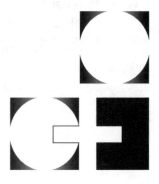

Asthma

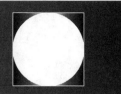

INTRODUCTION

Asthma is a reversible obstructive respiratory process, characterized by periods of exacerbation and remission, in which bronchial spasms obstruct the airways. One of the leading causes of chronic illness in childhood, this condition commonly appears before age 5 and, before adolescence, affects boys more than girls.

Although an asthma attack is commonly caused by an extrinsic factor (such as exercise or allergy to animal dander, pollen, smoke, or dust), such intrinsic factors as illness, stress, or fatigue also trigger attacks. Inflammation and edema accompany the bronchial spasms. Mucus cells produce thick secretions that are difficult to expectorate.

Treatment usually includes administration of steroids and bronchodilators, increased fluid intake, respiratory treatments (such as coughing and deep-breathing exercises and, if congestion is severe or pneumonia develops, chest physiotherapy), and nebulizer treatment. If an infection develops, treatment may also include antibiotics. Potential complications of the disorder include pneumothorax, heart failure, respiratory infections, emotional difficulties, and even death. In some cases, the child's condition can improve after adolescence or it can progress to emphysema later in adulthood.

ASSESSMENT

Respiratory
- Shortness of breath
- Prolonged expiratory wheezing
- Retractions
- Tachypnea
- Dry, hacking cough (most common sign)
- Rhonchi
- Nasal flaring

Cardiovascular
- Tachycardia

Neurologic
- Restlessness
- Anxiety
- Difficulty sleeping

Musculoskeletal
- Exercise intolerance

Integumentary
- Cyanosis
- Pallor

Psychosocial
- May not comply with treatment

NURSING DIAGNOSIS

Impaired gas exchange related to bronchial constriction

Expected outcome

The child will have improved gas exchange as evidenced by lack of wheezing and retractions, decreased coughing, pinkish skin color, capillary refill time of 3 to 5 seconds, and decreased restlessness.

Interventions

1. Encourage the child to perform coughing and deep-breathing exercises every 2 hours. Instruct him to take three or four deep breaths, then cough while in a sitting position.

2. Suction the child, as needed, to remove mucus from the airway.

Rationales

1. Coughing helps to clear mucus from the lungs, and deep breathing improves oxygenation. Sitting upright makes coughing easier.

2. Suctioning helps to remove secretions that the child cannot clear on his own.

3. If the child is severely congested or has pneumonia, perform chest physiotherapy three or four times each day.

3. Chest physiotherapy — a combination of postural drainage, chest percussion and vibration, and coughing and deep-breathing exercises — helps to loosen and eliminate secretions, reexpand lung tissue, and promote efficient use of respiratory muscles.

4. Assess the child's respiratory rate and auscultate for breath sounds.

4. This provides data to assess changes in breathing before and after treatment.

5. Place the child in high-Fowler's position or sitting with his chest forward.

5. These positions promote chest expansion.

6. Administer bronchodilators, such as albuterol, and steroids, such as methylprednisolone (Solu-Medrol), or inhaled steroids.

6. Bronchodilators relax bronchial smooth muscle; steroids reduce inflammation.

7. Administer humidified oxygen, as ordered.

7. Humidified oxygen improves oxygenation and helps loosen secretions.

8. Monitor the peak flow rate.

8. The peak flow rate indicates the degree of lung function impairment.

9. Remove potential allergens from the child's room.

9. Allergens can trigger asthma attacks.

NURSING DIAGNOSIS

Fatigue related to hypoxia

Expected outcome

The child will exhibit decreased restlessness and fatigue as evidenced by decreased agitation, uninterrupted sleep periods, no signs of respiratory distress, and increased ability to perform activities.

Interventions

1. Assess for signs of hypoxia or hypercapnia, including restlessness, agitation, cyanosis, increased heart rate, and increased respiratory rate.

2. Place the child in a supine position with the head of the bed elevated 45 degrees.

3. Provide adequate rest and quiet time. Cluster interventions accordingly.

Rationales

1. Early detection and prompt treatment of hypoxia and hypercapnia help prevent further restlessness and fatigue.

2. Placing the child in this position increases the lungs' ability to expand and improves oxygenation, thereby decreasing restlessness.

3. Rest and quiet time decrease the child's activity level, which decreases respiratory effort and lessens fatigue.

NURSING DIAGNOSIS

Altered nutrition: less than body requirements related to GI distress

Expected outcome

The child will have decreased GI distress as evidenced by decreased nausea and vomiting and improved nutritional intake (eating at least 80% of each meal).

(Text continues on page 6.)

Respiratory system

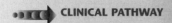

CLINICAL PATHWAY

Asthma

DRG: 98 (Pediatric asthma, ages 6 to 17)
Expected length of stay: 3 days

Plan	Preadmit/Emergency department	Day 1
Laboratory studies	• Blood chemistry studies	• Complete blood count and blood chemistry studies if not done in emergency department
Tests	• Pulse oximetry • Baseline peak flow meter	• Weight
Medications/I.V.		• Maintenance I.V. • I.V. steroids
Respiratory treatments	• Cool aerosol treatment • Oxygen administration	• Cool aerosol treatments • Continuous oximetry • Discontinue pulse oximetry if arterial oxygen saturation level by pulse oximetry (SpO_2) is greater than 93% on room air. • Oxygen therapy • Discontinue oxygen therapy if SpO_2 is greater than or equal to 93% and clinically stable. • Check peakflows and oxygen saturation level before treatments.
Osteopathic manipulative medicine (OMM)		• Rib raising • T_4 inhibition • Diaphragm release • OMM treatment daily • Documentation of severity of illness (asthma score)
Nutrition		• Diet for age • Encourage fluids.
Elimination		• Normal for age • Intake and output (I & O)
Activity		• As tolerated
Patient teaching		• Peak flow meter with asthma diary • Asthma education folder given and discussed • Patient guide
Discharge planning		• Consider case management to arrange home visit if needs identified.

Adapted with permission from Doctor's Hospital, Columbus, Ohio.

Day 2	Day 3	Outcome goals met
	• Check peakflows and oxygen saturation before OMM treatments.	
• Convert I.V. to normal saline well • I.V. steroids		• Respiratory rate appropriate for age
	• Begin oral steroids.	• Stable on discharge medications for 12 hr
• Re-evaluate for cool aerosol treatments per respiratory care professional. • Check peakflows and oxygen saturation before OMM treatment.	• Steroid/bronchodilators/cromolyn sodium (by cool aerosol treatments or metered-dose inhaler) • Treatment protocol has been followed.	• Peak flow: 80% predicted • Pulse oximetry greater than 97% on room air for 24 hr
• OMM treatment performed once a day		
• Diet for age • Encourage fluids.	• Regular diet	• Tolerates regular diet
• Normal for age • I & O	• Urine and stool output within normal limits	• Urine and stool output normal for age
• Up as tolerated • Evaluate exercise tolerance.	• Up as tolerated	• Maintain normal activity levels without shortness of breath.
• Proper use of inhaler with spacer • Disease process • Environmental triggers • Asthma booklet	• Review • Physical therapy: Family demonstrates proper use of inhaler and quantity to be used. • Provide learning pamphlet "Asthma Resources." • Drug education sheets – Albuterol – Intal • Asthma diary	• Patient/family verbalizes: – signs and symptoms of disease process and complications – medications (name, dose, adverse effects, purpose, schedule, food/drug interactions) – understanding of peak flow meter asthma zones and action – environmental control plan – asthma diary.
• Assess need for home nebulizer.	• Discharge day 3 • Instruct parents to bring asthma diary to all doctor's visits.	

Interventions

1. Serve the child small, frequent meals (five or six per day) consisting of foods he prefers.

2. Provide bland, low-fat foods. Use color as a guide; white-colored foods — such as toast, potatoes, and pudding made with low-fat milk — tend to be bland.

3. Avoid foods likely to cause an allergic response, such as eggs, wheat, and chocolate.

Rationales

1. Small, frequent meals require less energy to digest and do not overfill the stomach, which can decrease lung expansion. Providing the child with some of his favorite foods helps ensure adequate intake.

2. Spicy and high-fat foods cause GI distress and are not easily digested.

3. These foods may trigger an allergy attack in a child sensitive to them.

NURSING DIAGNOSIS

Risk for fluid volume deficit related to loss of fluid from the respiratory tract

Expected outcome

The child will maintain adequate hydration as evidenced by good skin turgor and a urine output of 1 to 2 ml/kg/hour.

Interventions

1. Assess the child's skin turgor, and monitor urine output every 4 hours.

2. Encourage the child to drink three to eight 8-oz (240-ml) glasses of fluid per day, depending on his age.

Rationales

1. Such assessment and monitoring helps to determine the level of hydration and the need for additional fluids.

2. The child needs enough fluid to maintain hydration and acid-base balance and to prevent shock.

NURSING DIAGNOSIS

Noncompliance related to loss of self-control

Expected outcome

The child will comply with medical treatment and nursing care as evidenced by taking all medications correctly and participating in routine treatment.

Interventions

1. As appropriate, allow the child to participate in decisions concerning routine treatment, such as times for chest physiotherapy and meals.

2. Explain to the child all procedures, such as laboratory workups and chest physiotherapy, and the reason he needs medication. Explain that laboratory workups allow the doctors and nurses to evaluate the effectiveness of medications and that chest physiotherapy helps loosen lung secretions to enable him to cough more effectively and breathe more easily.

Rationales

1. Giving the child some control over simple routines increases feelings of self-control and improves compliance with the overall treatment regimen.

2. Explanations help decrease fear and feelings of loss of control.

Nursing diagnosis

Knowledge deficit related to home care

Expected outcome

The child and parents will express an understanding of home care instructions.

Interventions

1. Explain the physiology of the disease to the child and parents.

2. Based on the child's history, teach about factors that may lead to asthma attacks, such as allergens, infections, exercise, weather changes, and stress.

3. Teach the child and parents about signs and symptoms of respiratory infection, including fever, respiratory distress, wheezing, and tachypnea.

4. Teach the child and family about the importance of taking all prescribed medications and about their possible adverse effects. Explain that:
• metaproterenol (Alupent), a bronchodilator, may cause some GI distress.
• albuterol (Proventil), a bronchodilator, should cause no adverse effects.
• corticosteroids (anti-inflammatory agents) may cause growth retardation, GI distress, altered immune response, and water retention (if given orally or I.V.).

5. Teach the child how to inhale medication through a metered-dose inhaler, a spacer device, or both, as appropriate.

6. Tell the parents and child to avoid antihistamines during an attack.

7. Teach the importance of maintaining activity levels appropriate for the child's condition.

8. Teach the parents and, if appropriate, the child how to monitor the peak flow rate and to report any decrease to the doctor.

Rationales

1. Understanding the disease may help the child and parents comply with the treatment regimen.

2. Such teaching may help decrease the number of future attacks.

3. Early detection and treatment of respiratory infection may prevent or lessen the respiratory distress associated with asthma attacks.

4. Compliance with the medication regimen ensures stable blood drug levels, thereby ensuring control over asthma attacks.

5. These devices promote delivery of the full dose of medication; a young child who is unable to use a metered-dose inhaler by itself can use a spacer device with the inhaler to help ensure the proper dosage.

6. Antihistamines make secretions thick and difficult to expectorate and can increase coughing.

7. Maintaining physical fitness is important to the child's normal development. Unless he is having an acute asthma attack, the child should maintain his usual activity level.

8. A drop in peak flow rate indicates the need for a change in medication and dosage.

Documentation checklist

During the hospital stay, document:
❑ child's status and assessment findings upon admission
❑ changes in the child's status
❑ pertinent laboratory and diagnostic findings
❑ child's and parents' abilities to manage an acute asthma attack
❑ fluid intake and output
❑ nutritional intake
❑ child's response to treatment
❑ child's and parents' reactions to chronic illness and hospital stay
❑ patient and family teaching guidelines
❑ discharge planning guidelines.

Bronchiolitis

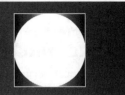

INTRODUCTION

Bronchiolitis, an inflammatory viral infection of the bronchioles, results in acute airway obstruction and decreased gas exchange in the alveoli. Commonly caused by respiratory syncytial virus (RSV), this disorder usually occurs in children ages 2 to 12 months, especially during the winter and early spring.

The infection is characterized by mucosal edema, increased mucus secretions, bronchiolar obstruction, and overdistention of the alveoli. Potential complications of the disorder include chronic lung disease and even death.

ASSESSMENT

Respiratory
- Tachypnea
- Retractions
- Nasal flaring
- Dyspnea
- Shallow respirations
- Decreased breath sounds
- Crackles
- Wheezing
- Prolonged expiration
- Cough

Cardiovascular
- Tachycardia

Neurologic
- Irritability
- Difficulty sleeping

Gastrointestinal
- Feeding difficulty

Integumentary
- Elevated temperature
- Cyanosis

Psychosocial
- Anxiety

NURSING DIAGNOSIS

Impaired gas exchange related to bronchiolar edema and increased mucus production

Expected outcome

The child will have improved gas exchange as evidenced by ease of respiration and pinkish skin.

Interventions

1. Provide a high-humidity environment by placing the child in a mist tent or cool humidification device.

2. Administer oxygen by face mask, nasal cannula, or oxygen tent, as ordered.

3. Position the child with his head and chest elevated and neck slightly extended.

4. Perform chest physiotherapy every 4 hours, as ordered.

5. Administer bronchodilators, as ordered.

6. Suction the child, as needed, to remove secretions.

7. Administer antiviral agents, as ordered.

Rationales

1. Cool mist from a mist tent or Croupette helps liquefy secretions and decreases bronchiolar edema.

2. Oxygen helps relieve the restlessness associated with respiratory distress and hypoxia.

3. This position maintains an open airway and eases respiration by decreasing pressure on the diaphragm.

4. Chest physiotherapy helps loosen and remove mucus that may be blocking the small airways.

5. Although commonly used to treat muscle spasms, bronchodilators also effectively treat bronchiolar edema.

6. Removing secretions helps clear the bronchioles, improving gas exchange.

7. Antiviral agents, such as respiratory syncytial virus immune globulin (RespiGam), are used to treat RSV; ribavirin (Virazole) has also been used, although its efficacy is questionable.

8. Promote adequate rest by decreasing noise and lights and providing warmth and comfort.

8. Adequate rest decreases the respiratory distress associated with bronchiolitis.

9. Assess the child's respiratory rate and rhythm hourly. If the child has increased respiratory distress, auscultate for breath sounds, perform chest physiotherapy, and inform the respiratory therapist.

9. Frequent assessments ensure adequate respiratory function.

10. Monitor the child's apical pulse; if you detect tachycardia (based on the child's age), notify the doctor at once.

10. Tachycardia may result from hypoxia or the effects of bronchodilator use.

NURSING DIAGNOSIS

Risk for fluid volume deficit related to increased water loss through exhalation and decreased fluid intake

Expected outcome

The child will maintain fluid balance as evidenced by a urine output of 1 to 2 ml/kg/hour and good skin turgor.

Interventions

1. Administer I.V. fluids, as ordered.

2. Ensure that the child receives adequate rest.

3. Monitor the child's fluid intake and output carefully.

4. Assess for signs of dehydration, including weight loss, pallor, poor skin turgor, dry mucous membranes, oliguria, and increased pulse rate.

5. Increase the child's oral fluid intake when the acute period has subsided.

Rationales

1. I.V. fluids are used to hydrate the child until the crisis has passed.

2. Resting allows the child's respiratory rate to return to baseline levels, decreasing the amount of water lost through exhalation.

3. Careful monitoring ensures adequate hydration. If urine output decreases, the child may require additional fluids.

4. These signs suggest that the child is not receiving enough fluids.

5. Fluids help to liquefy secretions.

NURSING DIAGNOSIS

Hyperthermia related to infection

Expected outcome

The child will maintain a body temperature of less than 100° F (37.8° C). (Specific temperature depends on method used to take temperature.)

Interventions

1. Maintain a cool environment by using lightweight pajamas and covers and maintaining the room temperature between 72° and 75° F (22° and 24° C).

2. Administer antipyretics, as ordered.

Rationales

1. A cool environment helps to reduce body temperature through radiant heat loss.

2. Antipyretics, such as acetaminophen (Tylenol), effectively reduce fever.

3. Monitor the child's temperature every 1 to 2 hours for sudden elevation.

4. Administer antimicrobials, if ordered.

5. Give the child tepid (98.6° F [37° C]) sponge baths to relieve fever.

3. Sudden elevation in temperature may result in a seizure.

4. Antimicrobials may be ordered to treat the underlying causative organism. Antibiotics usually are not ordered to treat RSV.

5. Sponge baths with tepid water effectively cool the body through conduction.

NURSING DIAGNOSIS

Social isolation related to isolation precautions

Expected outcome

The child will maintain social contacts despite being isolated because of his respiratory condition.

Interventions

1. Explain to the child (if appropriate) and parents the purpose and nature of isolation, including details about unfamiliar surroundings and the use of masks and gowns.

2. Introduce yourself upon entering the child's room.

3. Teach the parents and child (if appropriate) how to use the call system.

4. Assess the child at least hourly for any changes in his condition.

5. As appropriate, provide diversional activities, such as toys, books, television, and music. If the child is receiving oxygen, avoid toys that could emit sparks (for example, any electrical toy).

6. Encourage the parents to be with the child as much as possible and to take part in caregiving.

Rationales

1. Such explanations are necessary to avoid frightening the child.

2. The child and parents often have difficulty distinguishing staff personnel because of the required isolation clothing.

3. A call system lets the family communicate a need for assistance.

4. The child needs close monitoring to detect changes even though he is in isolation.

5. Such diversions keep the child stimulated and distracted when in isolation. Toys that could emit sparks could trigger a fire.

6. Parents provide a major source of socialization for the child in isolation.

NURSING DIAGNOSIS

Fatigue related to respiratory distress

Expected outcome

The child will rest at least 1 hour in the morning and afternoon.

Interventions

1. To help decrease the child's fatigue, provide rest periods every 2 hours. Also, bathe the child, change the bed linens, and perform neurologic checks during the same visit to allow for uninterrupted periods of rest.

2. Provide a quiet environment.

Rationales

1. The child needs adequate rest to prevent fatigue from increasing respiratory distress.

2. Unnecessary noise and activity may tire the child, increasing respiratory distress.

NURSING DIAGNOSIS

Altered nutrition: less than body requirements related to increased metabolic needs

Expected outcome

The child has improved nutritional intake as evidenced by consuming at least 80% of each meal.

Interventions

1. Provide small, frequent meals that include foods the child prefers.

2. Provide a diet high in calories and protein.

Rationales

1. Eating small, frequent meals requires less energy expenditure and respiratory use. The child will eat more of each meal if the meal includes favorite foods.

2. A high-protein, high-calorie diet is necessary to meet the child's increased metabolic needs.

NURSING DIAGNOSIS

Anxiety (child and parent) related to lack of knowledge about the child's condition

Expected outcome

The child and parents will be less anxious as evidenced by expressing an understanding of the child's condition.

Interventions

1. Assess the parents' and (if appropriate) the child's understanding of the child's condition and prescribed treatment regimen.

2. Encourage the parents to stay with the child.

3. Explain all procedures in developmentally appropriate terms.

4. Provide emotional support to the parents during the hospital stay.

Rationales

1. Such assessment serves as a basis on which to begin teaching.

2. Staying with the child allows the parents to provide support and helps decrease anxiety in both the child and his parents.

3. Providing explanations before procedures and throughout the hospital stay decreases anxiety from misunderstanding and a lack of knowledge.

4. Hospitalization poses a crisis situation. Listening to the parents' concerns and feelings helps them to deal with the crisis.

NURSING DIAGNOSIS

Knowledge deficit related to home care

Expected outcome

The parents will express an understanding of home care instructions.

Interventions

1. Teach the parents and child (if appropriate) how and when to administer medications, including details about dosages and adverse reactions.

2. Explain the signs and symptoms of respiratory distress and infection, including fever, dyspnea, tachypnea, a change in sputum color, and wheezing.

3. Explain the importance of adequate rest for the child.

4. Teach the importance of adequate nutrition and hydration, stressing the need for plenty of fluids and a high-calorie diet.

5. Teach the importance of providing a humidified environment with cool mist.

Rationales

1. Understanding the importance of maintaining a consistent medication regimen may help the parents to comply with the child's overall treatment. Knowing what adverse reactions to expect should prompt the parents to call for assistance when needed.

2. Such knowledge should prompt the parents to seek medical advice and attention when needed.

3. After infection, the child requires frequent rest periods to aid recovery and prevent a relapse of the infection.

4. Fluids help to liquefy secretions. A high-calorie diet helps to replace calories expended in fighting the disease.

5. Humidified air helps to thin secretions. Cool, humidified air from a mist tent is safer than the warm air of a vaporizer, which can cause burns.

Documentation checklist

During the hospital stay, document:

❏ child's status and assessment findings upon admission
❏ changes in the child's status
❏ pertinent laboratory and diagnostic findings
❏ fluid intake and output
❏ nutritional intake
❏ child's response to treatments
❏ child's and parents' reactions to the illness and hospital stay
❏ patient and family teaching guidelines
❏ discharge planning guidelines.

Bronchopulmonary dysplasia

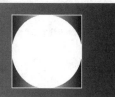

INTRODUCTION

Bronchopulmonary dysplasia (BPD) is a chronic, progressive pulmonary condition of unknown etiology characterized by pulmonary edema, bronchiolar and alveolar hypertrophy, and a prolonged need for oxygen. BPD typically occurs in premature infants with respiratory distress syndrome who have undergone endotracheal intubation, administration of high concentrations of oxygen, and high positive-pressure ventilation for prolonged periods. There is a 25% mortality rate up to age 1.

No cure exists, so treatment is supportive, usually focused on managing the symptoms. Potential complications include chronic respiratory disease, frequent respiratory infections, pneumothorax, heart failure, pulmonary hypertension, and sudden infant death syndrome.

ASSESSMENT

Respiratory
• Respiratory distress
• Retractions
• Dyspnea
• Crackles
• Rhonchi
• Wheezing
• Atelectasis

Cardiovascular
• Prolonged capillary refill time
• Right-sided heart failure

Gastrointestinal
• Difficulty feeding
• Weight gain or loss

Musculoskeletal
• Fatigue
• Delayed growth

Integumentary
• Pallor
• Circumoral cyanosis

Psychosocial
• Delayed development

NURSING DIAGNOSIS

Impaired gas exchange related to atelectasis

Expected outcome

The child will have improved gas exchange as evidenced by lack of wheezing, decreased retractions, pink skin color, and a capillary refill time of 3 to 5 seconds.

Interventions

1. Assess the child's respiratory and fluid status, noting skin color, respiratory effort, retractions, capillary refill time, breath sounds, secretions, vital signs, and edema every hour for 4 hours. Report any deviations from baseline data.

2. Perform chest physiotherapy every 4 hours for as long as tolerated and gentle suctioning four times daily or as needed.

3. Administer oxygen, as ordered. Monitor transcutaneous oxygen levels, if necessary (levels should be in the high 90s).

Rationales

1. Monitoring is essential because children with BPD are susceptible to lower respiratory tract infections, hypertension, and respiratory failure.

2. Chest physiotherapy helps loosen mucus in the lungs and assists with expectoration. Suctioning eliminates excess mucus from the airway.

3. BPD may cause intermittent or persistent hypoxia, requiring oxygen therapy.

4. Administer bronchodilators, as ordered.

4. Bronchodilators may be ordered to treat acute respiratory infections or to improve the passage of air to the alveoli.

5. Monitor the child's fluid intake and output carefully.

5. Monitoring fluid intake and output helps maintain adequate hydration, which is necessary to help liquefy secretions.

6. Administer diuretics, as ordered.

6. Diuretics help improve respiratory function by decreasing fluid retention and the risk of pulmonary edema.

7. Monitor electrolyte levels.

7. Such monitoring is essential, especially if diuretics are given; hypokalemia may occur.

8. Increase the child's fluid intake if not contraindicated.

8. Increased fluid intake helps liquefy secretions.

Nursing diagnosis

Altered nutrition: less than body requirements related to increased metabolic rate and high caloric demands

Expected outcome

The child will meet caloric requirements as evidenced by weight gain.

Interventions

1. Weigh the child daily at the same time (usually before the morning meal), without clothes and preferably with the same scale.

2. Consult the hospital dietitian when planning the child's meals, especially when the child needs high-calorie supplements or formulas.

3. Spend extra time with the child during feedings, as needed, to allow for frequent burping and resting.

4. Supplement oral feedings with nasogastric (NG) tube feedings, as needed and during the night.

5. Check placement of the NG tube before feeding (aspirate and inject air).

Rationales

1. Weighing the child on a daily basis detects any weight gain or loss.

2. A dietitian can help determine the child's nutritional needs based on age-appropriate developmental data. To increase the child's calorie intake, the dietitian may suggest small, frequent meals of high-calorie supplements and formulas, such as medium-chain triglyceride oil in formula, rather than increasing the total volume consumed.

3. Children with BPD sometimes tire during feedings and need extra time to complete feedings.

4. If the child cannot consume enough calories through oral feedings, NG tube feedings help ensure that he maintains weight.

5. Verifying that the NG tube is in the stomach helps prevent aspiration.

Nursing diagnosis

Altered growth and development related to chronic illness, prematurity, or prolonged hospital stay

Expected outcome

The child will achieve developmental milestones despite his prematurity or chronic illness.

Interventions

1. Assess the child's developmental status using standardized developmental tools, such as the Washington Guide or Denver Developmental Screening Test II. Consult a child development expert if one is available.

2. When possible, ensure that the same staff members care for the child.

3. Develop an individualized plan that includes visual, auditory, tactile, and social stimulation. Post the developmental plan at the child's bedside for all caregivers to see.

4. Assess the child's response to sound and to color and shapes at varying distances to determine if the child has any hearing or vision impairment. Report any evidence of such impairment immediately.

Rationales

1. Children with BPD are at risk for developmental delays because of prolonged hospitalization and decreased oxygen intake; they require careful assessment to identify any lags. A child development expert can help assess delays and plan therapy.

2. A child cared for by the same staff members is more likely to progress developmentally.

3. A specialized plan meets the child's unique developmental needs. Posting the plan ensures that all personnel who come in contact with the child can provide consistent stimulation.

4. Developmental delays can result from hearing or vision impairment, so early detection is essential.

NURSING DIAGNOSIS

Risk for altered parenting related to chronic illness

Expected outcome

The parents will bond effectively with the child as evidenced by expressing positive feelings and demonstrating positive interactive behaviors, such as touching, stroking, holding, and making direct eye contact.

Interventions

1. Encourage the parents to participate in the child's care.

2. Reinforce supportive behaviors, such as touching and holding the child.

3. Discuss with the parents what makes their child an individual. Allow them to express their concerns about the child's illness.

4. Help the parents to identify stressors (such as providing constant care for their child) and solve problems. Refer them to appropriate social service agencies or support groups, as needed.

Rationales

1. Direct participation in the child's care promotes bonding.

2. Reinforcement encourages the parents to repeat such behaviors.

3. Viewing the child as an individual helps to increase bonding between the parents and their child. Expressing concerns helps the parents vent their feelings and cope with the situation.

4. Because stressors may be overwhelming, the parents may need help to deal with the pressures brought on by the child's illness. Social service agencies and support groups provide emotional and financial support.

NURSING DIAGNOSIS

Risk for impaired skin integrity related to irritation from NG tube feedings

Expected outcome

The child will maintain skin integrity as evidenced by pinkish, intact skin around the nares and cheeks.

Interventions

1. Apply a skin barrier, such as Stomahesive, to both cheeks and secure tape to the barrier and cannula.

2. Assess and clean the skin by removing the skin barrier, as needed.

3. Change the child's body position every 2 hours.

Rationales

1. The skin barrier helps prevent the tape from irritating the child's skin.

2. Regular assessment and skin care help prevent skin breakdown.

3. Changing the child's body position helps to prevent skin breakdown.

NURSING DIAGNOSIS

Anxiety (parent) related to fear and lack of knowledge about the child's illness

Expected outcome

The parents will express less anxiety about the child's condition and less fear about procedures.

Interventions

1. Assess the parents' understanding of their child's condition — including that the condition is chronic — and prescribed treatment.

2. Explain all treatments, procedures, and equipment.

3. Provide emotional support to the parents during the child's hospital stay.

Rationales

1. Such assessment provides a basis to begin teaching and to provide ongoing teaching.

2. Explanations provided beforehand and throughout the hospital stay provide knowledge and help clear up misunderstanding, reducing anxiety.

3. Emotional support helps the parents cope with the crisis of hospitalization.

NURSING DIAGNOSIS

Knowledge deficit related to home care

Expected outcome

The parents will express an understanding of home care instructions and demonstrate home care procedures.

Interventions

1. Explain to the parents the importance of exposing the child to cool, humidified air.

2. Teach the parents the signs and symptoms of respiratory distress, including dyspnea, tachypnea, cyanosis, and retractions.

3. Teach the parents how to administer oxygen safely; include detailed instructions on rate and frequency.

4. Teach the parents how and when to administer medications; include information on dosages and adverse reactions.

Rationales

1. Humidified air liquefies secretions and promotes breathing. Cool, humidified air from a humidifier or nebulizer is safer than warm air from a vaporizer, which can cause burns or a buildup of mold.

2. Knowing such signs and symptoms should prompt the parents to seek medical help when needed.

3. Children with BPD usually require continuous oxygen administration. Parents must have firsthand knowledge to provide safe, appropriate care.

4. Parents need to know how to administer medications consistently and safely. Such knowledge also helps ensure compliance with the medication regimen.

5. Ensure that the parents attend a cardiopulmonary resuscitation class before the child is discharged.

6. Teach the parents how to administer feedings if the child is discharged with an NG tube. Include specific information about tube placement, feeding solutions, and indications of aspiration.

5. Because children with BPD are at increased risk for respiratory distress, parents must know how to provide prompt care in an emergency.

6. Because children with BPD are prone to aspiration, they often require feedings by an NG or, in some cases, a gastrostomy tube. Parents must know how to initiate feedings and monitor their progress and what to do if aspiration should occur.

Documentation checklist

During the hospital stay, document:
- ❏ child's status and assessment findings upon admission
- ❏ changes in the child's status
- ❏ pertinent laboratory and diagnostic findings
- ❏ fluid intake and output
- ❏ nutritional intake
- ❏ child's response to treatment
- ❏ child's and parents' reactions to the illness and hospital stay
- ❏ patient and family teaching guidelines
- ❏ discharge planning guidelines.

Respiratory system

Croup

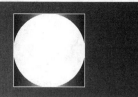

INTRODUCTION

Also known as laryngotracheobronchitis, croup is an infection of the upper and lower airways that causes subglottic edema and inflammation of the vocal cords, which sometimes results in respiratory distress (laryngospasm, dyspnea, and barking cough), stridor, retractions, and cyanosis. It usually follows an upper respiratory tract infection. The most common causes include respiratory syncytial virus, adenovirus, and parainfluenza virus.

Typically affecting children between ages 3 months and 3 years, croup can be life-threatening if not treated. Treatment usually includes administration of antibiotics and fluids and exposure to humidified air to maintain respiration. A child with severely compromised respiratory status may require intubation or tracheotomy.

ASSESSMENT

Respiratory
• History of cold symptoms lasting 1 to 2 days
• Signs and symptoms of respiratory distress
• Dyspnea
• Retractions
• Cyanosis
• Barking cough
• Whooping sound on inspiration

Cardiovascular
• Tachycardia

Neurologic
• Altered level of consciousness
• Restlessness
• Headache
• Confusion
• Disturbed sleep

Gastrointestinal
• Feeding difficulty

Integumentary
• Elevated temperature (usually less than 102° F [39° C], depending on method used to measure temperature)

Psychosocial
• Anxiety

NURSING DIAGNOSIS

Ineffective breathing pattern related to upper airway edema and thickened secretions

Expected outcome

The child will maintain a patent airway as evidenced by relief of respiratory distress.

Interventions

1. Assess the child's respiratory status frequently or continuously for signs and symptoms of increased respiratory distress and obstruction, including increased respiratory rate, stridor, retractions, nasal flaring, prolonged expirations, cyanosis, confusion, restlessness, decreased breath sounds, tachycardia, and barking cough.

2. Provide cool, humidified air with a mist tent, cool humidification device, or face mask.

3. Administer oxygen, as ordered.

Rationales

1. Signs and symptoms of increased respiratory distress may indicate that the obstruction is worsening. A rapid, rising respiratory rate with an increased heart rate may be the first sign of hypoxia.

2. Cool mist helps to liquefy secretions.

3. Oxygen may be ordered to alleviate hypoxia and restlessness. However, because oxygen use may mask the early signs of hypoxia and increasing obstruction with subsequent hypercapnia, it should only be used to treat known hypoxia.

4. Administer aerosolized racemic epinephrine, as ordered; watch for signs of rebound obstruction.	**4.** Racemic epinephrine reduces swelling of the subglottic mucosa. Because the drug's effects are short term, it may result in rebound obstruction.
5. If the child can tolerate it, place him in high-Fowler's position.	**5.** This position increases lung capacity by decreasing diaphragmatic pressure on the lungs.

NURSING DIAGNOSIS

Risk for fluid volume deficit related to decreased oral intake

Expected outcome

The child will maintain fluid balance as evidenced by good skin turgor and a urine output of 1 to 2 ml/kg/hour.

Interventions

1. Assess the child's ability to tolerate fluids (swallowing, choking, or coughing).

2. Administer and monitor I.V. fluids, as ordered.

3. Carefully monitor the child's fluid intake and output.

4. Assess the child for signs of dehydration, including poor skin turgor, dry mucous membranes, sunken fontanels, and sunken eyes.

Rationales

1. The child's ability to tolerate fluids may be complicated by throat discomfort, increased respiratory rate, or vomiting.

2. I.V. fluids may be ordered to decrease the physical effort associated with oral feeding. If the child has severe respiratory distress, oral fluids are contraindicated because of the risk of aspiration and vomiting.

3. Careful monitoring allows detection of early signs of dehydration, such as decreased urine output.

4. The child's fluid intake may need to be adjusted if signs of dehydration appear.

NURSING DIAGNOSIS

Anxiety (child) related to respiratory distress and hospital stay

Expected outcome

The child will be less anxious as evidenced by restful sleep periods and a stable respiratory status.

Interventions

1. Allow the child to assume a comfortable position during treatment with humidified air or oxygen. For example, place the child on his side or elevate the head of the bed.

2. Postpone all tests and procedures that are not urgent until the child's respiratory status has improved.

3. Encourage the parents to stay with the child.

Rationales

1. The child should be made as comfortable and secure as possible to alleviate anxiety during treatment because discomfort may increase the child's respiratory rate and cause stridor. The child may tolerate a mist tent or cool humidification device better than a face mask.

2. The child's anxiety level may already be high because of his increased respiratory distress; unfamiliar tests and procedures may compound the problem.

3. The parents' presence can help reduce anxiety, helping to stabilize the child's respiratory rate.

4. Provide familiar objects, such as toys and blankets, for the child to keep with him in the mist tent or Croupette. Avoid toys that emit sparks if the child is receiving oxygen.

4. Familiar objects provide a sense of security and help relieve some of the anxiety associated with the new and strange environment.

5. Provide a quiet, calm atmosphere.

5. A quiet, calm atmosphere helps to decrease anxiety and promote normal respirations.

NURSING DIAGNOSIS

Anxiety (parent) related to fear and lack of knowledge about the child's condition.

Expected outcome

The parents will express less anxiety about and greater understanding of their child's condition and less fear about procedures.

Interventions

1. Assess the parent's understanding of their child's condition and treatments as well as their possibly fearful reaction to the sounds their child makes when in respiratory distress.

2. Explain to the parents all procedures, treatments, and equipment.

3. Provide emotional support to the parents during the child's hospital stay.

Rationales

1. Such assessment allows you to develop a teaching plan to help the parents understand their child's condition and treatments, relieving some of their fear.

2. Explanations provided beforehand and throughout the hospital stay provide knowledge and help clear up misunderstanding, reducing the parents' anxiety.

3. Emotional support helps the parents cope with the crisis of hospitalization.

NURSING DIAGNOSIS

Knowledge deficit related to home care

Expected outcome

The parents will express an understanding of home care instructions.

Interventions

1. Teach parents how and when to administer medications; include information on dosages and adverse reactions.

2. Explain to the parents the signs and symptoms of respiratory distress and infection, including fever, dyspnea, tachypnea, yellowish or greenish sputum, and wheezing.

3. Explain the importance of adequate rest for the child.

Rationales

1. Understanding the medication regimen may help parents to comply with the child's overall treatment. Knowing what adverse reactions may result from the medications allows the parents to seek medical help when necessary.

2. Knowing how to recognize signs and symptoms allows the parents to seek medical help when necessary.

3. After infection, the child needs frequent rest periods to promote recovery and prevent relapses.

4. Teach about the importance of adequate hydration and nutrition. Explain that the child will need to drink two to four 8-oz (240-ml) glasses of fluid daily (depending on the child's renal and cardiovascular status) and eat high-calorie meals.

5. Teach about the importance of providing a humidified environment using cool mist.

6. If the child has an attack during cold weather, suggest the parents wrap the child in a warm blanket or coat and take him outside.

4. Fluids help liquefy secretions. A high-calorie diet helps replace calories expended to fight the disease.

5. Humidified air helps to thin secretions. Cool, humidified air from a nebulizer is safer than the warm air of a vaporizer, which can cause burns and promote mold buildup.

6. Cold air decreases swelling and croup-like cough.

Documentation checklist

During the hospital stay, document:
- ❏ child's status and assessment findings upon admission
- ❏ changes in the child's status
- ❏ pertinent laboratory and diagnostic findings
- ❏ fluid intake and output
- ❏ nutritional intake
- ❏ child's response to treatment
- ❏ child's and parents' reactions to the illness and hospital stay
- ❏ patient and family teaching guidelines
- ❏ discharge planning guidelines.

Cystic fibrosis

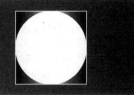

INTRODUCTION

An autosomal recessive disease, cystic fibrosis (CF) is the most common life-threatening genetic disease of white children in the United States. CF affects the function of the respiratory and other body systems, causing the mucus-secreting exocrine glands to produce increased, thickened secretions. Typically, these thick secretions obstruct the functioning and decrease cell membrane transfer of such organs as the lungs, pancreas, and liver, resulting in difficult breathing, chronic respiratory infections, nutritional deficits, and cirrhosis.

The disease, which varies in severity, is associated with many complications, including chronic respiratory infections, meconium ileus (at birth), pancreatitis, gallstones, pneumothorax, rectal prolapse, and male infertility. Treatment includes pulmonary therapy, administration of pancreatic enzymes and vitamins, and a diet high in calories and protein. Although many children survive into adulthood (median survival age is 28 years), more males survive than females.

ASSESSMENT

Respiratory
- Wheezing
- Nonproductive cough
- Hemoptysis
- Atelectasis
- Dyspnea
- Barrel chest
- Tracheobronchitis
- Tachypnea

Gastrointestinal
- Failure to thrive
- Foul-smelling, bulky, loose stools or chronic diarrhea
- Increased appetite
- Ulcers

Genitourinary
- Vaginal infections

Musculoskeletal
- Fatigue
- Short stature

Eye, ear, nose, and throat
- Sinusitis
- Nasal polyps

Integumentary
- Bruising
- Cyanosis
- Salty-tasting skin
- Digital clubbing (in severe cases)

Psychosocial
- Delayed development
- Anxiety
- Anger (potential)
- Depression (potential)

NURSING DIAGNOSIS

Impaired gas exchange related to increased mucus production

Expected outcome

The child will have increased mobilization of mucus secretions as evidenced by decreased respiratory distress, cyanosis, and coughing.

Interventions

1. Perform chest physiotherapy as needed, up to every 4 hours.

2. Administer humidified oxygen by face mask; do not use a mist tent.

Rationales

1. Chest physiotherapy helps mobilize secretions, maintain lung capacity, and increase oxygenation.

2. Humidity loosens and thins secretions and oxygen increases tissue aeration. Because the child's stimulus to breathe often depends on low oxygen levels, highly concentrated oxygen should not be used. The warm, moist environment of a mist tent may promote bacterial growth.

3. Assess the child's respiratory status every 4 hours.

3. Frequent respiratory assessments allow for early detection of changes in the child's condition.

4. Instruct the child to perform deep-breathing exercises every 4 hours.

4. Deep-breathing exercises help to increase lung expansion.

5. Administer bronchodilators by mouth, nebulizer, or metered-dose inhaler with a spacer device, as ordered.

5. Bronchodilators help thin secretions and promote lung expansion. A spacer device ensures the child inhales the full dose of medication.

NURSING DIAGNOSIS

Risk for infection related to increased mucus production

Expected outcome

The child will have no signs of infection as evidenced by lack of fever, chills, and increasing respiratory distress.

Interventions

1. Administer antibiotics, as ordered.

2. Assess vital signs for evidence of increased respiratory rate, dyspnea, and cyanosis.

3. Monitor the white blood cell (WBC) count.

Rationales

1. Antibiotics may be ordered to help fight infection.

2. These changes indicate a worsening infection.

3. An elevated WBC count indicates infection.

NURSING DIAGNOSIS

Altered nutrition: less than body requirements related to reduced absorption of nutrients

Expected outcome

The child will have an improved nutritional status as evidenced by minimal weight loss, good skin turgor, and increased intake (eating more than 80% of meals).

Interventions

1. Weigh the child at the same time each day, using the same scale.

2. Administer pancreatic enzymes before meals and with snacks; provide supplements of vitamins A, D, E, and K, as ordered.

3. Provide a diet high in calories, protein, and carbohydrates; if necessary, monitor the child's carbohydrate intake.

4. Give respiratory treatments before meals.

Rationales

1. Daily weighing helps assess the child's nutritional status.

2. Pancreatic enzymes aid digestion and absorption of nutrients. Children with CF do not absorb fat-soluble vitamins normally.

3. This type of diet helps replace nutrients lost through decreased absorption in the GI tract. A diet too high in carbohydrates may increase diarrhea.

4. Respiratory treatments given after meals may cause coughing and vomiting, increasing the risk for aspiration

Nursing diagnosis

Anxiety (child) related to respiratory distress and hospital stay

Expected outcome

The child will have decreased anxiety as evidenced by restful sleeping periods and a stable respiratory status.

Interventions	Rationales
1. Allow the child to assume a comfortable position.	**1.** Forcing the child to assume a particular position may increase anxiety and respiratory distress.
2. Postpone all tests and procedures until the patient has a patent airway.	**2.** Tests and procedures may increase the child's anxiety level, increasing respiratory distress.
3. Encourage the parents to stay with the child and participate in his care.	**3.** The parents' presence and participation in care provides security and reduces anxiety

Nursing diagnosis

Anxiety (parent) related to lack of knowledge about the child's condition

Expected outcome

The child's parents will be less anxious as evidenced by their ability to support the child and explain the condition.

Interventions	Rationales
1. Assess the parent's understanding of the child's condition and prescribed treatment.	**1.** Such assessment serves as a basis for teaching.
2. Provide explanations about the medical condition, procedures, and required treatments.	**2.** Explanations provided beforehand and throughout the hospital stay improve knowledge and dispel any misunderstanding, decreasing anxiety.
3. Reinforce supportive behaviors, such as talking to and touching the child.	**3.** Reinforcement encourages the parents to repeat such behaviors.
4. Provide emotional support to the parents during the child's hospital stay.	**4.** Listening to the parents' concerns and feelings helps them to deal with the crisis of hospitalization.
5. Refer the parents and child to such organizations as the Cystic Fibrosis Foundation; encourage them work with a center that has experience in treating CF.	**5.** Such organizations can provide support and information. A center that has experience in treating CF can provide high-quality, up-to-date care.

Nursing diagnosis

Knowledge deficit related to home care

Expected outcome

The parents will express an understanding of home care instructions and demonstrate home care procedures.

Interventions

1. Teach the parents about antibiotic administration and potential adverse reactions, including rash, GI distress, vomiting, and respiratory distress.

2. Explain the rationale for long-term antibiotic therapy.

3. Teach the parents the signs and symptoms of respiratory distress, including dyspnea, tachypnea, cyanosis, wheezing, and tachycardia.

4. Stress the importance of encouraging the child to drink two to four 8-oz (240-ml) glasses of fluid each day (depending on the child's renal and cardiovascular status).

5. Teach the parents how to give their child enzymes before meals — not mixed with the food — and how to provide a diet high in calories, protein, and carbohydrates.

Rationales

1. Parents need to know how to administer medications safely and consistently. Knowing what adverse reactions may occur should prompt the parents to seek medical help when necessary.

2. Long-term therapy helps limit lung damage from repeated infections.

3. Recognizing the signs and symptoms of respiratory distress should prompt parents to seek medical help when necessary.

4. Adequate fluids liquefy secretions and replace water lost through the lungs, preventing dehydration that can result in electrolyte imbalances.

5. Such a diet helps replace some of the nutrients lost through nonabsorption; enzymes given before meals help digestion.

Documentation checklist

During the hospital stay, document:
- ❏ child's status and assessment findings upon admission
- ❏ changes in the child's status
- ❏ pertinent laboratory and diagnostic findings
- ❏ fluid intake and output
- ❏ nutritional intake
- ❏ respiratory therapy
- ❏ medication administration
- ❏ child's response to treatment
- ❏ child's and parents' reaction to the illness and hospital stay
- ❏ patient and family teaching guidelines
- ❏ discharge planning guidelines.

Epiglottitis

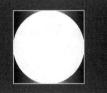

INTRODUCTION

Epiglottitis is an obstructive airway infection characterized by rapidly occurring acute respiratory distress and inflammation of the epiglottis. The infection, which often is caused by *Haemophilus influenzae* type b, has a rapid onset. Typically, the child exhibits no signs at bedtime but awakens with swallowing difficulty and a sore throat. Fever and lethargy occur rapidly, followed by dyspnea.

This condition usually affects children between ages 2 and 5 and may be life-threatening if not treated immediately. Treatment includes mechanical ventilatory support or tracheostomy. Antibiotics also may be used. The prognosis is generally good if the child receives immediate treatment.

ASSESSMENT

Respiratory
• History of sore throat with sudden onset of respiratory distress (dyspnea, tachypnea, retractions, wheezing)
• Mouth breathing
• Inspiratory stridor
• Hypoxia

Cardiovascular
• Tachycardia
• Thready pulse

Gastrointestinal
• Drooling
• Inability to swallow

Musculoskeletal
• Erect, chin-thrust posturing
• Restlessness

Integumentary
• Elevated temperature

Psychosocial
• Anxiety
• Fear

NURSING DIAGNOSIS

Ineffective breathing pattern related to upper airway edema

Expected outcome

The child will maintain a patent airway as evidenced by no signs of acute respiratory distress.

Interventions

1. Assess the child for signs and symptoms of respiratory distress, including dyspnea, tachypnea, cyanosis, drooling, and wheezing.

2. Keep emergency intubation and tracheostomy equipment at the child's bedside at all times.

3. Avoid direct stimulation of the airway with a tongue depressor, culture swab, suction catheter, or laryngoscope.

4. Allow the child to assume a comfortable position other than the horizontal position (elevate the head of the bed).

Rationales

1. Such assessment is necessary to determine the severity of the child's condition and to prevent complete respiratory failure.

2. Emergency intubation and tracheostomy equipment should be on hand in case complete obstruction occurs.

3. Any manipulation of the epiglottis may cause laryngospasm and swelling, possibly causing complete obstruction. Direct examination should be performed in surgery or the emergency department.

4. Allowing the child to assume a position he finds comfortable helps ease anxiety and decreases the risk of increased respiratory distress. Placing the child in a horizontal position may cause rapid tissue deterioration.

5. Continuously monitor the child's skin color, respiratory status, and heart rate until a patent airway is ensured.

5. Continuous monitoring allows detection of complete obstruction, which can occur at any time.

Nursing diagnosis

Ineffective airway clearance related to inflammation and edema

Expected outcome

The child will maintain a patent and secure airway as evidenced by absence of respiratory distress.

Interventions

1. Assess the adequacy of the child's respirations, noting especially any sign of increased respiratory rate, rhonchi, wheezing, retractions, and restlessness.

2. Restrain the child with soft wrist or elbow restraints. Be sure to check the circulation in the hands and fingers every 4 hours.

3. Maintain endotracheal tube placement by taping the tube securely to the child's maxilla.

4. Maintain the child's head and neck in a neutral position (with the head and neck in complete alignment). During positioning, move the head and trunk together as a unit.

5. Carefully suction the child with an endotracheal tube, as needed, when secretions appear in the airway.

6. Administer humidified oxygen by face mask, nasal cannula, or ventilator, as ordered.

Rationales

1. Such changes in respiratory status usually indicate respiratory distress.

2. Because reintubation can be difficult, traumatic, and potentially life-threatening, restraints may be necessary to prevent the child from pulling out the endotracheal tube.

3. Proper taping will ensure minimal movement and decrease the incidence of extubation.

4. This ensures minimal movement of the tube in the trachea, decreasing the risk of trauma and later stenosis.

5. The child may need frequent suctioning because the artificial airway interferes with his ability to clear secretions. Careful suctioning avoids increased trauma to the airway, which could lead to hypoxia and atelectasis.

6. Humidified oxygen prevents secretions from drying and thickening in the airway

Nursing diagnosis

Risk for fluid volume deficit related to decreased fluid intake

Expected outcome

The child will maintain fluid balance as evidenced by good skin turgor, a urine output of 1 to 2 ml/kg/hour, and a capillary refill time of 3 to 5 seconds.

Interventions

1. Do not give the child oral fluids before intubation.

2. Administer and monitor I.V. fluids, as ordered.

3. Carefully monitor the child's fluid intake and output.

Rationales

1. Oral fluids before intubation may cause swallowing difficulty and the increase the risk of aspiration.

2. I.V. fluids keep the child hydrated.

3. Decreased urine output may be an early indication of dehydration.

4. Assess the child for signs of dehydration, including poor skin turgor, dry mucous membranes, and sunken fontanels and eyes.

4. Dehydration indicates that the child needs increased fluid intake.

Nursing diagnosis

Hyperthermia related to infection

Expected outcome

The child will maintain a body temperature of less than 100° F (37.8° C).

Interventions

1. Monitor the child's temperature every 2 to 4 hours for elevation.

2. Administer antipyretics (acetaminophen or ibuprofen, not aspirin), as ordered.

3. Administer tepid (98.6° F [37° C]) sponge baths if medication does not bring the child's temperature down.

4. Obtain blood cultures, as ordered.

5. Administer antimicrobials, as ordered.

Rationales

1. Temperatures higher than 101.3° F (38.5° C) usually are associated with *Haemophilus influenzae,* the most common causative agent in epiglottitis.

2. Antipyretics help reduce fever and allow the child to rest more comfortably; aspirin given to children under age 12 has been linked to Reye's syndrome.

3. Tepid sponge baths cool the body surface, constrict blood vessels, and lower the overall metabolism, thereby lowering the body temperature.

4. Cultures are necessary to identify and treat septic infections, which occur in up to 70% of all children with epiglottitis.

5. Antimicrobials, such as cefuroxime (Ceftin), ampicillin (Omnipen), and chloramphenicol (Chloromycetin), are effective against *H. influenzae.*

Nursing diagnosis

Anxiety and fear (child) related to respiratory distress and hospital stay

Expected outcome

The child will be less anxious and fearful as evidenced by restful sleep and even, unlabored breathing.

Interventions

1. Allow the child to assume a comfortable position.

2. Postpone all testing until a patent airway is ensured.

3. Encourage the parents to stay with the child and participate in his care.

4. Explain all procedures and treatments to the child in terms he can understand.

Rationales

1. Forcing the child into a specific position increase the child's anxiety, resulting in increased respiratory distress.

2. Testing may further compound the child's anxiety, thereby increasing respiratory distress.

3. The child should be made as comfortable as possible to decrease his anxiety. The parents' presence and participation provide the child with a sense of security.

4. Explanations offered beforehand can help lessen the anxiety associated with certain procedures and treatments.

5. Provide the child with familiar objects, such as toys and blankets. If the child is receiving oxygen, make sure the toys cannot emit sparks.

5. Familiar objects help the child feel more secure in the strange hospital environment. Toys that emit sparks may ignite oxygen.

NURSING DIAGNOSIS

Anxiety (parent) related to lack of knowledge concerning the child's condition

Expected outcome

The parents will be less anxious as evidenced by their ability to support their child and explain his condition.

Interventions

1. Assess the parents' understanding of the child's condition and prescribed treatment.

2. Explain the child's medical condition, any procedures, and the prescribed treatment.

3. Reinforce supportive behaviors, such as talking to and touching the child.

4. Provide emotional support to the parents during the hospital stay.

Rationales

1. Such assessment serves as a basis for a teaching plan.

2. Providing explanations beforehand and throughout the hospital stay improves knowledge and dispels any misunderstanding, decreasing anxiety.

3. Reinforcement encourages the parents to continue supportive behaviors.

4. Listening to the parents' concerns and feelings helps them to deal with the crisis of hospitalization.

NURSING DIAGNOSIS

Knowledge deficit related to home care

Expected outcome

The parents will express an understanding of home care instructions.

Interventions

1. Teach about antibiotic administration, including information about such potential adverse reactions as GI distress, rash, and respiratory distress (dyspnea, tachypnea, cyanosis, wheezing, and tachycardia). If the child has a fever, tell the parents to use acetaminophen or ibuprofen instead of aspirin to bring down the fever.

2. Explain the importance of encouraging the child to drink two to four 8-oz (240-ml) glasses of fluid each day.

Rationales

1. Parents need to know how and when to administer antibiotics safely and consistently. Knowing the potential adverse reactions should prompt them to seek medical help when necessary. Giving aspirin to children under age 12 has been linked to Reye's syndrome.

2. Fluids replace water lost through expiration and ease difficult swallowing. Inadequate fluid intake can lead to dehydration and eventual electrolyte imbalance.

Documentation checklist

During the hospital stay, document:
❏ child's status and assessment findings upon admission
❏ changes in the child's status
❏ pertinent laboratory and diagnostic findings
❏ intubation efforts
❏ fluid intake and output
❏ child's response to treatments
❏ child's and parents' reactions to the illness and hospital stay
❏ patient and family teaching guidelines
❏ discharge planning guidelines.

Pneumonia

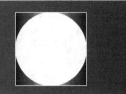

INTRODUCTION

Pneumonia is an inflammation of the lungs usually caused by bacterial (staphylococcus, pneumococcus, or streptococcus) or viral (respiratory syncytial virus) infection. Less common causes include mycoplasmas, foreign body aspiration, and fungi. Occurring as a primary disease or as a complication of another illness, pneumonia is characterized by thick exudate that blocks the alveoli and decreases oxygen exchange. The bacterial or viral form of pneumonia may have a rapid onset.

Common in infants and young children, pneumonia may occur at any age, with highest incidence during the late fall, winter, and early spring. Treatment includes primary respiratory support for the viral form and antibiotics and respiratory support for the bacterial form.

ASSESSMENT

Respiratory
• Increased respiratory rate
• Retractions
• Chest pains
• Crackles
• Decreased breath sounds
• Nasal flaring
• Cyanosis
• Productive cough
• Rhonchi

Cardiovascular
• Tachycardia

Neurologic
• Headache
• Irritability
• Difficulty sleeping

Gastrointestinal
• Decreased appetite
• Stomach pain

Musculoskeletal
• Restlessness
• Fatigue

Integumentary
• Elevated temperature
• Circumoral cyanosis

NURSING DIAGNOSIS

Impaired gas exchange related to exudate accumulation and increased mucus production

Expected outcome

The child will have improved gas exchange as evidenced by ease of respiration, improved skin color, and decreased restlessness.

Interventions

1. Allow the child to assume a comfortable position.

2. Provide a cool mist environment with a face mask, oxygen hood, or oxygen tent.

3. Administer oxygen by face mask, oxygen hood, or oxygen tent, as ordered.

4. Encourage the child to perform coughing and deep-breathing exercises every 2 hours.

5. Suction the child, as needed. Keep suction equipment at the child's bedside.

Rationales

1. Assuming a comfortable position, such as a semi-erect position, makes breathing easier.

2. Cool mist humidifies the airways, helps thin secretions, and reduces bronchial edema.

3. Oxygen helps decrease the restlessness associated with respiratory distress and hypoxemia.

4. Coughing helps remove secretions; deep breathing encourages lung expansion.

5. Suctioning may be necessary to maintain airway patency, especially if the child's cough is ineffective.

6. Perform chest physiotherapy every 4 hours, as ordered.

6. Chest physiotherapy helps loosen exudate and secretions for easy removal through coughing and suctioning.

7. Assess the child's respiratory status for evidence of dyspnea, tachypnea, wheezing, crackles, rhonchi, and cyanosis.

7. These signs may indicate that the treatment is ineffective and that the child's condition may be worsening.

8. Encourage oral fluid intake, if not contraindicated.

8. Fluids generally liquefy secretions.

9. Provide frequent rest periods.

9. Rest conserves the energy needed to fight infection.

10. Turn the child every 1 to 2 hours.

10. Regular turning helps mobilize secretions.

NURSING DIAGNOSIS

Hyperthermia related to infection

Expected outcome

The child will maintain a body temperature of less than 100° F (37.8° C).

Interventions

1. Maintain a cool environment.

2. Administer antipyretics (acetaminophen or ibuprofen, not aspirin), as ordered.

3. Monitor the child's temperature every 1 to 2 hours for sudden elevation.

4. Obtain a sputum specimen for culturing.

5. Administer antimicrobials, as ordered.

6. Administer tepid (98.6° F [37° C]) sponge baths, as needed, to relieve fever.

Rationales

1. A cool environment helps to reduce temperature through radiant heat loss.

2. Antipyretics usually reduce fever effectively by returning the set point to normal.

3. Sudden elevation in temperature may cause a seizure.

4. A sputum specimen helps identify the causative agent.

5. Antimicrobials attack the causative organism.

6. Tepid sponge baths cool the body surface through conduction.

NURSING DIAGNOSIS

Risk for fluid volume deficit related to fluid loss through hyperthermia or hyperpnea (or both)

Expected outcome

The child will maintain fluid balance as evidenced by a urine output of 1 to 2 ml/kg/hour, good skin turgor, and a capillary refill time of 3 to 5 seconds.

Interventions

1. Carefully monitor the child's fluid intake and output.

2. Assess the child for increased respiratory rate and fever every 1 to 2 hours.

Rationales

1. Careful monitoring detects decreased urine output, which may indicate dehydration.

2. Increases in respiratory rate and body temperature typically result in increased fluid loss.

3. Assess the child for signs of dehydration, including oliguria, poor skin turgor, dry mucous membranes, and sunken fontanels and eyes.

3. Such signs indicate the need for increased fluid intake.

4. Administer I.V. fluids, as ordered.

4. I.V. fluids may be necessary to keep the child adequately hydrated.

5. Encourage oral fluid intake every 1 to 2 hours, if not contraindicated.

5. Increased fluid intake helps prevent dehydration and liquefies secretions.

NURSING DIAGNOSIS

Ineffective airway clearance related to inflammation

Expected outcome

The child will have less respiratory difficulty as evidenced by restful sleeping periods and age-appropriate respiratory and heart rates.

Interventions

1. Auscultate the child's lungs for signs of increased airway swelling and impending obstruction, including dyspnea, tachypnea, and wheezing, and assess for drooling.

2. Avoid direct stimulation of the airway with a tongue depressor, culture swab, suction catheter, or laryngoscope.

3. Allow the child to assume any comfortable position except the horizontal position.

4. Monitor the child's respiratory status and vital signs continuously until a patent airway is ensured. Keep emergency intubation equipment at the bedside.

Rationales

1. Early recognition of these signs is essential because swelling usually progresses rapidly and can be fatal.

2. Any manipulation of the airway tissue may cause laryngospasm and swelling, possibly leading to complete obstruction.

3. A horizontal position may cause rapid tissue deterioration, possibly leading to complete obstruction.

4. Continuous monitoring is mandatory because increasing edema can cause complete obstruction at any time, requiring emergency intubation.

NURSING DIAGNOSIS

Altered nutrition: less than body requirements related to increased metabolic needs

Expected outcome

The child will have improved nutritional intake as evidenced by eating at least 80% of meals by the end of the hospital stay.

Interventions

1. Maintain the child on a high-protein, high-calorie diet.

2. Serve small, frequent meals that include foods the child prefers.

3. Avoid milk and full-strength formula.

Rationales

1. The child needs a diet high in protein and calories to meet increased energy needs.

2. Eating small, frequent meals decreases respiratory effort. Serving favorite foods helps ensure that the child will eat most of each meal.

3. Milk and formula thicken secretions.

NURSING DIAGNOSIS

Anxiety (parent) related to lack of knowledge about the child's condition

Expected outcome

The parents will be less anxious as evidenced by their ability to support the child and explain his condition.

Interventions	Rationales
1. Assess the parents' understanding of the child's condition and prescribed treatment.	**1.** Such an assessment provides a basis on which to begin teaching.
2. Allow the parents to stay with the child throughout the hospital stay.	**2.** Allowing the parents to stay provides the child with support.
3. Explain all procedures to the child and parents.	**3.** Providing explanations beforehand and throughout the hospital stay improves knowledge and dispels any misunderstanding, decreasing anxiety.
4. Provide emotional support to the parents throughout the child's hospital stay.	**4.** Listening to the parents' feelings and concerns helps them to deal with the crisis of hospitalization.

NURSING DIAGNOSIS

Knowledge deficit related to home care

Expected outcome

The parents will express an understanding of home care instructions.

Interventions	Rationales
1. Instruct the parents on how and when to administer medications; provide details on dosages and adverse reactions.	**1.** Understanding the importance of consistent medication administration may help the parents to comply with the medication regimen. Knowing the potential adverse reactions should prompt them to seek medical help when necessary.
2. Explain the signs and symptoms of respiratory distress and infection, including fever, dyspnea, tachypnea, yellowish or greenish sputum, and wheezing.	**2.** Knowing the signs and symptoms should prompt the parents to seek medical help when necessary.
3. Explain the importance of adequate rest for the child.	**3.** After infection, the child requires frequent rest periods to help recovery and prevent a relapse.
4. Explain the importance of encouraging fluid intake and maintaining the child on a high-calorie diet.	**4.** Fluids help liquefy secretions; a diet high in calories helps replace calories used to fight the disease.
5. Instruct the parents to provide a humidified environment with a cool mist humidifier.	**5.** Humidified air helps thin secretions. Cool air is safer than warm air, which can cause burns.
6. Take steps to prevent further respiratory infections.	**6.** Repeated respiratory infections increase long-term problems.

Documentation checklist

During the hospital stay, document:

❏ child's status and assessment findings upon admission
❏ changes in the child's status
❏ pertinent laboratory and diagnostic findings
❏ fluid intake and output
❏ nutritional intake
❏ child's response to treatment
❏ child's and parents' reactions to the illness and hospital stay
❏ patient and family teaching guidelines
❏ discharge planning guidelines.

Tuberculosis

INTRODUCTION

Tuberculosis (TB) results from infection with *Mycobacterium tuberculosis*. A child who has a positive skin reaction to the TB screening test receives chest X-rays to determine the presence and extent of active lesions. Children are the most vulnerable during their first 3 years of life and again in the years just before, during, and just after puberty.

Recently, the number of TB cases has increased, most notably in the homeless, those in lower income groups, and those infected with human immunodeficiency virus. Patients with TB generally receive care on an outpatient basis; in severe cases, hospitalization may be necessary. All cases are reported to the local health department. This plan focuses on care provided during hospitalization.

ASSESSMENT

Integumentary
• Fever
• Chills
Gastrointestinal
• Weight loss
Respiratory
• Cough
• Pleural effusion
• Calcifications on X-ray
Neurologic
• Meningitis
Musculoskeletal
• Bone infections

NURSING DIAGNOSIS

Impaired gas exchange related to infective process

Expected outcome

The child will experience reduced coughing and dyspnea.

Interventions

1. Provide humidified oxygen for the child with dyspnea.

2. Elevate the head of the bed.

3. Administer cough expectorants as appropriate.

Rationales

1. Dyspnea may occur until chemotherapeutic agents begin to take effect; humidified oxygen helps decrease dyspnea and improves oxygenation.

2. Elevation allows the diaphragm muscles to expand.

3. Expectorants help loosen mucus.

NURSING DIAGNOSIS

Knowledge deficit related to disease process

Expected outcome

The family will express an understanding of the disease process and treatment.

Interventions

1. Teach the parents and child (if appropriate) about the transmission and treatment of TB.

2. Teach the parents and child (if appropriate) how to administer medications (for example, antibiotics), how long medication therapy should last, and what could happen if the child does not receive the full course of medication.

Rationales

1. Understanding how TB is transmitted and treated helps alleviate anxiety and increases compliance with treatments, isolation procedures, and medication administration.

2. Understanding how to administer medication and the risks of stopping the medication early improves compliance.

NURSING DIAGNOSIS

Noncompliance related to long-term therapy

Expected outcome

The parents and child will adhere to therapy guidelines.

Interventions

1. Assess how much the parents and child (if appropriate) know about TB and what misunderstandings they may have.

2. Teach the parents and child (if appropriate) about the medication regimen and the reasons for completing the full course of drug treatment, and reinforce your teaching as necessary.

3. Identify alternative caregivers who can give the child his medication if necessary.

Rationales

1. Assessment helps you determine what the parents and child need to learn to help them comply with long-term drug therapy.

2. Teaching and reinforcement give the parents and child the information they need to follow the complete drug regimen and decrease the risk of failure because of a knowledge deficit.

3. This reduces the risk of the child missing any doses during therapy.

NURSING DIAGNOSIS

Risk for altered parenting related to patient isolation

Expected outcome

The child will not experience separation anxiety related to decreased parental contact.

Interventions

1. Teach the parents about proper isolation technique.

2. Encourage the parents and other family members to visit frequently.

Rationales

1. Understanding and following isolation technique helps prevent the spread of TB while allowing the parents to be with the child as much as possible, decreasing separation.

2. Frequent family contact decreases the child's separation anxiety.

Documentation checklist

During the hospital stay, document:
- ❑ child's status and assessment finding upon admission
- ❑ changes in the child's status, especially changes in respiratory status
- ❑ pertinent laboratory and diagnostic findings
- ❑ fluid intake and output
- ❑ nutritional intake
- ❑ compliance with medication regimen
- ❑ child's response to treatment
- ❑ child's and parents' reactions to the illness and hospital stay
- ❑ patient and family teaching guidelines
- ❑ discharge planning guidelines.

Part 2

Cardiovascular system

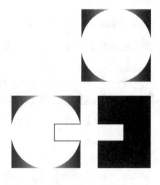

Arrhythmias

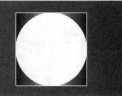

INTRODUCTION

Any deviation in the normal heart rate or rhythm, arrhythmias are directly related to disturbances in the conduction pathways of the heart. Generally classified according to their site of origin (ventricular or supraventricular), arrhythmias in children are usually congenital or related to cardiac surgery. Their clinical significance depends on cardiac output, blood pressure, and site of origin.

Arrhythmias are not common in children. Treatment usually involves the use of antiarrhythmic medications, such as digitalis glycosides and verapamil (Calan).

ASSESSMENT

Cardiovascular
- Abnormal heart rate for age
- Irregular R-R intervals
- Absence of P wave before each QRS complex
- Long PR interval
- Abnormally shaped P wave or QRS complex
- Signs of decreased cardiac output (prolonged capillary refill time, peripheral edema, crackles, rhonchi, and tachycardia)

NURSING DIAGNOSIS

Decreased cardiac output related to cardiac arrhythmia

Expected outcome

The child will maintain effective cardiac output as evidenced by a capillary refill time of 3 to 5 seconds, pinkish mucous membranes, increased energy levels, and improved feeding.

Interventions

1. Monitor the child's cardiovascular status using a cardiac monitor.

2. Assess and record the child's apical heart rate, peripheral pulses, blood pressure, capillary refill time, fluid intake and output, and skin characteristics (such as mottling, color, edema, temperature, and diaphoresis).

3. Administer cardiovascular medications, as ordered.

4. Help the child conserve energy by clustering nursing care.

Rationales

1. Cardiac monitoring indicates and documents any deviation from the child's normal heart rate and rhythm.

2. Such assessment provides data on any changes from the child's baseline measurements, possibly indicating arrhythmia.

3. Cardiovascular medications may be prescribed to help interrupt the electrical disturbances associated with the arrhythmia.

4. Clustering care allows for longer periods of rest.

NURSING DIAGNOSIS

Risk for injury related to medication dosage or physiologic response to medication

Expected outcome

The child will suffer no injuries from medication dosages or physiologic response to medication.

Interventions

1. After medication administration, monitor the child's heart rate and rhythm using a cardiac monitor.

2. Monitor the child's potassium and calcium levels. Watch for clinical signs of potassium and calcium imbalance.

3. Double-check the accuracy of all dosages before administration; make sure the patient receives the ordered amount.

Rationales

1. Antiarrhythmic medications may produce arrhythmias, which can be detected by cardiac monitoring.

2. The effectiveness of antiarrhythmic medications depends on proper adjustment of the intracellular electrolytes. Potassium imbalances can cause arrhythmias; calcium imbalances can cause cardiac arrest.

3. Giving too much or too little of the medication can cause arrhythmias.

NURSING DIAGNOSIS

Risk for infection related to I.V. access site and use of cardiac electrodes

Expected outcome

The child will have no sign of infection as evidenced by the absence of erythema, tenderness, and swelling at the I.V. or electrode sites; a body temperature of 97.6° to 99° F [36.4° to 37.2° C]); and age-appropriate vital signs.

Interventions

1. Check the I.V. site hourly for signs of erythema or infiltration and for possible dislodgment of the I.V. line.

2. Change the I.V. tubing every 24 to 72 hours, as appropriate.

3. Check electrode sites every shift for signs of rash or erythema.

Rationales

1. Assessing the I.V. site hourly helps to detect skin burns from chemical infiltration or the interruption of antiarrhythmic medications caused by dislodgment of the I.V. line — both possible sources of infection.

2. Changing the tubing regularly helps prevent bacterial growth; an I.V. site that was difficult to start may be changed less frequently.

3. Electrode gel can cause skin irritation, possibly leading to infection. Removing electrode adhesive pads can cause skin breakdown, creating a potential site for bacterial infiltration. Use of needle electrodes also provides a potential site for bacterial infiltration.

NURSING DIAGNOSIS

Diversional activity deficit related to restricted activity from attachment to the cardiac monitor

Expected outcome

The child will participate in child-life activities despite attachment to a cardiac monitor.

Interventions

1. Consult a child-life worker (play therapist) about appropriate play activities and stimulation.

2. Encourage the child to interact with other children on the unit, providing the other children are free from respiratory infections.

Rationales

1. A child-life worker can plan appropriate activities based on the child's developmental level and physical restrictions.

2. Such contact with peers helps prevent feelings of isolation and encourages the child to participate in activities.

Cardiovascular system

3. Provide toys, games, and books appropriate for the child's developmental level.

3. These activities help divert the child's attention from his condition and help decrease boredom. They also provide stimulation to help the child grow developmentally.

NURSING DIAGNOSIS

Knowledge deficit related to the child's illness, hospital stay, and home care

Expected outcome

The parents will express an understanding of the child's illness, reason for hospitalization, and home care instructions and demonstrate home care procedures.

Interventions

1. Teach the parents the following:

• the cause of the child's arrhythmias

• signs and symptoms of heart failure, including tachypnea, tachycardia, diaphoresis, fatigue, difficulty feeding, peripheral edema, rapid weight gain, dyspnea, and cyanosis
• the action, dosage, and administration of and potential adverse reactions to antiarrhythmic medications.

2. Explain the purpose and use of the cardiac monitor to the parents and child (if age-appropriate). If the child requires home monitoring, explain how the system works, how to set the alarms, and the type of problems they may encounter when using the monitor at home. If problems develop, tell the parents to contact the hospital or the doctor.

3. Make sure the parents attend a cardiopulmonary resuscitation (CPR) class before the child is discharged from the hospital.

Rationales

1. Understanding the nature and seriousness of the child's condition helps the parents comply with the treatment and monitor the child's progress.
• Understanding the cause of the child's illness helps the parents to regain a sense of control over the situation.
• Recognizing the signs and symptoms of heart failure should prompt the parents to seek medical help when necessary, helping to avert serious complications.

• Knowing the action, correct dosage, and administration of antiarrhythmic medications helps parents to comply with the child's treatment; recognizing adverse reactions should prompt them to seek medical attention when necessary.

2. Such explanations help alleviate the parents' fears and prevent unnecessary preoccupation with the operation of the monitor, allowing the parents to concentrate on other aspects of the child's care.

3. The parents need to know when and how to initiate CPR to sustain the child's circulation and respiration in the event of cardiac arrest related to the arrhythmia.

Documentation checklist

During the hospital stay, document:
☐ child's status and assessment findings upon admission
☐ changes in the child's status
☐ pertinent laboratory and diagnostic findings
☐ fluid intake and output
☐ nutritional intake
☐ growth and development status
☐ child's response to treatment
☐ child's and parents' reactions to the illness and hospital stay
☐ patient and family teaching guidelines
☐ discharge planning guidelines.

Congenital heart defects

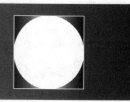

INTRODUCTION

Congenital heart defects, the second leading cause of death in infancy, result from abnormal cardiovascular development during fetal life that obstruct or alter blood-flow patterns. Defects are classified as either acyanotic or cyanotic.

In acyanotic defects, oxygenated blood is shunted from the left to the right side of the heart but is not mixed with unoxygenated blood in the systemic circulation. The major acyanotic defects that affect children include the following:

• *Ventricular septal defect (VSD),* the most common of all congenital heart defects, refers to an abnormal opening in the ventricular septum that allows oxygenated blood from the left ventricle to mix with unoxygenated blood in the right ventricle. It usually requires surgical repair.

• *Coarctation of the aorta* refers to the narrowing of the aorta near the remnant of the fetal ductus arteriosus. This defect usually requires surgical repair.

• *Atrial septal defect (ASD)* refers to an opening in the septum of the atria that allows blood to shunt from the left to the right. If ASD does not close spontaneously, surgery is necessary.

• *Patent ductus arteriosus (PDA)* is a persistent opening between the aorta and the pulmonary artery that failed to close at birth. Although PDA, which predominantly affects premature infants, may close spontaneously, surgery may be necessary.

In cyanotic defects, blood is shunted from the right to the left side of the heart, where unoxygenated blood flows from the left ventricle to all parts of the body, resulting in cyanosis. The major cyanotic defects that affect children include the following:

• *Transposition of the great vessels* is a condition in which the pulmonary artery and the aorta are reversed: the aorta is attached to the right ventricle, and the pulmonary artery is attached to the left ventricle. This creates two separate circulatory systems that cannot sustain life. Surgery is necessary to correct the defect.

• *Tetralogy of Fallot* consists of four separate defects — VSD, overriding aorta, pulmonary stenosis, and right ventricular hypertrophy — requiring surgical repair.

ASSESSMENT

VSD
Cardiovascular
• Mild: holosystolic murmur at the left lower sternal border
• Moderate to severe: holosystolic murmur (same as for mild defect), signs of heart failure (tachypnea, tachycardia, restlessness, increased central venous pressure, weight gain, decreased urine output, diaphoresis), failure to thrive, enlarged liver, decreased energy, feeding difficulties, and weight gain from fluid retention
Pulmonary
• Severe: pulmonary edema

Coarctation of the aorta
Cardiovascular
• Mild: 1+ or absent femoral, popliteal, and pedal pulses; mild hypertension (increased bilaterally in the arms and decreased in the legs)
• Moderate: absent femoral, popliteal, and pedal pulses; moderate to severe hypertension (detected bilaterally in the arms; decreased in the legs)
• Severe: same as for moderate defect, plus signs of heart failure

ASD
Cardiovascular
• Quiet systolic ejection murmur (best heard by a highly trained practitioner)
• Enlarged heart
Respiratory
• Increased incidence of upper respiratory tract infections
Musculoskeletal
• Exercise intolerance

PDA
Cardiovascular
• Mild: 4+ bilateral peripheral pulses, wide pulse pressure, and a continuous murmur in the left upper anterior midclavicular thorax
• Moderate: signs of heart failure
• Severe: left-sided heart enlargement
Respiratory
• Mild: frequent upper respiratory tract infections

(Text continues on page 49.)

Cardiovascular system

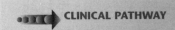

Open heart surgery

	Day1/Preop/Floor
Consults	• Cardiac service • Anesthesia
Tests	• Complete blood count (CBC), platelets, blood chemistry studies, clotting studies, fibrinogen levels • Type and crossmatch • Electrocardiogram (ECG), chest X-ray, echocardiogram • Urinalysis
Treatments	• Pulse oximetry • Vital signs (VS) q 4 hr • Antiseptic bath or shower • I.V. fluid management as needed, intake and output (I & O) • Developmental appropriate interventions provided
Medication	• Aspirin discontinued 2 weeks prior to admission when necessary
Diet	• Age appropriate, as ordered • Nothing by mouth after midnight
Activity	• Age appropriate, as ordered
Team process	• Patient history/assessment admission form • Systems assessment • Growth cure by doctor • Preop checklist completed
Teaching C = class H = handout R = reference V = video	• Orient to unit routine. • On-going pre-op teaching • Visit intensive care unit (ICU). • Review plan of care.
Discharge planning	• Assess support network. • Reinforce length of stay.
Needs and outcomes	• Patient/parent verbalizes concerns about surgery and hospitalization. • Patient maintains developmental level. • Patient/parent verbalizes an understanding of floor routine and policies. • Patient/parent verbalizes an understanding of preop teaching.

Day 2/OR/PICU	Day 3/POD #1/PICU
• Respiratory therapy	• Respiratory therapy
• Lab work as ordered	• ECG, chest X-ray • Reassess frequency of blood work.
• Cardiac/respiratory (CR) monitors, neuro checks, pulse oximetry • VS q 15 min to 1 hr • Maintain pressure lines, hypothermia blanket, I.V.s, pacing wires (covered and secured), chest tubes to pleur-evac low wall suction, ventilatory support (hold if left atrium [LA] line), pulmonary care q 2 hr and as needed. • 4 point restraints • Strict I & O q hr, eye care • Transfusions as needed • Indwelling urinary catheter • Daily weight (hold if LA line) • Nasogastric (NG) tube to low gomco, check Ph and guaiac	• CR monitors, neuro checks, pulse oximetry • VS q hr • Maintain pressure lines, pacing wires (covered and secured), chest tubes to pleur-evac low wall suction; wean ventilatory support. • Pulmonary toilet q 2 hr and when necessary • Indwelling urinary catheter • Daily weight (hold if LA line) • NG tube to low gomco, check pH and guaiac • Strict I & O q hr • I.V.
• I.V. vasoactive drugs, pain management • I.V. sedation, I.V. antibiotics, histamine$_2$ blockers, diuretics	• I.V. sedation • Pain management • Wean vasoactive drugs. • I.V. antibiotic, histamine$_2$ blockers • Diuretics, digitalize
• Age appropriate, as ordered	• Age appropriate, as ordered
• Age appropriate, as ordered	• Age appropriate, as ordered
• Systems assessment	• Systems assessment
• Orient to ICU routine. • Postop care instructions: interventions, medications • Cardiac education flowsheet	• Reinforce postop care instructions.
• Assess support network.	
• Patient displays no evidence of arrythmias. • Patient is adequately perfused as evidenced by palpable pulses to extremities, warmth, and urine output. • Patient's gas exchange is maintained through ventilatory support as evidenced by arterial blood gas (ABG) and oxygen saturation levels within acceptable parameters. • Patient's pain is adquately controlled as evidenced by non-verbal communication, ability to rest, and VS. • Patient remains free from harm. • Patient/parent uses appropriate developmental supportive services. • Parent verbalizes understanding of unit routine and policies and postop care instructions.	• Patient shows no signs of bleeding as evidenced by chest tube drainage; CBC and VS are within acceptable parameters. • Patient demonstrates adequate perfusion as evidenced by tolerance of vasoactive weaning. • Patient demonstrates improved gas exchange as evidenced by tolerance of ventilatory weaning. • Patient's skin integrity is maintained. • Patient's pain is adequately controlled as evidenced by non-verbal communication, ability to rest, and VS.

Cardiovascular system

(continued)

Open heart surgery *(continued)*

	Day 4/POD#2/PICU	Day 5/POD #3/PICU
Consults	• Child life • Social work	
Tests		• Chest X-ray after chest tubes discontinued
Treatments	• CR monitors, neuro checks, pulse oximetry • VS q 1 hr, pulmonary toilet q 2 hr and p.r.n. • Maintain pressure lines, I.V.s, disconnect LA line. • Chest tubes to pleur-evac low wall suction • Extubate to oxygen, remove sternal dressing • Strict I & O q 1 hr, eye care • Indwelling urinary catheter • Daily weight • Discontinue NG tube	• Wean oxygen as tolerated • Pulmonary toilet q 2 hr and p.r.n. • Pulse oximeter • CR monitors, VS q 2 hr • I.V. • Daily weight • Discontinue chest tubes • I & O
Medication	• Discontinue vasoactive drugs. • Pain management • I.V. antibiotic, histamine-2 blockers • Diuretics • Maintenance lanoxin	• Pain management • Maintenance lanoxin and diuretic • Discontinue antibiotics after chest tube discontinued. • Discontinue histamine-2 blockers.
Diet	• Age appropriate, as ordered	• Age appropriate, as ordered
Activity	• Age appropriate, as ordered	• Age appropriate, as ordered
Team process	• Systems assessment	• Systems assessment
Teaching C = class H = handout R = reference V = video	• Reinforce postop care instructions.	• Start medication teaching with preprinted medication instruction sheets.
Discharge planning		
Needs and outcomes	• Patient tolerates discontinuation of vasoactive medications as evidenced by maintenance of perfusion. • Patient is afebrile. • Patient tolerates extubation as evidenced by ABGs and oxygen saturation levels; breathing effort is within acceptable parameters. • Patient's incision is intact without swelling or drainage. • Patient does not have vomiting after eating. • Patient's pain is adequately controlled as evidenced by verbalization/use of pain scale. • Patient/parent verbalizes an understanding of patient's current condition and intervention changes.	• Patient tolerates chest tube removal with no evidence of pneumothorax or bleeding. • Patient is hemodynamically stable as evidenced by rhythm, perfusion, and VS. • Patient's respiratory status is stable as evidenced by oxygen saturation levels, breath sounds, and effort within acceptable parameters. • Patient's chest tube/line sites are intact without redness, swelling, or drainage. • Patient voids spontaneously after catheter removal. • Patient tolerates increased activity. • Patient/parent verbalizes an understanding of initial medication teaching.

Cardiovascular system

Day 6/POD#4/Transfer to pediatrics

Day 7/POD #5/Pediatrics

- Pulmonary toilet q 2 hr and p.r.n.
- Pulse oximeter q 4 hr
- VS q 4 hr
- Discontinue I.V.s.
- Daily weight
- Remove pacing wires.

- Pulmonary toilet q 4 hr
- Pulse oximeter q 4 hr
- VS q 4 hr
- Daily weight
- Remove chest tube dressing.

- Pain management
- Maintenance lanoxin and diuretic

- Pain management
- Maintenance lanoxin and diuretic

- Age appropriate, as ordered

- Age appropriate, as ordered

- Age appropriate, as ordered

- Age appropriate, as ordered

- Systems assessment

- Systems assessment

- Orient to pediatric floor
- Medication teaching with preprinted medication instruction sheets

- Assess/reinforce all prior discharge teaching.

- Patient's respiratory status is stable as evidenced by oxygen saturation levels within acceptable parameters; lungs aerating fully, clearly bilaterally.
- Patient tolerates increased activity.
- Patient/parent verbalizes an understanding of floor routine and policies.
- Patient/parent verbalizes an understanding of medications, interventions, and treatments.

- Patient/parent verbalizes an understanding of medications, interventions, and treatments as evidenced by active participation.

(continued)

Open heart surgery (continued)

	Day 8/POD #6/Pediatrics	Day 9/POD #7/Pediatrics
Consults		
Tests	• Chest X-ray, ECG, echocardiogram	
Treatments	• Pulmonary toilet q 4 hr • Pulse oximeter q 4 hr • VS q 4 hr • Daily weight	• Pulmonary toilet q 4 hr • Pulse oximeter q 4 hr • VS q 4 hr • Daily weight • Check/remove sutures.
Medication	• Pain management • Maintenance lanoxin and diuretic	• Pain management • Maintenance lanoxin and diuretic
Diet	• Age appropriate, as ordered	• Age appropriate, as ordered
Activity	• Age appropriate, as ordered	• Age appropriate, as ordered
Team process	• Systems assessment	• Systems assessment
Teaching C = class H = handout R = reference V = video	• Reinforce all prior discharge teaching.	• Reinforce all prior discharge teaching.
Discharge planning	• 24-hour written discharge notice given	• Discharge instructions with pre-printed sheets • Follow-up appointment with doctor • Discharge by 11 a.m.
Needs and outcomes	• Patient/parent verbalizes and displays confidence and readiness for discharge.	• Patient/parent verbalizes and displays confidence and readiness for discharge today. • Patient/parent verbalizes an understanding of the discharge instructions.

Adapted with permission from North Shore Health System, Manhasset, N.Y. (Revised 6/95)

Transposition of the great vessels
Cardiovascular
- Heart murmur (if VSD is present)
- Egg-shaped heart on X-ray
- 3+ or 4+ pulses (depending on whether ductus arteriosus is patent)
- No increase in oxygen saturation with oxygen administration

Integumentary
- Severe cyanosis

Tetralogy of Fallot
Cardiovascular
- Systolic murmur along the upper left sternal border
- Boot-shaped heart on X-ray
- Normal peripheral pulses
- Tendency toward cyanotic spells (dyspnea, deep sighing respirations, bradycardia, fainting, seizures, and loss of consciousness)
- Thrill along upper left sternal border

Neurologic
- Loss of consciousness

Musculoskeletal
- Exercise intolerance
- Squatting position (if patient is child rather than infant)

Hematologic
- Polycythemia
- Elevated hemoglobin and hematocrit values

Integumentary
- Cyanosis
- Digital clubbing

Psychosocial
- Anxiety

NURSING DIAGNOSIS

Anxiety (parent) related to child's congenital heart defect

Expected outcome

The parents will have decreased anxiety as evidenced by their ability to express feelings, ask appropriate questions about the child's condition, and interact with the child.

Interventions

1. Explain the heart defect using an illustration, and answer any questions the parents may have; if appropriate, discuss any genetic component of the defect.

2. Update the parents regularly on the child's condition.

3. Allow the parents to hold or cuddle the infant as soon and as often as possible.

Rationales

1. Explaining the defect and answering the parents' questions helps reduce anxiety by allowing them to visualize and better understand the defect; some defects have a genetic component.

2. Regular updates allow the parents to maintain some contact with the child, alleviating some of their anxiety.

3. Holding and cuddling promote bonding and a sense of security, alleviating anxiety.

NURSING DIAGNOSIS

Knowledge deficit related to impending surgery

Expected outcome

The parents and child (if appropriate) will demonstrate an understanding of the impending surgery as evidenced by their ability to explain the purpose of surgery and ask appropriate questions.

Cardiovascular system

Interventions

1. Assess the parents' and child's knowledge of the impending surgery and the child's developmental level (see appendix A, Normal growth and development).

2. Instruct the child and parents on the perioperative events that require their direct participation, including:
• bathing the child with povidone-iodine solution (Betadine) or hexachlorophene (pHisoHex) the night before surgery
• touring the intensive care unit (ICU) before surgery
• making sure the child receives nothing by mouth before surgery (the actual time will depend on the child's age)
• attending teaching sessions on postoperative procedures and equipment, such as chest tubes, oxygen masks, incentive spirometers, dressings, endotracheal tubes, I.V. lines, central venous pressure and arterial monitoring, electrocardiogram (ECG) monitoring, and postural drainage.

3. Teach the child coughing, deep-breathing, and splinting techniques, if appropriate.

Rationales

1. Such assessment serves as a basis on which to begin teaching.

2. The child and parents need to anticipate the events surrounding the surgery. The surgeon will explain the actual procedure and associated risks to the parents.

3. Coughing, deep breathing, and splinting help to loosen and remove secretions from the respiratory tract and increase oxygenation. Familiarity with these techniques promotes compliance after surgery.

NURSING DIAGNOSIS

Risk for injury related to positioning, electrical current, blood loss, and surgical procedure

Expected outcome

The child will suffer no injuries during the surgical procedure.

Interventions

1. Assess the child's pressure points hourly during the surgical procedure for evidence of skin breakdown. Look for redness, blanching of the skin, abrasions, and open wounds.

2. Calculate the child's total fluid volume, based on fluid intake and expected blood loss.

3. If the child is undergoing surgery to repair coarctation of the aorta, monitor the blood pressure in the leg during the surgery.

4. Monitor the child's heart rhythm. Have temporary pacing wires and a temporary pacemaker available in case of an emergency.

5. Check the electrical ground pad and ECG electrode sites for evidence of burns.

Rationales

1. Skin breakdown, which can occur within 1 hour of the start of surgery, places the child at risk for infection.

2. Adequate fluid replacement is necessary to maintain cardiac output.

3. During surgery to repair coarctation, an aortic cross clamp is required. Monitoring the blood pressure in the leg helps ensure the proper return of blood flow to the lower body.

4. Monitoring the heart rhythm is essential because the surgical procedure may temporarily or permanently interrupt the normal conduction of the heart.

5. Electrical grounding at these sites may cause first-degree burns.

NURSING DIAGNOSIS

Decreased cardiac output related to surgical procedure

Expected outcome

The child will maintain adequate cardiac output after surgery as evidenced by age-appropriate heart and respiratory rates; strong, regular pulses; and a capillary refill time of 3 to 5 seconds.

Interventions

1. After surgery, assess the child's cardiac status hourly as follows:
• Measure and record the child's hemodynamic monitor readings (arterial line, central venous pressure [CVP] line, intracardiac catheter, and thermistor cardiac output). Normal left atrial pressure is 0 to 8 mm Hg; normal CVP is 0 to 5 mm Hg.
• Monitor laboratory blood studies, including prothrombin time, arterial blood gas (ABG) measurements, and complete blood count. (See appendix E, Normal laboratory values.)

• Assess the child for signs of heart failure, such as dyspnea, crackles, tachycardia, and tachypnea; look for periorbital edema and weight gain in an infant.
• Assess the child's heart sounds for muffling or a friction rub.

2. Assess the child's renal function by:
• measuring and recording fluid intake and output hourly (normal output should be greater than 1 ml/hour)
• monitoring specific gravity at every voiding or every 2 to 4 hours if the child has a catheter in place
• monitoring blood urea nitrogen (BUN) and serum creatinine levels.

3. Assess the child's fluid and electrolyte status by:
• monitoring electrolyte levels (see appendix E, Normal laboratory values)

• measuring and recording fluid intake and output hourly

• looking for evidence of edema and poor skin turgor

• weighing the child daily.

Rationales

1. Surgery can cause severe trauma to the child's body.

• Hemodynamic instability may result from the trauma of surgery. Specifically, changes in CVP can indicate right-sided heart failure, changes in arterial line pressure can indicate changes in blood pressure, and changes in cardiac output can indicate heart failure.
• Cardiac bypass can damage the blood cells and cause hemolysis of red cells, possibly leading to anemia. Anticoagulants may be ordered to prevent clots. ABG measurements indicate the level of oxygen perfusion in the blood.
• Because of the stress of surgery, the child may be at risk for heart failure from the increased workload of the heart and increased sodium and water retention.
• Bleeding may occur in the pericardial sac and restrict the heart's ability to function. Muffled heart sounds may indicate cardiac tamponade. Friction rub may indicate postpericardiotomy syndrome (delayed pericardial or pleural reaction characterized by fever, chest pain, and signs of pericardial or pleural inflammation).

2. Surgery may compromise normal renal function.
• Measuring and recording the fluid intake and output helps determine fluid status and kidney function.

• Specific gravity indicates hydration status and the kidneys' ability to concentrate urine.
• Decreased BUN and creatinine levels may indicate kidney failure.

3. Surgery may cause fluid and electrolyte imbalances.
• Monitoring electrolyte levels helps determine the child's hydration status and potassium level. (Decreased potassium levels may result in arrhythmias.)
• Measuring intake and output helps determine fluid status and kidney functioning and helps prevent fluid overload.
• Evidence of edema and poor skin turgor may indicate poor hydration and heart failure.
• Weight gain is an early sign of heart failure.

Cardiovascular system

4. Assess the child's respiratory status by:

• monitoring and recording the child's respiratory rate and patterns, breath sounds, skin color, and capillary refill time; also monitor ventilator settings, intracardiac catheter and oximeter readings, and carbon dioxide levels
• checking if the endotracheal (ET) tube is securely taped and noting tube placement on X-ray to assess the patency of the ET tube
• monitoring and recording the amount of chest tube drainage hourly (normal output is less than 3 ml/hour); also check for excessive bleeding, proper placement of the chest tube, and signs of infection at the site
• monitoring ABG levels every 4 to 8 hours

• ventilating the child with 100% oxygen for 1 minute before and after ET suctioning.

5. Assess the child's neurologic status, noting pupillary reactions, muscle tone, and reflexes (grasp, sucking, and swallow).

4. Surgery may compromise the child's respiratory status.
• Immobility, pain, and the use of anesthetic gases alter normal pulmonary function.

• An improperly positioned ET tube can hamper respiratory function.

• Excessive drainage may indicate hemorrhage; infection stresses the child's immune system.

• ABG levels directly measure the effectiveness of respiratory status.
• Ventilation with 100% oxygen relaxes the alveoli and prevents severe hypoxia and respiratory arrest.

5. Impaired neurologic status can occur as a result of decreased cardiac output, hypoxia, acidosis, electrolyte imbalance, or cerebral thrombosis.

NURSING DIAGNOSIS

Risk for infection related to immobility and numerous incision sites

Expected outcome

The child will have no signs of infection as evidenced by a body temperature of 97.6° to 99° F (36.4° to 37.2° C), a stable white blood cell count, and age-appropriate vital signs.

Interventions

1. Assess the incision and I.V. sites hourly for evidence of bleeding, erythema, infiltration, and excess drainage.

2. Monitor the child's temperature and check for leukocytosis.

3. Assess the child's pressure points hourly for the first 2 or 3 hours, then every 2 hours thereafter.

4. Administer antibiotics, as ordered.

5. Change dressings, as ordered, using sterile technique.

Rationales

1. The child's immunologic system has already been stressed by surgery. Any further stress caused by infection of the incision site could lead to septic shock. Fluid loss by infiltration or bleeding could alter cardiac output.

2. Elevated temperature and leukocytosis may indicate infection.

3. Such assessments are necessary to avoid skin breakdown.

4. Antibiotics may be prescribed to help prevent infection.

5. Sterile technique helps prevent the introduction of bacteria into the incision.

NURSING DIAGNOSIS

Risk for injury related to indomethacin administration (in premature infants with PDA)

Expected outcome

The infant will demonstrate no signs of injury as evidenced by age-appropriate heart and respiratory rates and a urine output of 1 to 2 ml/kg/hour.

Interventions	Rationales
1. Administer indomethacin (Indocin), as ordered. Be sure to check and double-check all dosages before administering the medication (0.2 mg/kg initially).	**1.** Indomethacin constricts the ductus to promote closure. Double-checking dosages helps prevent overdosage.
2. Assess and record the infant's cardiac, respiratory, renal, GI, and neurologic status every 4 hours; if the infant is unstable, assess every 1 to 2 hours.	**2.** Such assessment is necessary to detect any possible complications (such as hemorrhage) after indomethacin administration.

NURSING DIAGNOSIS

Decreased cardiac output related to spasm of pulmonary infundibulum (in children with tetralogy of Fallot)

Expected outcome

The child will have no evidence of cyanotic spells.

Interventions	Rationales
1. Recognize the signs and symptoms of cyanotic spells, including dyspnea, deep sighing respirations, bradycardia, fainting, seizures, and eventual loss of consciousness.	**1.** Early recognition allows for intervention before the anoxia becomes severe enough to cause loss of consciousness.
2. Place the child in a prone knee-to-chest position.	**2.** This position decreases the workload on the heart by decreasing peripheral blood return.
3. Speak in quiet tones and gently rub the child's back.	**3.** Soothing tones and touch comfort the child and help relax the spasm.
4. Ventilate the child with 100% oxygen using a face mask, nasal cannula, or blow device.	**4.** Ventilation with 100% oxygen increases the amount of oxygen in inspired air and in the circulation.
5. Administer morphine sulfate I.M. (0.1 to 0.2 mg/kg) or I.V. (0.5 to 0.1 mg/kg), as ordered.	**5.** Morphine helps relax the spasm and causes peripheral vasodilation.
6. Teach the parents how to perform interventions 1 through 4.	**6.** Knowing how to perform these interventions helps the parents to cope with the crisis brought on by the spasm and allows them to participate in the child's care.
7. Teach the parents how to administer a beta blocker, such as propranolol hydrochloride (Inderal).	**7.** Beta blockers interrupt the mechanism involved in spasms of the pulmonary infundibulum. Teaching parents how to administer such medications helps promote compliance with the home care regimen.

Cardiovascular system

Nursing diagnosis

Risk for infection (bacterial endocarditis) related to high-flow shunt (in children with VSD)

Expected outcome

The child will have no signs of bacterial endocarditis and bacteremia.

Interventions	Rationales
1. Explain to the parents the causes of bacterial endocarditis, particularly dental and surgical procedures. Explain that, to prevent infection, the child typically receives prophylactic antibiotic therapy.	**1.** Understanding the causes of bacterial endocarditis promotes compliance with the prescribed antibiotic therapy.
2. Give the parents written instructions for antibiotic therapy prescribed for specific procedures.	**2.** Having such information promotes compliance with the medication regimen.

Nursing diagnosis

Anxiety (child) related to ICU environment, separation from parents, parental anxiety, surgery, and immobility

Expected outcome

The child will be less anxious as evidenced by cooperating with the procedures and treatment and demonstrating age-appropriate play.

Interventions	Rationales
1. Encourage the parents to visit the child and participate in his care as often as possible.	**1.** Parental contact provides the child with feelings of safety and security.
2. Explain to the child and parents each step in postoperative care.	**2.** Familiarity with procedures and nursing measures decreases anxiety and increases cooperation.
3. Consult a child-life worker or play therapist about providing the child with toys and activities appropriate for his developmental level.	**3.** Toys and activities help divert the child's attention from his environment and provide developmental stimulation.

Nursing diagnosis

Knowledge deficit related to home care

Expected outcome

The parents will express an understanding of home care instructions and will demonstrate home care procedures.

Interventions	Rationales
1. Teach the parents the signs of wound infection, including purulent drainage, fever, and a foul-smelling odor.	**1.** Because infection can occur up to 3 weeks after surgery, parents need to know which signs to report.

2. Teach the parents how to administer medications while the child is still in the hospital.

2. Practice promotes comfort with the procedure and ensures compliance. Having the parents practice while the child is still in the hospital lets you assess the parents' ability to administer medications correctly.

3. Teach the parents how to monitor the child's pulse rate, and tell them to report persistent deviations of 15 to 20 beats above or below the baseline level.

3. Knowing how to monitor the child's pulse rate allows the parents to detect and report any significant changes that could indicate complications.

4. Instruct the parents to feed the child small, frequent meals.

4. Eating small, frequent meals decreases the workload on the heart while maintaining adequate caloric intake.

5. Teach the parents the signs and symptoms of postpericardiotomy syndrome, including fever, chest pain, and dyspnea.

5. Postpericardiotomy syndrome, a potentially life-threatening condition, can occur up to 3 weeks after major heart surgery. Parents need to know what signs and symptoms to report in case of an emergency.

Documentation checklist

During the hospital stay, document:
- ❏ child's status and assessment findings upon admission
- ❏ changes in the child's status
- ❏ pertinent laboratory and diagnostic findings
- ❏ fluid intake and output
- ❏ nutritional intake
- ❏ growth and development status
- ❏ child's response to treatment
- ❏ child's and parents' reactions to the illness and hospital stay
- ❏ patient and family teaching guidelines
- ❏ discharge planning guidelines.

Cardiovascular system

Heart failure

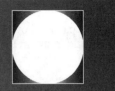

INTRODUCTION

Heart failure develops when the heart cannot pump sufficient amounts of blood into the systemic circulation to meet work demands. Usually differentiated into left-sided or right-sided failure, heart failure commonly results from congenital heart defects during infancy.

Complications of this disorder include hepatomegaly, ascites, and cyanosis. Treatment may include diuretics (to treat edema and prevent the reabsorption of sodium) and digoxin (to increase cardiac contractility and slow the heart rate), a low-sodium diet, fluid restrictions, and decreases in activities and stress.

ASSESSMENT

Infants
Cardiovascular
• Mild: resting tachycardia (greater than 160 beats/minute)
• Severe: decreased peripheral pulses (1+ or 2+; if patent ductus arteriosus is the cause, 4+)
Respiratory
• Mild: resting tachypnea (greater than 60 breaths/minute)
• Compensatory: excessive respiratory effort (resting tachypnea, substernal and intercostal retractions, nasal flaring, crackles, dry cough, dyspnea, and orthopnea)
Gastrointestinal
• Mild: slow weight gain
Genitourinary
• Severe: decreased urine output (less than 1 ml/hour)

Musculoskeletal
• Mild: fatigue with feedings, failure to thrive, developmental delays
Integumentary
• Mild: diaphoresis (head and face), pallor, duskiness
• Compensatory: orbital edema, peripheral edema, cold extremities, scrotal edema (in male infants with severe heart failure)

Children and adolescents
Cardiovascular
• Mild: resting tachycardia
• Severe: decreased peripheral pulses (1+ or 2+; if patent ductus arteriosus is the cause, 4+)
Respiratory
• Mild: resting tachypnea, exertional dyspnea
• Compensatory: excessive respiratory effort (including resting tachypnea, substernal and intercostal retractions, nasal flaring, crackles, and dry cough), wheezes, orthopnea
Gastrointestinal
• Mild: loss of appetite, rapid weight gain ("water weight")
Genitourinary
• Severe: decreased urine output (less than 1 ml/hour)
Musculoskeletal
• Mild: exertional fatigue
Integumentary
• Mild: diaphoresis (forehead)
• Compensatory: orbital edema, dependent edema of the arms and legs, pallor, duskiness, cold extremities

NURSING DIAGNOSIS

Fluid volume excess related to increased blood flow to the lungs (as in ventricular septal defect, patent ductus arteriosus, atrioventricular fistula, cardiac valvular insufficiency, renal failure, or excessive I.V. fluid administration)

Expected outcome

The child will maintain a stable cardiac status as evidenced by age-appropriate heart and respiratory rates and no crackles or rhonchi.

Interventions

1. Assess and record the child's cardiovascular status by noting apical heart rate and rhythm, peripheral pulses, blood pressure, capillary refill time, and skin changes (mottling, edema, increased or decreased temperature, diaphoresis).

2. Use a cardiac monitor to assess the child's status. Assess his vital signs and notify the doctor immediately of any significant changes.

3. Administer digoxin (Lanoxin), the drug of choice, or other cardiovascular medications, as ordered. Give half of the total digitalizing dosage in the initial dose, then a quarter of the total dosage in two subsequent doses. Give digoxin every 12 hours in infants and children.

4. Provide frequent rest periods.

5. When treating the child, approach him in a calm manner, provide consistency in care, and perform procedures that may seem threatening in a treatment room, not in the child's room.

6. Monitor serum digoxin levels (therapeutic levels range from 0.5 to 2 ng/ml).

7. Assess for signs of digoxin toxicity, such as vomiting and blurred vision.

Rationales

1. Such assessment provides essential data on changes in the child's cardiac status, including tachycardia, bradycardia, hypotension, and irregular heart rate — all indications of cardiac decompensation.

2. Cardiac monitoring immediately detects changes in the child's heart rate and rhythm, such as tachycardia (an early sign of heart failure) and arrhythmias (a possible adverse effect of some heart failure medications).

3. Such medications slow and strengthen heart contractions.

4. Frequent rest decreases the heart's workload.

5. These interventions can help decrease stress and anxiety, decreasing the heart's workload.

6. Monitoring is necessary to maintain therapeutic levels.

7. Digoxin can cause severe adverse reactions.

NURSING DIAGNOSIS

Impaired gas exchange related to pulmonary edema

Expected outcome

The child will maintain adequate oxygenation as evidenced by pinkish skin color and mucous membranes and a capillary refill time of 3 to 5 seconds.

Interventions

1. Assess and record the child's respiratory status by:
• noting the rate, character, and regularity of respirations
• auscultating for breath sounds
• noting the presence and character of cough.

2. Place the child in semi-Fowler's position.

3. Administer oxygen by face mask, oxygen hood (for an infant), or nasal cannula, as ordered.

4. Administer diuretics, as ordered; note the child's intake and output.

Rationales

1. This assessment provides essential data on changes in the child's respiratory status, such as evidence of respiratory distress (dyspnea, crackles, tachypnea, retractions, and cyanosis).

2. Semi-Fowler's position allows gravity to relieve pressure on the heart and lungs.

3. This increases the amount of oxygen in inspired air, which helps to compensate for impaired oxygen exchange in the alveoli from pulmonary congestion.

4. Diuretics cause tissues to release fluid and the kidneys to flush out the excess fluid.

Cardiovascular system

5. Monitor serum electrolyte levels, especially potassium (see appendix E, Normal laboratory values).

5. Electrolyte imbalances may result from edema or diuretic use; decreased or elevated potassium levels can cause arrhythmias.

6. Monitor oximeter readings, which should be in the high 90s.

6. An oximeter measures changes in the child's oxygenation, which can become compromised because of pulmonary congestion and impaired gas exchange in the alveoli.

Nursing diagnosis

Altered nutrition: less than body requirements related to decreased energy reserves

Expected outcome

The child will maintain adequate nutritional intake as evidenced by eating 80% of all meals and maintaining a stable weight and good skin turgor.

Interventions

1. Schedule feedings or meals after rest periods, and provide a calm environment.

2. Serve small, frequent feedings or meals (five to six per day).

3. Place the child in semi-Fowler's position during feedings.

4. Feed the child his favorite formula or meals that include some of his favorite foods; if the child is taking a potassium-depleting medication, try to include potassium-rich foods.

5. If ordered, administer oxygen during feedings.

6. Increase the child's caloric intake by offering high-calorie formulas or foods.

7. If the child tires before taking in enough food or formula, initiate nasogastric feeding, as ordered.

8. Assess and record the child's fluid intake and output daily.

9. Restrict the child's fluid intake, as ordered.

Rationales

1. The child has more energy after rest for the work of sucking or chewing and swallowing. A calm environment helps relax the child, improving intake.

2. Small, frequent meals help prevent stomach distention from eating too much at one time and use up less of the child's energy at any one feeding.

3. Semi-Fowler's position promotes swallowing; gravity helps relieve pressure on the heart and lungs.

4. Feeding the child his favorite formula or foods helps ensure increased intake; decreased potassium levels can trigger arrhythmias.

5. Because pulmonary congestion has decreased the child's oxygen uptake, increasing the oxygen concentration of inspired air can help increase the child's energy level while he is eating.

6. The child must take in more calories to meet the increased metabolic demands resulting from tachypnea, tachycardia, and respiratory distress.

7. Nasogastric feeding ensures that the child receives adequate nutrition.

8. Fluid retention may indicate worsening heart failure.

9. Fluid restrictions may be ordered to decrease the circulatory volume associated with fluid retention.

NURSING DIAGNOSIS

Risk for injury related to medication dosage or physiologic response to medication

Expected outcome

The child will suffer no injuries from medication dosages or physiologic response to medication.

Interventions	Rationales
1. Monitor the child's heart rate and rhythm using a cardiac monitor.	**1.** Cardiac monitoring detects disturbances in the child's heart rate or rhythm related to medication use. For example, first-degree heart block or sinus bradycardia may indicate digoxin toxicity, and ventricular arrhythmias may be caused by hypokalemia from diuretic use.
2. Monitor the child's electrolyte levels.	**2.** Electrolyte imbalance may result from medication use. For example, diuretics can cause hypokalemia, which can potentiate the action of digoxin to toxic levels.
3. Double-check all dosage calculations for accuracy; make sure the order is correct and that the child is receiving the correct amount.	**3.** Verifying the accuracy of all dosages ensures that the child receives the correct medication in the exact amount necessary for therapeutic effectiveness.

NURSING DIAGNOSIS

Anxiety (parent) related to the child's illness, hospital stay, and eventual home care

Expected outcome

The parents will be less anxious as evidenced by asking appropriate questions about the child's condition.

Interventions	Rationales
1. Explain to the parents the nature of the child's illness and the reason for the hospital stay. Also explain all procedures and treatments, and begin discharge instructions at the start of the hospital stay.	**1.** Knowing this information should help the parents understand the child's condition and expected treatment and help ease their anxiety.
2. Encourage the parents to participate in the child's care by helping to administer medications and by bathing, feeding, and monitoring the child.	**2.** Participating in the child's care decreases the parents' anxiety about the treatment and hospital stay. It also allows them to begin practicing home care procedures while under your supervision.
3. Provide emotional support to the parents.	**3.** Providing emotional support helps relieve anxiety.

NURSING DIAGNOSIS

Knowledge deficit related to the disease process and home care

Expected outcome

The parents will express an understanding of the disease and home care instructions.

Interventions

1. Teach the parents the signs and symptoms of heart failure, including tachypnea, tachycardia, fatigue, poor feeding, restlessness, diaphoresis, rapid weight gain, dyspnea, cyanosis, wheezing, and peripheral edema.

2. Teach the parents about the prescribed medication regimen; include details on dosages and potential adverse reactions, especially for digoxin, and provide information on poison control.

3. Teach the parents the purpose and use of home monitoring devices.

4. Explain to the parents the importance of feeding the child a high-calorie, low-sodium diet; if the child is taking a potassium-depleting medication, explain the importance of adding potassium-rich foods to the child's diet.

Rationales

1. Knowing the signs and symptoms of heart failure should prompt the parents to seek medical help when needed.

2. Explaining this information helps ensure correct medication administration and compliance with the overall treatment plan; the parents need to know what steps to take if another child accidentally takes the medication.

3. The child may require home monitoring to detect episodes of bradycardia, tachycardia, or apnea.

4. The child will need extra calories to grow and low sodium levels to prevent fluid retention and hypertension; the child taking potassium-depleting medications is at risk for arrhythmias from decreased potassium levels. Knowing this information should encourage compliance with the dietary regimen.

Documentation checklist

During the hospital stay, document:
- ❏ child's status and assessment findings upon admission
- ❏ changes in the child's status
- ❏ pertinent laboratory and diagnostic findings
- ❏ fluid intake and output
- ❏ nutritional intake
- ❏ child's response to treatment
- ❏ child's and parents' reactions to the illness and hospital stay
- ❏ patient and family teaching guidelines
- ❏ discharge planning guidelines.

Part 3

Neurologic system

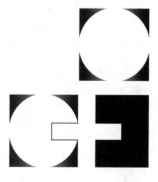

Head injury

INTRODUCTION

Head injury refers to any trauma to the scalp, skull, or brain, including concussion (most common), cerebral contusion or laceration, fracture, and vascular injuries (epidural or subdural hematoma). Types of skull fracture include linear (most common in children), depressed, compound (communication between lacerated scalp and brain), and basilar (involving either the base of the brain or the vault of the skull).

Complications of head injury may include increased intracranial pressure (ICP), epidural or subdural hemorrhage, and cerebral edema. The prognosis depends on the severity of the injury and the duration of coma. Treatment includes the administration of I.V. fluids, anticonvulsants, and steroids.

ASSESSMENT

Because children do not always exhibit signs at the time of injury, they require close monitoring for 24 to 48 hours after any suspected head injury. Documentation of a fall or accident constitutes an important part of assessment. Children treated for head injuries should also be assessed and treated for spinal injury.

Concussion
Neurologic
- Impaired consciousness for a variable period
- Headache (postconcussion syndrome)
- Vertigo
- Depressed reflexes
- Anxiety
- General malaise

Respiratory
- Decreased respirations

Cardiovascular
- Bradycardia
- Hypotension

Cerebral contusion
The severity of the contusion will depend on the extent of cranial injury, the amount of cerebral edema, and the amount of bleeding.
Neurologic
- Possible loss of consciousness
- Mild motor or sensory weakness
- Headache
- Vertigo
- Posttraumatic seizures (later sign)

- Coma
- Irritability
- Restlessness

Skull fracture
Neurologic
- Altered skull contour
- Conjunctival hemorrhage (associated with fracture of the anterior fossa)
- Cerebrospinal fluid (CSF) rhinorrhea
- Periorbital ecchymosis (raccoon eyes)
- CSF otorrhea
- Palsies of C1, C7, and C8 nerves
- Posttraumatic seizures (later sign)
- Coma

Cardiovascular
- Hypovolemia (associated with fractures over the sagittal or lateral sinus)

Integumentary
- Ecchymosis at the base of the neck (associated with basilar skull fracture and fractures over the mastoid process)

Epidural hematoma
The following signs and symptoms of epidural hematoma occur after initial awakening and alertness.
Neurologic
- Brief loss of consciousness
- Sudden headache
- Decreased level of consciousness (LOC)
- Unilateral pupillary dilation; bilateral pupillary dilation (if not decompressed)
- Decerebrate posturing (later sign)
- Hemiparesis
- Irritability
- Lethargy

Respiratory
- Respiratory depression
- Apnea

Cardiovascular
- Bradycardia

Gastrointestinal
- Vomiting

Acute subdural hematoma
Acute subdural hematoma usually presents with diffuse symptoms; however, signs and symptoms of cerebral laceration, contusion, or intracerebral hematoma also may be noted.

Neurologic
- Headache
- Loss of consciousness
- Focal seizures
- Unilateral pupillary dilation
- Hemiparesis
- Agitation
- Drowsiness with confusion
- Progressive slowness of thinking

Chronic subdural hematoma
Neurologic
- Headache
- Progressive decrease in LOC (may be over weeks or months resulting from a relatively minor injury)

- Nuchal rigidity
- Ipsilateral pupillary dilation
- Hemiparesis
- Tight or bulging fontanels (in infants)
- Increased head circumference
- Hyperactive reflexes
- Irritability
- Low-grade fever

Gastrointestinal
- Anorexia
- Vomiting

Eye, ear, nose, and throat
- Retinal hemorrhage

NURSING DIAGNOSIS

Ineffective breathing pattern (with potential for respiratory failure) related to increased ICP

Expected outcome

The child will maintain adequate respiratory effort and gas exchange as evidenced by age-appropriate respiratory patterns, Pao_2 of 80 to 100 mm Hg, $Paco_2$ of 25 to 30 mm Hg, and pink mucous membranes.

Interventions

1. Establish an open airway by extending the child's neck after cervical vertebral fracture has been ruled out. Do not hyperextend the neck.

2. Insert an oral airway.

3. Anticipate the need for endotracheal intubation in a child with increasing dyspnea.

4. Raise the head of the child's bed 30 degrees after spinal cord injury has been ruled out.

5. Insert a nasogastric tube or an orogastric tube.

6. Suction only as needed; oxygenate before and after suctioning.

7. Monitor the child's respiratory effort for rate, depth, and pattern hourly until he is stable.

Rationales

1. Extending the neck helps to decrease upper airway obstruction. Hyperextension can compress the trachea.

2. An oral airway helps prevent airway obstruction in a child with a decreased LOC.

3. Intubation may be necessary to provide mechanical ventilation to maintain adequate gas exchange.

4. Raising the head of bed helps to maximize diaphragmatic excursion, assisting ventilatory effort.

5. Insertion of either of these tubes decompresses the stomach, which decreases the potential for vomiting and aspiration. For suspected basilar skull fracture, only an orogastric tube should be used because of the risk of infection from an open pathway to the brain, especially if the child has a nasal CSF leak.

6. Suctioning should be kept to a minimum because it can increase ICP. (*Note:* Nasal suctioning is contraindicated in suspected basilar skull fracture because of the risk of an open pathway to the brain.)

7. Abnormal breathing patterns may decrease breathing efficiency and adversely affect gas exchange.

Neurologic system

8. Monitor arterial blood gas (ABG) results for abnormal levels.

8. Paco$_2$ levels should be kept at 25 to 30 mm Hg to induce vasoconstriction to lower the brain's blood volume, which will decrease increased ICP. (Levels less than 20 mm Hg may cause severe vasoconstriction, leading to lactic acidosis and secondary brain ischemia.)

NURSING DIAGNOSIS

Altered peripheral tissue perfusion related to hypotension secondary to hypovolemic shock

Expected outcome

The child will maintain adequate tissue perfusion as evidenced by strong peripheral pulses, warm extremities, body temperature less than 100° F (37.8° C), a capillary refill time of 3 to 5 seconds, and age-appropriate blood pressure.

Interventions

1. Monitor the child's vital signs hourly, and check his extremities for warmth, brisk capillary refill, strong pulses, and pink nail beds.

2. Monitor central venous pressure and systemic arterial pressure hourly if the child is undergoing invasive monitoring.

3. Administer blood products, colloid solutions, or I.V. fluids, as ordered.

Rationales

1. An increase in tympanic or rectal temperature and a decrease in skin temperature can indicate poor systemic perfusion, possibly a sign of hypovolemia. Fever may indicate an epidural hematoma. Cold stress increases oxygen consumption and produces peripheral vasoconstriction. Shock can result in hypotension, tachycardia followed by bradycardia, and increased respiratory rate.

2. Hypotension may cause brain injury secondary to cerebral ischemia. Central venous pressure and systemic arterial pressure decrease with hypotension.

3. Such fluids help increase the circulating fluid volume. Hypotonic fluids usually are not administered because they can increase extracellular water uptake. Hypovolemia may be secondary to hemorrhage.

NURSING DIAGNOSIS

Risk for fluid volume deficit related to nausea and vomiting

Expected outcome

The child will maintain adequate hydration as evidenced by moist mucous membranes, good skin turgor, and age-appropriate electrolyte levels.

Interventions

1. Monitor the child's fluid intake and output every 2 to 8 hours, depending on the outcome of specific gravity levels taken every 8 hours.

2. Weigh the child daily, and assess his skin turgor and mucous membranes every 8 hours.

Rationales

1. An increased urine concentration may indicate a fluid deficit.

2. Weight loss, poor skin turgor, and dry mucous membranes indicate a fluid deficit.

NURSING DIAGNOSIS

Risk for injury related to altered LOC secondary to head injury or increased ICP (or both)

Expected outcome

The child will have no signs of further injury.

Interventions

1. Assess the child's neurologic status hourly for the first 8 hours, then as ordered for the following:
• altered LOC, such as lack of response to painful stimuli, altered pupillary response, decreased reflexes, and seizures
• unilaterally dilated, sluggish, or fixed pupils
• decreased motor activity

2. Monitor the child's vital signs hourly (until stable) for signs of tachycardia, bradycardia, hypotension, widened pulse pressure, and decreased respiratory rate.

3. Ensure that the child maintains a cerebral perfusion pressure greater than 50 mm Hg by draining CSF fluid through the intracranial pressure line to reduce pressure.

4. Provide rest periods between nursing interventions or treatment.

5. Administer I.V. lidocaine (Xylocaine) or another analgesic, as ordered, before performing such uncomfortable interventions as suctioning.

6. Administer diuretics, including mannitol (Osmitrol) and furosemide (Lasix), as ordered. Monitor electrolyte balance, especially potassium level.

7. Monitor for drainage from the nose and ears. Test any drainage for glucose with a reagent strip.

Rationales

1. Altered LOC may indicate increasing ICP. Unilaterally dilated, sluggish, or fixed pupils may precede an emergency, such as brain anoxia. Inappropriate motor responses, such as decreased reflexes, decreased response to stimuli, or seizures, may indicate brain damage.

2. These signs may indicate Cushing's syndrome (rare in children), which can result from the use of steroids to treat cerebral edema.

3. Cerebral perfusion pressure, which measures the blood flow to the brain, must be maintained to prevent ischemia.

4. Adequate rest helps prevent a cumulative rise in ICP.

5. Administering an analgesic before suctioning or other uncomfortable procedures reduces the risk of stimulating the child, which could lead to increased ICP.

6. These agents help reduce ICP by controlling the fluid volume in the cerebral spaces. Osmotic diuretics, such as mannitol, act to pull fluid from cerebral extracellular space into the bloodstream. However, a rebound effect may occur approximately 6 hours after the medication is stopped. Nonosmotic diuretics, such as furosemide, lower systemic blood flow through action on the kidneys, decreasing cerebral fluid volume. Diuretics can cause electrolyte imbalance, especially a drop in potassium level, which can trigger arrhythmias.

7. CSF, which tests positive for glucose, may drain from the nose or ears.

NURSING DIAGNOSIS

Decreased cardiac output related to hemorrhage

Expected outcome

The child will maintain adequate cardiac output as evidenced by age-appropriate heart rate, blood pressure, and hematocrit; pink mucous membranes; a strong pulse; and capillary refill time of 3 to 5 seconds.

Neurologic system

Interventions

1. Monitor the child's vital signs hourly for the first 8 hours, then as ordered.

2. Assess the child every 8 hours for physical evidence of hemorrhage, such as an alteration in skull contour, bruising or external hematoma, bleeding from an ear, or a change in LOC. Report these signs immediately.

Rationales

1. The child may have tachycardia or hypotension, both of which are physiologic responses to hemorrhage.

2. Physical findings of hemorrhage may signify a decrease in circulatory volume.

NURSING DIAGNOSIS

Risk for injury secondary to seizures

Expected outcome

The child will have no signs of further injury as evidenced by maintaining neurologic function despite seizure activity. (About 10% of children with cerebral contusions exhibit seizure activity beginning hours to years after the initial injury.)

Interventions

1. Take necessary seizure precautions, including keeping an artificial airway and suctioning equipment within easy reach and keeping side rails up and padded.

2. Administer anticonvulsant medications, as ordered.

Rationales

1. Because seizures can result in falls, head injuries, anoxia, choking, and possible death, these precautions are necessary to help prevent injury and the risk of further complications.

2. Anticonvulsant medications help control seizures.

NURSING DIAGNOSIS

Pain related to head injury

Expected outcome

The child will demonstrate minimal discomfort as evidenced by expressing reduced or no pain and maintaining vital signs within age-appropriate limits.

Interventions

1. Assess the child's complaints of pain, noting the pain's location, duration, and severity. Also assess vital signs, noting increased pulse rate, increased or decreased respiratory rate, and diaphoresis. To relieve pain, change the child's position, decrease stimulation, and administer pain medication.

2. Decrease the amount of light, noise, and other environmental stimuli in the child's room.

Rationales

1. Pain assessment is necessary, especially in the child too young to express his discomfort. Pain may result in increased ICP secondary to hypoventilation and Valsalva's maneuver. Increased pulse rate, increased or decreased respiratory rate, or diaphoresis may reflect discomfort.

2. Such stimuli may be disturbing to a child with a head injury because stimulation increases neurologic irritability, which decreases pain tolerance. Stimulation also may lead to increased ICP.

NURSING DIAGNOSIS

Anxiety (child and parent) related to traumatic head injury

Expected outcome

The child and parents will demonstrate minimal anxiety as evidenced by exhibiting decreased agitation and asking appropriate questions about the illness and treatment.

Interventions	Rationales
1. Explain to the child and parents the purpose of all nursing measures and how those measures will be carried out.	**1.** Knowing beforehand what procedures will be performed, and why, helps reduce anxiety.
2. Allow the parents to stay with the child, depending on the child's status.	**2.** This allows the parents to give the child emotional support, decreasing the child's anxiety. It also reduces the parents' anxiety by allowing them to see and participate in the child's care.

NURSING DIAGNOSIS

Risk for infection related to injury

Expected outcome

The child will have no signs or symptoms of infection as evidenced by a body temperature less than 100° F (37.8° C), absence of drainage from the wound, and age-appropriate white blood cell count.

Interventions	Rationales
1. Assess the amount and character of any drainage from the child's nose, mouth, or auditory canal.	**1.** Assessing such drainage may indicate a CSF leak, which suggests an open pathway to the brain. (Testing for CSF leakage may involve use of a reagent strip to detect the amount of glucose present in CSF; decreased amounts may indicate infection.) An open pathway to the brain may increase the child's risk of infection.
2. Monitor the child's temperature every 4 hours.	**2.** Hyperthermia may signal infection.
3. Assess for signs and symptoms of meningitis, including nuchal rigidity, irritability, headache, fever, vomiting, and seizures.	**3.** CSF leakage increases the risk of meningitis because of the open pathway to the brain.
4. Change all wound dressings using sterile technique.	**4.** Sterile technique helps prevent the introduction of bacteria into the open wound, decreasing the risk of infection.

Neurologic system

NURSING DIAGNOSIS

Risk for impaired skin integrity related to physical immobility

Expected outcome

The child will have no signs of impaired skin integrity as evidenced by increased joint mobility and the lack of skin breakdown and pressure ulcers.

Interventions

1. Perform passive range-of-motion (ROM) exercises every 4 hours.

2. Place the child's feet on a footboard or in high-top sneakers when not performing ROM exercises.

3. Maintain the child in proper body alignment, and change his position every 2 hours.

Rationales

1. Passive ROM exercises help maintain joint mobility, which decreases the risk of skin breakdown.

2. A footboard prevents footdrop and skin breakdown; high-top sneakers maintain the same joint angle as a footboard.

3. Using hand and leg rolls and proper back support helps prevent muscle strain sometimes caused by proper alignment and improved positioning. Changing position helps prevent skin breakdown.

NURSING DIAGNOSIS

Knowledge deficit related to home care

Expected outcome

The parents will express an understanding of home care instructions and will demonstrate home care procedures.

Interventions

1. Instruct the parents on the nature and expected course of the child's head injury.

2. Teach the parents to recognize signs of potential complications, including altered LOC, changes in the child's gait, fever, seizures, repeated vomiting, and speech changes.

3. Teach the parents the purpose and use of medications; include details on administration and potential adverse reactions.

4. Teach the parents about seizure precautions, including having the child wear a protective helmet, maintaining the child's airway during a seizure episode, and putting side rails on the child's bed.

5. Emphasize the importance of the child performing activities of daily living himself; as appropriate, he should exercise daily or regularly, feed himself, perform activities that provide stimulation, and take care of his hygiene needs.

Rationales

1. Such knowledge helps the parents better understand the need for treatment and the possible long-term effects of the injury.

2. Knowing how to recognize signs of potential complications should prompt the parents to seek medical help when necessary.

3. The child must receive all medications — whether for infection or seizures — consistently to ensure effectiveness. Knowing potential adverse reactions should prompt parents to seek medical help when necessary.

4. These precautions help prevent injury to the child during seizures.

5. The child may have lost his ability to perform certain activities of daily living and may need retraining and continual encouragement.

6. Provide safety-related information on the use of seat belts, car restraints, and safety helmets.

6. This helps ensure that the parents and child follow necessary safety precautions to decrease the chance of another head injury.

Documentation checklist

During the hospital stay, document:
❒ child's status and assessment findings upon admission
❒ changes in the child's status
❒ pertinent laboratory and diagnostic findings
❒ child's neurologic status
❒ fluid intake and output
❒ child's response to treatment
❒ child's and parents' reactions to the injury and hospital stay
❒ patient and family teaching guidelines
❒ discharge planning guidelines.

Hydrocephalus

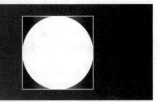

INTRODUCTION

Hydrocephalus—characterized by head enlargement, prominence of the forehead, brain atrophy, and mental deterioration—is caused by failure of circulating cerebrospinal fluid (CSF) to drain from cerebral ventricles. An obstruction or impaired absorption results in increased fluid buildup and intracranial pressure (ICP), which, if unrelieved, may lead to brain damage and death. Hydrocephalus may be congenital or result from a tumor, infection, or hemorrhage.

Treatment involves surgical placement of a shunt to relieve the ICP. Possible complications include infection, blockage, and subdural hematoma.

ASSESSMENT

Shunt malfunction
Neurologic
Infants
- Split cranial sutures
- Swelling along shunt tract
- High-pitched cry
- Bulging fontanels
- Prominent scalp veins
- Irritability when awake
- Increased frontal occipital circumference
- Sunset eyes (setting-sun sign)

Toddlers
- Headaches
- Seizures
- Swelling along the shunt tract
- Irritability
- Sunset eyes (occurs if hydrocephalus remains uncorrected)

School-age children
- Headaches
- Resplitting of cranial sutures
- Seizures
- Papilledema
- Sunset eyes (occurs if hydrocephalus remains uncorrected)

Adolescents
- Papilledema
- Sunset eyes (occurs if hydrocephalus remains uncorrected)
- Seizures
- Deterioration in level of consciousness (LOC)
- Cushing's triad (bradycardia, widened pulse pressure, and apnea)
- Pupil dilation

Gastrointestinal
Infants
- Vomiting
- Change in appetite

Toddlers
- Vomiting

School-age children
- Vomiting

Musculoskeletal
Infants
- Lethargy
- Lower extremity spasticity

Toddlers
- Lethargy

School-age children
- Lethargy

Psychosocial
School-age children
- Decreased school performance
- Change in attention span

Respiratory
Adolescents
- Cheyne-Stokes respiration

Shunt infection
Neurologic
- Swelling or redness along shunt tract
- Signs and symptoms of shunt dysfunction (headaches, seizures, bulging fontanels [in infants], decreased LOC)

Gastrointestinal
- Poor appetite

Integumentary
- Elevated temperature

NURSING DIAGNOSIS

Altered cerebral tissue perfusion related to increased ICP

Expected outcome

The child will maintain brain function and will develop no further signs of ICP.

Interventions

1. Perform a neurologic assessment every 2 to 4 hours of the child's pupillary response, grip, grasp, pain response, interactive responses (smiling, talking, babbling), and disposition (pleasantness or irritability).

2. Assess the child's vital signs every 2 to 4 hours, noting irregularities in respiration and heart rate and rhythm and widening pulse pressures.

3. Perform a cranial nerve assessment every 2 to 4 hours.

4. Elevate the head of the bed 30 degrees.

5. If the child is an infant, assess his fontanels every 4 hours for bulging. Be sure to perform the assessment during quiet periods because the fontanels usually bulge during crying.

6. If the child is under age 2, measure the head circumference daily.

7. Assess for and report any swelling along the shunt tract every 8 hours.

8. Keep oxygen and suction equipment readily available at the child's bedside during periods of altered LOC.

9. Document the parents' recollection of the child's previous experiences with shunt malfunction.

10. Note the quality and pitch of the child's cry.

11. If the child is an infant, keep his body in proper alignment when holding him.

Rationales

1. Frequent assessments provide data for determining changes in the child's baseline neurologic status that indicate ICP. However, by the time clinical manifestations occur, the child already may have significant ICP.

2. Frequent vital sign assessments help detect early signs of ICP (such as tachycardia, blood pressure fluctuation, and Cheyne-Stokes respiration) or later signs of advancing ICP (Cushing's triad: widened pulse pressure, bradycardia, and apnea).

3. Changes in cranial nerve function are a direct reflection of ICP. Most commonly, C3 and C6 are affected as demonstrated by pupillary changes and extraocular eye movement. C7, C9, and C10 also may be affected as evidenced by asymmetrical facial movement, inability to speak and swallow, and stridor or crowing sounds on inspiration.

4. Elevating the head of the bed allows gravity to increase cerebral venous drainage, which helps decrease ICP.

5. Full, bulging fontanels directly reflect increased ICP.

6. Abnormal head enlargement in children under age 2, especially infants, indicates increased ICP. Normally, an infant's head grows an average of 3/4" (2 cm) per month until age 3 months, then about 1/8" (0.3 cm) per month until age 1 year.

7. Swelling along the shunt tract or around the shunt pump may indicate that the shunt is clogged.

8. Oxygen and suction equipment are necessary in case seizures develop or the child becomes apneic.

9. Because each child experiences highly individual signs and symptoms of shunt malfunction, the parents' recollection helps the nursing and medical staff to determine whether the shunt is working properly.

10. A high-pitched cry usually indicates increased ICP.

11. Because of his enlarged head, the infant may be difficult to hold; however, body alignment should be maintained to avoid putting a strain on his neck.

Neurologic system

NURSING DIAGNOSIS

Risk for infection related to surgical placement of shunt

Expected outcome

The child will have no signs of infection related to shunt placement as evidenced by a body temperature less than 100° F (37.8° C) and no signs of incisional swelling or drainage, irritability, lethargy, or loss of appetite.

Interventions

1. Assess the child for temperature instability, decreased LOC, loss of appetite, vomiting, increased white blood cell count, and swelling or redness along the shunt tract.

2. Monitor the child's temperature every 4 hours.

3. Position the child so that no weight is placed on the valve site for the first 24 to 48 hours after surgery.

4. Assess the child's incision site every 4 hours, looking for drainage or swelling. Note the amount and type of any drainage.

5. Administer antibiotics, as ordered.

Rationales

1. These signs signal shunt infection, which usually occurs within the first month after shunt insertion.

2. Decreased temperature is an early sign of infection in a neonate, and elevated temperature is an early sign of infection in a child.

3. Positioning the head in this manner helps prevent skin breakdown on or around the shunt pump, alleviating the risk of infection. Neonates, who are especially susceptible to shunt infection, may require special positioning for a longer time.

4. Swelling around the pump, shunt tract, or surgical incision—with or without drainage—may be an early sign of shunt infection.

5. Prophylactic antibiotics usually are ordered at the time of surgery and continued for 48 to 72 hours after surgery.

NURSING DIAGNOSIS

Risk for fluid volume deficit related to altered nutritional status in the preoperative and postoperative phases

Expected outcome

The child will demonstrate no signs of dehydration as evidenced by stable weight, good skin turgor, stable electrolyte levels, adequate tearing, moist mucous membranes, and a urine output of 1 to 2 ml/kg/hour.

Interventions

1. Carefully monitor the child's fluid intake and output.

2. Weigh the child at the same time each day.

3. Note the frequency and amount of vomiting.

4. Monitor the child's serum electrolyte levels daily if vomiting occurs. Pay particular attention to sodium and potassium levels.

Rationales

1. Careful monitoring detects fluid losses.

2. Weight gain or loss reflects hydration status.

3. Vomiting, a common sign of increased ICP, may substantially affect the child's hydration status. Parenteral nutrition may be needed to help correct fluid losses, especially in infant who cannot tolerate oral feedings.

4. Large amounts of sodium, potassium, and other electrolytes are lost through vomiting.

5. Initiate parenteral nutrition, as ordered, and monitor administration hourly.

6. If the child has undergone surgery for placement of a ventriculoperitoneal shunt, wait at least 24 hours after the return of active bowel sounds to begin giving clear liquids.

5. Administration of parenteral fluids helps restore normal fluid and electrolyte balance.

6. Waiting at least 24 hours after the return of bowel sounds ensures that the child does not have a paralytic ileus resulting from the surgery.

Nursing diagnosis

Risk for injury related to onset of seizures

Expected outcome

The child will suffer no injury resulting from seizures.

Interventions

1. Determine whether the child has a history of seizures.

2. Institute seizure precautions for a child with increasing ICP or shunt malfunction. Keep suction equipment on hand.

3. During a seizure episode, take the following measures:
• Help the child lie on his side, either on the bed or floor, and remove any obstacles from the area.
• Do not attempt to restrain the child, but remain at his side.
• Do not attempt to place anything in the child's mouth.
• Assess the child's respiratory status.
• Note any body movements and the duration of the seizure.

Rationales

1. Seizures occur in up to 40% of children within 2 years after shunt placement.

2. Seizures are a later sign of increased ICP. Seizure precautions are necessary to prevent injury to the child.

3. These measures help protect the child and aid in medical follow-up.
• These steps help prevent injuries from falling and from convulsive or jerking seizure activity.
• Restraining or forcefully moving the child may cause trauma.
• Trying to force an object into the child's mouth may damage the teeth and gums.
• The child may need respiratory resuscitation if he becomes apneic during or after a seizure.
• The types of movement and the duration of the seizure helps define what type of seizure the child had.

Nursing diagnosis

Fluid volume excess related to placement of ventriculoatrial shunt

Expected outcome

The child will develop no signs or symptoms of cardiac overload as evidenced by absence of dyspnea, crackles, tachypnea, tachycardia, and cyanosis.

Interventions

1. Assess the infant's or child's respiratory and cardiovascular status every 2 to 4 hours for signs of decreased cardiac output and respiratory distress, including tachypnea, tachycardia, dyspnea, and arrhythmias (this assessment is especially important in infants).

Rationales

1. During ventriculoatrial shunt placement, the distal end of the shunt is placed in the right atrium, where the CSF will drain. Because of the increased fluid volume in the right atrium, cardiac overload and respiratory distress may occur.

Neurologic system

2. Weigh the child daily.

2. Weight gain may indicate fluid retention, which is associated with cardiac overload.

3. Monitor the child's fluid intake and output.

3. Such monitoring evaluates the child's fluid status.

Nursing diagnosis

Anxiety (parent and child) related to lack of understanding about the child's condition and treatment

Expected outcome

The parents and child (if appropriate) will express an understanding of hydrocephalus, the necessity of shunt placement, and the usual operative routine.

Interventions

1. Explain to the parents and child (if appropriate) the definition of *hydrocephalus,* the anatomy of the ventricles, and the basic purpose of the shunt. Use diagrams and a sample shunt, if available, to help clarify your explanation. Also explain the purpose of any diagnostic tests ordered and the procedure that will be followed.

2. Describe the usual perioperative events, including:
• nothing-by-mouth status
• consent form signing
• establishment of an I.V. access
• transport of the child to the operating room
• waiting facilities for parents
• scheduled time of surgery
• expected length of surgery
• recovery room
• vital sign monitoring
• placement of incision
• dressings.

3. Allow time for the parents to ask questions and express their fears and concerns.

4. Help the child to prepare the hospital stay and surgery, using a doll, actual hospital equipment, and diagrams and videos as appropriate for the child's developmental level.

5. Reinforce the surgeon's explanations.

6. Refer the parents to a social worker or other social services personnel, as needed.

Rationales

1. Such explanations help decrease fear and anxiety and promote acceptance of the child's condition.

2. Explaining these events to the parents ensures that they are aware of what the child will undergo and helps encourage their participation in routine preoperative preparation, as allowed.

3. Parents need time to assimilate all the information so that they can form questions and express fears and concerns.

4. Doll demonstration is extremely useful in helping a child deal with events that occur during a hospital stay. Diagrams, videos, books, and discussion may be more appropriate for the older child.

5. Parents and children often receive large amounts of information in a short period of time. Repeated explanations help them understand the child's condition.

6. A social worker can provide intense counseling to help the parents cope with their child's condition and hospital stay and can assist in discharge planning and referrals to community organizations

Nursing diagnosis

Knowledge deficit related to disease and home care

Expected outcome

The parents will express an understanding of the disease and home care instructions and will demonstrate home care procedures.

Interventions

1. Assess the parents' understanding of the disease and how the shunt functions.

2. Instruct the parents on how to care for the shunt, including details on signs and symptoms of shunt malfunction and infection and on the specific care for the shunt.

3. Emphasize the importance of continued neurologic follow-up examinations.

4. Allow time for the parents to ask questions and express concerns.

5. Explain that the shunts will be modified as the child grows.

6. Explain any seizure medications prescribed, such as carbamazepine (Tegretol) or phenytoin (Dilantin). Review potential adverse effects.

Rationales

1. Such assessment serves as a basis on which to begin teaching.

2. The parents need to know how to care for the child's shunt and what signs and symptoms to report.

3. The child will require lifelong follow-up studies to assess shunt and tubing function and the child's general well-being.

4. Asking questions and expressing concerns helps the parents understand the discharge instructions.

5. Shunt length must be extended as the child grows.

6. Brain injury may make the child susceptible to seizures; medications can help control seizures.

Documentation checklist

During the hospital stay, document:
- ☐ child's status and assessment findings upon admission
- ☐ an changes in the child's status
- ☐ pertinent laboratory and diagnostic findings
- ☐ fluid intake and output
- ☐ shunt functioning
- ☐ growth and development status
- ☐ child's and parents' reactions to the illness and hospital stay
- ☐ patient and family teaching guidelines
- ☐ discharge planning guidelines.

Neurologic system

Intraventricular hemorrhage

INTRODUCTION

Intraventricular hemorrhage (IVH) refers to bleeding into the ventricles of the cerebrum. This type of bleeding affects only premature infants; those of less than 34 weeks' gestation are at greatest risk for IVH. Physical signs can range from acute to subtle to no observable signs.

Possible complications include increased intracranial pressure (ICP), brain anoxia and damage, developmental delays, and even death. Treatment usually is supportive and includes administration of anticonvulsants, vitamin E, and steroids and ventilatory support.

ASSESSMENT

Neurologic
Acute signs and symptoms
• Seizures (generalized or focal)
• Unresponsiveness to stimuli
• Bulging or tautness of anterior fontanel
Subtle signs and symptoms
• Slight unresponsiveness to stimuli
Respiratory
• Apnea
Cardiovascular
• Hypotension
Musculoskeletal
Acute signs and symptoms
• Hypotonicity
Subtle signs and symptoms
• Slight hypotonicity
Integumentary
Acute signs and symptoms
• Ashen color
• Temperature instability
Subtle signs and symptoms
• Pallor

NURSING DIAGNOSIS

Risk for injury related to fragility of the capillary beds in the cerebrum

Expected outcome

The infant will have no further signs of hemorrhage as evidenced by a stable hemodynamic status, normal ICP, absence of seizures, and cerebral perfusion pressure above 50 mm Hg.

Interventions

1. Monitor and maintain the infant's partial pressure of arterial oxygen (PaO_2), partial pressure of arterial carbon dioxide, oxygen saturation, and pH by maintaining a patent airway and using an oxygen-delivery device, such as an oxygen hood, continuous positive airway pressure, or a mechanical ventilator.

2. Monitor the infant's blood pressure every 4 hours.

3. Assess the infant's neurologic status every 2 to 4 hours, noting any seizure activity or increased tension in the fontanels. Document the anterior fontanel and head circumferences every 4 to 8 hours initially, then every 24 hours.

Rationales

1. Maintaining the infant's blood gas levels prevents hypoxic episodes, which may lead to circulatory failure and increased cerebral perfusion. Increased cerebral perfusion increases the pressure in vessels, making rupture more likely.

2. Adequate cerebral blood flow depends on normal systemic blood pressure.

3. Seizure activity may decrease cerebral blood flow. The fontanels may bulge or become taut. Increased head circumference may indicate IVH.

4. To decrease the risk of hypothermia or hyperthermia, do not expose the infant to drafts, keep him covered unless he is in a self-contained incubator unit or on a warming table, and use a thermal sensor patch or probe to monitor his body temperature.

4. Extreme changes in temperature increase the stress on the infant's cardiovascular system, possibly increasing ICP.

5. If sodium bicarbonate is ordered to correct metabolic acidosis, administer a diluted 1:1 solution over 20 to 30 minutes.

5. A hyperosmolar solution may increase intravascular pressure, which may dilate cerebral vessels and cause hemorrhage.

6. Assess serial hemoglobin and hematocrit levels every 1 to 2 days.

6. Sudden, dramatic decreases in hemoglobin and hematocrit levels may indicate IVH.

7. Carefully monitor the infant's fluid intake and output.

7. Careful monitoring helps prevent fluid overload or depletion, either of which could alter the infant's systemic pressure and cause hemorrhage.

8. Cluster nursing care measures to help minimize stress on the infant.

8. Stressful stimuli may decrease the infant's PaO_2 levels.

9. Elevate the head of the crib or the self-contained incubator unit 15 to 30 degrees.

9. Elevating the head of the bed helps prevent increased blood flow and brain congestion.

10. Assist with ultrasonography or computed tomography scans, as necessary.

10. These diagnostic tests help assess the infant's condition.

NURSING DIAGNOSIS

Knowledge deficit related to the infant's condition and home care

Expected outcome

The parents will express an understanding of the infant's condition and home care instructions.

Interventions

1. Assess the parents' understanding of the infant's illness.

2. Provide explanations about the infant's medical condition, procedures, and required treatment.

3. Explain the purpose and use of prescribed medications; include details on dosages and potential adverse reactions.

4. To promote normal development, tell the parents to stimulate the baby by exposing him to bright colors, giving him developmental toys, exercising his muscles, and talking to him.

5. Teach the parents seizure precautions and what to do if a seizure occurs; include positioning the infant on his side, maintaining respiratory status, protecting the infant from injury, and recording seizure activity.

Rationales

1. Such assessment serves as a basis on which to begin teaching.

2. This information helps the parents understand the infant's condition and need for hospitalization and decreases their anxiety about the infant's well-being.

3. This information helps the parents correctly administer the prescribed medications. Understanding what adverse reactions may occur allows the parents to seek medical help when necessary.

4. IVH can delay development and cause brain damage, so the infant needs stimulation to grow normally. Approximately 20% of infants with IVH have developmental disorders.

5. Parents need to know how to cope with a seizure because IVH increases the risk for seizures.

Neurologic system

Documentation checklist

During the hospital stay, document:

❏ infant's status and assessment findings upon admission
❏ changes in the infant's status
❏ pertinent laboratory and diagnostic findings
❏ fluid intake and output
❏ nutritional intake
❏ growth and development status
❏ ICP monitoring
❏ ventilator settings
❏ parents' reactions to the infant's illness and hospital stay
❏ family teaching guidelines
❏ discharge planning guidelines.

Meningitis

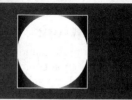

INTRODUCTION

Meningitis is inflammation of the meninges of the brain, spinal cord, or both. Bacterial or viral in origin, meningitis is often preceded by a respiratory infection, sore throat, or flulike signs and symptoms. *Neisseria meningitidis* accounts for most cases of meningitis. It has the highest incidence in children under age 5, with peak incidence in children ages 3 to 5 months. A severe form of meningitis, meningococcemia has a rapid onset and can cause death. Signs and symptoms include high fever, lethargy, chills, and a rash.

ASSESSMENT

Neurologic
• Seizures
• Increased intracranial pressure (ICP)
• Sunset eyes (setting-sun sign)
• Nuchal rigidity
• Positive Kernig's sign
• Positive Brudzinski's sign
• Decreased pupil reactivity
• Irritability
• Opisthotonos
• Headache
• High-pitched cry

Respiratory
• Recent history of infection, sore throat, or flulike signs and symptoms

Gastrointestinal
• Vomiting

Integumentary
• Bulging fontanels
• Petechiae
• Cool extremities
• Rash
• Cyanosis
• Fever

NURSING DIAGNOSIS

Altered cerebral tissue perfusion related to increased ICP

Expected outcome

The child will not develop signs of increased ICP.

Interventions

1. Assess the child's neurologic status every 2 to 4 hours, noting any signs of lethargy, bulging fontanels (in infants), pupillary changes, or seizures.

2. Monitor the child's fluid intake and output every shift.

3. Monitor the child's vital signs every 2 to 4 hours.

4. Note the quality and pitch of the child's cry.

Rationales

1. Frequent neurologic assessments establish a baseline that allows identification of early signs of increasing ICP.

2. Increased fluid volume can increase ICP.

3. Vital signs change with increased ICP.

4. A high-pitched cry usually indicates increased ICP.

NURSING DIAGNOSIS

Risk for injury secondary to seizures

Expected outcome

The child will have no injuries from seizures.

Interventions

1. Take seizure precautions, such as having an artificial airway and suction equipment within reach and keeping the side rails up and padded.

2. Administer anticonvulsant medications, as ordered.

3. During a seizure, take the following measures:

• Help the child lie on his side, either on the bed or floor, and remove any obstacles from the area.
• Do not attempt to restrain the child, but remain at his side.
• Do not attempt to place anything in the child's mouth.
• Assess the child's respiratory status.

• Note any body movements and the seizure's duration.

Rationales

1. These precautions help prevent falls, head injuries, anoxia, choking, and death and reduce the risk of further complications.

2. Anticonvulsant medications help control seizures.

3. These measures help protect the child and aid in medical follow-up.
• These steps help prevent injuries from falling and from jerking motions during the seizure.
• Restraining or forcefully moving the child may cause injury.
• Trying to force an object into the child's mouth may damage the teeth and gums.
• The child may need respiratory resuscitation if he becomes apneic during or after a seizure.
• The types of movement and the duration of the seizure helps define what type of seizure the child had.

NURSING DIAGNOSIS

Hyperthermia related to infection

Expected outcome

The child's body temperature will remain less than 100° F (37.8° C).

Interventions

1. Monitor the child's temperature every 2 to 4 hours.

2. Administer antipyretics, as ordered.

3. Administer antimicrobials, as ordered.

4. Maintain a cool environment.

5. Administer tepid (98.6° F [(37° C]) sponge baths, as needed.

Rationales

1. Monitoring detects elevations.

2. Antipyretics reduce fever by reducing the set point to normal.

3. Antimicrobials treat the underlying infection.

4. A cool environment reduces fever through radiant heat loss.

5. Tepid sponge baths cool the body surface through conduction.

NURSING DIAGNOSIS

Knowledge deficit related to home care

Expected outcome

The parents will express an understanding of home care instructions.

Interventions

1. Teach the parents how and when to administer prescribed medications; include details on dosages and adverse reactions.

2. Teach the parents the importance of providing adequate rest for the child.

Rationales

1. Understanding the importance of consistent medication administration may improve compliance. Knowing what potential adverse reactions may occur allows the parents to seek medical help when necessary.

2. After infection, frequent rest periods promote recovery.

Documentation checklist

During the hospital stay, document:
- ❐ child's status and assessment findings upon admission
- ❐ changes in the child's status
- ❐ pertinent laboratory or diagnostic findings
- ❐ child's neurologic status
- ❐ fluid intake and output
- ❐ nutritional intake
- ❐ growth and development status
- ❐ child's response to treatment
- ❐ child's and parents' reactions to the illness and hospital stay
- ❐ patient and family teaching guidelines
- ❐ discharge planning guidelines.

Neurologic system

Myelomeningocele

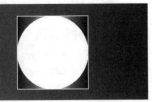

INTRODUCTION

In myelomeningocele, the most common form of spina bifida, the spinal column does not completely close, and a thin sac containing a portion of the spinal cord, meninges, and spinal fluid protrudes from the back. Hydrocephalus also develops in 70% to 90% of all infants born with myelomeningocele, either in utero or during the neonatal period.

Measuring alpha-fetoprotein levels in amniotic fluid can help detect the defect, which occurs in about 1 in 1,000 live births. The location of the defect helps determines its severity. Because myelomeningocele and other neural tube defects have been linked to folic acid deficiency, women of childbearing age may be able to decrease the risk of such defects by increasing their intake of folic acid.

Potential complications include paralysis, joint deformities, meningitis, and lack of bladder or bowel control. Treatment involves surgery, antibiotic administration, physical therapy, and bladder and bowel retraining. Many children are able to walk with the use of crutches or braces.

ASSESSMENT

Neurologic
• Decreased level of consciousness
• Increased head circumference
• Bulging fontanels
• Lethargy
• Irritability

Respiratory
• Apnea

Gastrointestinal
• Vomiting
• Poor sucking reflex

Genitourinary
• Dysuria
• Urine retention
• Dribbling
• Incontinence

Integumentary
• Leakage of cerebrospinal fluid (CSF) from the sac
• Temperature instability
• Skin breakdown

NURSING DIAGNOSIS

Impaired skin integrity related to presence of sac and surgical procedure

Expected outcome

The infant will have no signs of postoperative infection as evidenced by a body temperature less than 100° F (37.8° C), age-appropriate white blood cell (WBC) count, and no purulent drainage.

Interventions

1. During the preoperative and early postoperative periods, maintain the infant in a prone position with the buttocks elevated higher than the head.

2. Use blanket rolls or sandbags to keep the infant from moving from side to side.

3. During the preoperative period, cover the sac with a sterile dressing soaked in normal saline solution. Reinforce the site frequently with new dressings; however, do not remove dressing that adheres to the lesion.

4. Test any drainage from the sac for glucose. Notify the doctor immediately if any CSF leaks from the sac.

Rationales

1. The prone position minimizes pressure on the sac, decreasing the risk of rupture.

2. This helps keep the infant in the prone position.

3. A moist covering over the sac keeps the membrane moist, helping to prevent tearing or rupture of the sac, which could lead to CSF leakage.

4. CSF tests positive for glucose. CSF leakage places the child at risk for meningitis.

5. During the postoperative period, place a transparent occlusive (Op-Site) dressing over the infant's buttocks distal to the sac.

5. The plastic covering helps prevent contamination of the sac or surgical incision.

6. Every 4 hours, assess the infant for signs of infection (including fever, increased white blood cell count, and purulent drainage from the sac) or seizure.

6. Frequent assessments allow for early detection and treatment of infection or seizure.

7. Emphasize the importance of good hand-washing technique to all visitors.

7. Good hand-washing technique minimizes the risk of infection.

NURSING DIAGNOSIS

Hypothermia related to heat loss through the sac

Expected outcome

The infant will maintain a body temperature less than 100° F (37.8° C).

Interventions

1. During the initial preoperative and early postoperative periods, place the infant in a self-contained incubator unit or a radiant warmer.

2. Monitor the infant's temperature every 4 hours for instability.

Rationales

1. Because of the sac protrusion, the infant has an increased amount of exposed skin surface area. A self-contained incubator unit or radiant warmer minimizes heat loss from convection and evaporation from the skin surface.

2. Temperature instability may be a sign of a central dysfunction or an early sign of infection, such as sepsis or meningitis.

NURSING DIAGNOSIS

Altered cerebral tissue perfusion related to hydrocephalus and increased intracranial pressure (ICP)

Expected outcome

The infant does not develop signs of increased ICP (bulging fontanels, increasing head size, vomiting, and high-pitched cry).

Interventions

1. Assess the infant's neurologic status every 2 to 4 hours, noting any signs of lethargy, bulging fontanels, pupillary changes, or seizures.

2. Measure the infant's head circumference daily.

3. Assess the infant's anterior fontanel every 4 to 8 hours.

4. Report any swelling around or leakage of clear fluid from the infant's back incision.

Rationales

1. Frequent neurologic assessments establish a baseline, allowing identification of early signs of hydrocephalus.

2. An increase beyond the normal limits is a sign of hydrocephalus.

3. Normally, the anterior fontanel closes around age 12 to 15 months. Until then, any bulging at the site may indicate increased ICP.

4. Swelling or leakage may indicate progressive hydrocephalus or surgical infection (or both).

Neurologic system

Arnold-Chiari syndrome

Arnold-Chiari syndrome, an elongation or tonguelike downward projection of the cerebellum and medulla through the foramen magnum into the spinal canal, occurs in all infants with the myelomeningocele form of spina bifida. Hydrocephalus commonly accompanies the defect, resulting from impaired drainage of cerebrospinal fluid.

Besides the signs and symptoms of hydrocephalus, other indications of Arnold-Chiari syndrome include nuchal rigidity, noisy respirations, irritability, vomiting, weak sucking reflex, and hyperextension of the neck.

Treatment requires surgical placement of a shunt like that used in hydrocephalus. Surgical decompression of the cerebellar tonsils at the foramen magnum sometimes is indicated.

5. Assess the infant's respiratory rate and rhythm every 2 to 4 hours for signs of apnea, stridor, or an ineffective or weak sucking reflex.

5. Such signs indicate Arnold-Chiari syndrome, a malformation of the hindbrain. All infants with myelomeningocele have Arnold-Chiari syndrome; however, only about 10% of these infants become symptomatic. Hydrocephalus aggravates this problem. (See *Arnold-Chiari syndrome.*)

NURSING DIAGNOSIS

Altered urinary elimination related to injury of spinal cord nerves

Expected outcome

The infant will develop no signs of urinary tract infection (UTI) as evidenced by a body temperature less than 100° F (37.8° C) and an age-appropriate WBC count.

Interventions

1. Carefully note frequency and amount of the infant's urine.

2. Monitor and record the infant's fluid intake and output carefully.

3. Maintain or implement intermittent catheterization every 4 hours. Teach the parents how to perform catheterization using clean technique or Credé's maneuver.

4. Catheterize the infant after he voids.

5. Weigh the infant daily.

6. Encourage increased fluid intake.

Rationales

1. Neurogenic bladder and sphincter commonly occur in children with myelomeningocele. Function depends on the integrity of the sacral nerve roots. Often, voiding only occurs when urine overflows the bladder.

2. Such monitoring ensures early detection of inadequate voiding, which can lead to UTI.

3. Intermittent catheterization completely empties the bladder, and Credé's maneuver uses gentle pressure below the umbilicus to the symphysis pubis to empty the bladder; both decrease the risk of UTI.

4. This helps determine how well the infant is emptying the bladder on his own. Overdistention of the bladder causes ischemia to the bladder wall and weakens its resistance to infection. Also, residual urine provides a medium for bacterial growth in the bladder.

5. Weight changes can reflect hydration status.

6. Increased fluid intake increases renal blood flow and helps flush bacteria from the urinary tract.

7. Observe, report, and record any signs of urinary tract infection, including foul-smelling urine, elevated temperature, and cloudy urine.

7. Myelomeningocele increases the risk for UTIs; recognizing signs early promotes early treatment.

NURSING DIAGNOSIS

Constipation related to level of spinal cord injury

Expected outcome

The infant will maintain regular bowel movements.

Interventions

1. Observe, report, and record characteristics of the infant's anal opening and bowel movement pattern.

2. Assess for abdominal distention, vomiting, and difficulty feeding.

Rationales

1. Anal sphincter assessment may reveal the presence of anal "wink," a reflex that indicates abnormal bowel function. Assessment of the infant's bowel movement pattern ensures early recognition of constipation and lack of sphincter control.

2. These signs may indicate constipation.

NURSING DIAGNOSIS

Risk for impaired skin integrity related to contact with urine or feces

Expected outcome

The infant will develop no signs of skin breakdown or excoriation in the perineal region.

Interventions

1. After each soiling, clean the infant's perineum as soon as possible and pat the area dry.

2. Apply an appropriate ointment or cream, such as A&D Ointment, around the perineal region.

3. Expose excoriated areas to air as much as possible.

Rationales

1. Cleaning the perineum helps prevent irritation from urine and feces. Rubbing the area dry instead of patting can cause further irritation.

2. Ointments and creams provide a protective barrier for the skin.

3. This keeps the area dry and promotes healing.

NURSING DIAGNOSIS

Risk for impaired skin integrity related to altered mobility

Expected outcome

The infant will develop no signs of pressure ulcers (redness over bony prominences or skin breakdown).

Neurologic system

Interventions

1. Place the infant on a sheepskin surface, waterbed pad, or convoluted foam mattress.

2. Keep bed linens clean and dry at all times. Place a soft nonirritating pad or cloth under the infant's face.

3. Change the infant's position at least every 2 hours.

4. Massage the infant's pressure points with lotion every 2 hours.

5. Protect the infant from exposure to excessive heat or cold.

6. Assess for swelling, erythema, and skin breakdown.

7. Assess for altered sensation in the infant's arms and legs.

Rationales

1. These surfaces help prevent pressure ulcers.

2. Clean, dry linens and a soft, nonirritating pad help minimize irritation to the infant's skin.

3. Maintaining the same position for prolonged periods can lead to skin breakdown.

4. Massage increases blood flow to tissues, preventing skin breakdown.

5. The defect may interfere with the infant's ability to sense temperature extremes that can cause skin damage.

6. Early recognition and treatment help prevent pressure ulcers and infection.

7. Altered sensation interferes with the ability to sense pain, increasing the risk for skin breakdown.

NURSING DIAGNOSIS

Risk for injury related to decreased mobility

Expected outcome

The infant will maintain good muscle tone and full range of motion (ROM) and remains free from contractures and hip dislocation.

Interventions

1. When changing the infant's diapers after surgery, lift him by his buttocks rather than his feet.

2. Use sandbags or small blanket rolls to align the infant's extremities during positioning.

3. Perform ROM exercises on the infant's legs and arms as instructed by the physical therapist.

Rationales

1. This helps prevent hip dislocation.

2. Because of the defect and level of spinal cord involvement, the infant may have contractures, which impair muscle movement and proper body alignment. Proper positioning helps maintain alignment and prevent further contractures.

3. ROM exercises stretch out contractures the infant may have and help prevent further contractures. The physical therapist and doctor carefully evaluate alignment, movement, and integrity of the infant's extremities, joints, and muscle groups. This evaluation serves as the basis for an individualized exercise plan. Because of the potential for injury to the infant, the nurse should never initiate ROM exercises without first consulting the physical therapist.

NURSING DIAGNOSIS

Altered nutrition: less than body requirements related to surgery

Expected outcome

The infant will maintain adequate nutrition as evidenced by weight gain.

Interventions

1. Maintain the infant on an I.V. dextrose solution during the preoperative and early postoperative phase.

2. If the infant will receive formula, advance him to formula within 48 hours of surgery by either bottle-feeding or gavage.

3. While the infant is in the prone position after surgery, turn his head and elevate his chin slightly to feed him with a bottle.

4. Assess the infant's sucking abilities.

5. If the infant will be breast-fed, take the following measures:

Rationales

1. Maintaining the infant on an I.V. infusion ensures that he receives adequate fluids when he cannot receive anything by mouth.

2. As long as infant has no respiratory difficulties, he should be able to tolerate formula within 48 hours of surgery, ensuring adequate nutritional intake.

3. This ensures adequate nutritional intake and promotes the sucking reflex.

4. A poor sucking reflex may be related to increased ICP.

5. In most cases, an infant with myelomeningocele may be breast-fed despite his medical condition.
• If the mother is available, place the infant prone on the mother's lap on at least two pillows.
• This position minimizes pressure on the infant's back incision and brings his head to the level of the breast, promoting intake.
• If the mother is unavailable, store pumped breast milk properly in the refrigerator or freezer. Teach the parents how to pump and transport the milk.
• Proper storing and transportation preserve the milk's nutritional value.

NURSING DIAGNOSIS

Altered parenting related to separation from the infant at birth

Expected outcome

The parents will bond with the infant before discharge as evidenced by stroking, touching, and talking to the infant and by taking over some of the routine caregiving activities.

Interventions

1. Explain to the parents the nature of the defect and what they may expect during the hospital stay, using diagrams and written information as appropriate.

2. Help the father or significant other to schedule his activities so he can spend time with the infant and mother.

Rationales

1. A basic understanding the defect and what to expect helps the parents through the stages of grieving and establishes a foundation for home care instruction.

2. In most cases, the father or significant other is the nurse's first contact while the mother is recovering from recent delivery. Helping him to schedule activities helps promote parental bonding.

Neurologic system

3. Model attachment behaviors for the parents by moving from simple touching and stroking of the infant to more complex caregiving tasks, such as changing diapers, bathing, and clothing the infant.

3. Parents normally begin the attachment process through touching, stroking, and talking to the infant immediately after birth. The urgency of the situation at the time of delivery usually disrupts this process, so you may need to serve as a role model and demonstrate that touching and stroking are good for the infant. Later, helping the parents progress to more complex tasks reinforces the parent-infant bond.

4. Teach home care instructions after the parents begin demonstrating attachment behaviors.

4. The parents can better learn and retain home care instructions after they progress through the grieving process and begin demonstrating attachment behaviors.

NURSING DIAGNOSIS

Altered growth and development related to the hospital stay

Expected outcome

The infant will develop at an appropriate rate despite the hospital stay.

Interventions

1. Provide the infant with auditory, tactile, and sensory stimulation (such as touching, stroking, and talking to the infant; hanging a black and white mobile over the crib; playing soft music or a recording of the mother's voice; and changing the infant's position) during nursing care procedures.

2. Refer the parents to an appropriate developmental program at discharge.

3. Teach the parents about the stages of normal infant development and the importance of infant stimulation.

Rationales

1. Such stimulation enhances the infant's physical, emotional, and mental development.

2. Myelomeningocele and hydrocephalus put the infant at risk for developmental delay.

3. Knowing the stages of development helps parents to provide the infant with appropriate developmental activities, maximizing the child's potential intellectual achievement.

NURSING DIAGNOSIS

Knowledge deficit related to home care

Expected outcome

The parents will express an understanding of the infant's condition, treatment, follow-up appointments, and home care instructions.

Interventions

1. Assess the parents' stage in the grieving process and their understanding of the infant's defect and treatment.

Rationales

1. Such an assessment helps determine the parents' readiness to learn complex caregiving tasks.

2. Provide several short teaching sessions on catheterization, feeding, medication administration, skin care, and the signs and symptoms of increased ICP. Give the parents a chance to practice caregiving skills.

3. Provide appropriate education materials on caregiving skills, including booklets, videotapes, and diagrams.

4. Help the family obtain the community services they need after discharge, including:
• support groups, such as a spina bifida association or parent support group
• babysitting for other children
• financial assistance
• home health care
• durable medical equipment
• occupational and physical therapy
• follow-up care from a center experienced in the long-term effects of myelomeningocele.

2. Short teaching sessions improve comprehension by focusing the parents' attention for a limited time. Practicing caregiving skills reinforces the parents' understanding of what they learned.

3. These materials allow the parents to review information at their convenience and offer other perspectives on caregiving skills.

4. The child will need comprehensive follow-up throughout his life. By age 10, the child will have had an average of 11 other surgeries, causing a financial and emotional drain on the family.

Documentation checklist

During the hospital stay, document:
❐ infant's status and assessment findings upon admission
❐ changes in the infant's status
❐ pertinent laboratory and diagnostic findings
❐ fluid intake and output
❐ nutritional intake
❐ infant's preoperative and postoperative status
❐ infant's neurologic status
❐ infant's response to treatment
❐ parents' reactions to the infant's illness and hospital stay
❐ growth and development status
❐ patient and family teaching guidelines
❐ discharge planning guidelines.

Neurologic system

Reye's syndrome

INTRODUCTION

A form of acute encephalopathy that follows a viral infection, Reye's syndrome usually affects children ages 2 months to 18 years. Classic characteristics, which are stage-dependent, include rash, confusion, and vomiting with possible progression to coma. Researchers have linked the development of Reye's syndrome with viral infection and aspirin use; however, the exact cause of the condition remains unknown.

Potential complications include seizures, coma, and even death (about 40% of all children die). Treatment includes administration of corticosteroids, dextrose 10% solution, mannitol, and urea. Additional measures include monitoring for increased intracranial pressure (ICP) and stabilizing respirations.

ASSESSMENT

General
Respiratory
• History of recent viral illness (such as influenza or chickenpox)
Gastrointestinal
• History of salicylate (aspirin) ingestion as treatment for viral illness

Stage 1
Neurologic
• Responsiveness to commands
• Lethargy
• Irritability
Gastrointestinal
• Vomiting
Musculoskeletal
• Fatigue
• Sleepiness

Stage 2
Neurologic
• Disorientation
• Delirium
• Combativeness
• Hyperactive reflexes
• Responsiveness to noxious stimulus
Respiratory
• Hyperventilation
Hepatic
• Hepatic dysfunction

Stage 3
Neurologic
• Obtundation
• Coma
• Decorticate posturing
• Preserved pupillary light reflexes
• Possible dilated pupils
• Intact oculovestibular and doll's eyes reflexes
Respiratory
• Hyperventilation

Stage 4
Neurologic
• Deepening coma
• Decerebrate posturing
• Loss of oculocephalic reflexes
• Large, fixed pupils
• Dysconjugate eye movements

Stage 5
Neurologic
• Flaccid paralysis
• Loss of deep tendon reflexes
• Respiratory arrest

NURSING DIAGNOSIS

Altered cerebral tissue perfusion related to increased ICP

Expected outcome

The child will be responsive and will maintain a normal level of consciousness.

Interventions

1. Perform a neurologic assessment every 2 to 4 hours, or as needed.

2. Raise the head of the bed 30 to 45 degrees, and maintain the child's head in a neutral position (with the head and neck in complete alignment) to avoid neck flexion and rotation.

3. Monitor the child's respiratory status every 2 to 4 hours for hyperventilation.

4. Monitor the child hourly for decreased blood and pulse pressures and increased heart rate.

Rationales

1. Frequent assessments provide data for early detection of neurologic deterioration.

2. This position helps maintain cerebral blood flow and oxygenation.

3. Hyperventilation may result from carbon dioxide retention and increased ICP.

4. Such changes in vital signs signal increased ICP. However, specific changes vary with each child.

NURSING DIAGNOSIS

Altered cerebral tissue perfusion related to increased cerebral edema

Expected outcome

The child will maintain adequate cerebral perfusion as evidenced by a cerebral perfusion pressure above 50 mm Hg.

Interventions

1. Continuously monitor ICP and cerebral perfusion pressure. Notify the doctor if the child's pressure increases.

2. Hyperventilate the child to maintain ICP below 20 mm Hg, or as ordered.

3. Monitor arterial blood gas (ABG) levels, as ordered.

4. Administer diuretics, as ordered, and monitor the child's fluid intake and output.

5. Closely monitor the child's vital signs and perform neurologic assessments every 2 hours.

Rationales

1. Cerebral perfusion pressure measures blood flow to the brain. Increased pressure may signal a worsening of the child's condition.

2. Hyperventilation helps decrease ICP.

3. ABG levels should be maintained at a constant level to prevent cerebral edema from worsening.

4. Diuretics help decrease fluid retention. Monitoring fluid intake and output helps determine the effectiveness of diuretic therapy.

5. Vital signs and neurologic status change with changes in ICP.

NURSING DIAGNOSIS

Risk for injury (hypoglycemia) related to decreased calorie intake or possible metabolic dysfunction or both

Expected outcome

The child will have no signs of injury as evidenced by maintaining a serum glucose level between 100 and 200 mg/dl.

Interventions

1. Administer a dextrose solution to the child, as ordered.

2. Monitor the child's blood glucose level every 2 to 4 hours, or as ordered.

Rationales

1. Dextrose will increase the blood glucose level to prevent brain damage.

2. Such monitoring helps prevent hypoglycemic brain damage.

Neurologic system

NURSING DIAGNOSIS

Altered cardiopulmonary, cerebral, and renal tissue perfusion related to increased ICP

Expected outcome

The child maintains adequate circulatory volume as evidenced by a central venous pressure of 0 to 5 mm Hg, age-appropriate hematocrit values, and a urine output of 1 to 2 ml/kg/hour.

Interventions

1. Monitor the child's vital signs (pulse rate, blood pressure, peripheral pulses, and temperature) and central venous pressure every 1 to 2 hours.

2. Monitor electrolyte and hematocrit values, as ordered.

3. Carefully monitor the child's fluid intake and output (including nasogastric feedings).

Rationales

1. Changes in vital signs signal changes in the child's perfusion status. An increase in temperature may indicate a malfunction in the central nervous system.

2. Electrolyte imbalances may result from the disease (such as phosphaturia or hypoglycemia) or treatment (such as diuretic therapy). Hyponatremia and hyposmolarity may occur with inappropriate secretion of antidiuretic hormone. A fall in hematocrit may result from hemodilution, signaling fluid overload.

3. Careful monitoring allows for accurate fluid replacement and lowers the risk of dehydration or cerebral edema.

NURSING DIAGNOSIS

Ineffective breathing pattern (with the potential for respiratory failure) related to cerebral edema

Expected outcome

The child will maintain adequate gas exchange as evidenced by normal partial pressure of arterial oxygen (PaO_2) and partial pressure of arterial carbon dioxide ($PaCO_2$) levels.

Interventions

1. Auscultate for the child's breath sounds every 2 to 4 hours or as needed.

2. Monitor the child's ABG levels for adequate gas exchange (PaO_2 of 80 to 100 mm Hg and $PaCO_2$ of 35 to 45 mm Hg).

Rationales

1. Auscultation provides data respiratory assessment.

2. Decreasing PaO_2 and increasing $PaCO_2$ indicate poor gas exchange.

3. If the child requires endotracheal intubation, take the following steps:
• After intubation, monitor the ventilator readings for fraction of inspired oxygen and respiratory rate hourly.
• Perform chest physiotherapy, as needed. Hyperventilate and sedate the child 4 hours before chest physiotherapy.

• Administer muscle relaxants, as ordered, to maintain ventilatory control.
• Use soft restraints, as needed, to prevent the child from removing the tube. Check limb circulation hourly.

3. Endotracheal intubation may be ordered to control respiratory effort.
• Such monitoring detects signs of respiratory failure.

• Chest physiotherapy helps clear the airway and improve gas exchange. Hyperventilation and sedation beforehand help prevent dangerous increases in ICP that can result from suctioning performed during chest physiotherapy.
• Muscle relaxants reduce agitation and ensure that the child does not fight the ventilator.
• Soft restraints help limit the child's movement, preventing access to the mouth and nose. Color, warmth, and capillary refill time must be checked because the restraints can restrict circulation in the limbs.

NURSING DIAGNOSIS

Risk for impaired skin integrity related to physical immobility

Expected outcome

The child will maintain skin integrity as evidenced by the lack of skin breakdown and pressure ulcers.

Interventions

1. Move and position the child carefully, as ordered, depending on the degree of increased ICP.

2. Place the child on a convoluted foam, air, or bead mattress.

3. Turn and reposition the child every 2 hours.

4. Assess pressure points with every position change, noting areas of increased redness or shininess.

5. Massage pressure points with every turning.

6. Bathe the child daily using water alone or a moisturizing soap.

Rationales

1. Movement may increase ICP.

2. These mattresses reduce or eliminate the risk of pressure ulcers.

3. Turning and repositioning help relieve pressure areas. However, because movement may increase ICP, turning and repositioning depends on the child's ICP.

4. Increased redness or shininess indicates increased pressure, possibly leading to skin breakdown.

5. Massage increases circulation to the area and decreases the risk of skin breakdown.

6. Bathing helps increase circulation, preventing skin breakdown. Harsh soaps can dry the skin.

NURSING DIAGNOSIS

Anxiety and fear (child) related to hospital stay

Expected outcome

The child will show minimal anxiety and fear as evidenced by age-appropriate blood pressure, pulse rate, and ICP.

Neurologic system

Interventions

1. If the child is placed in a drug-induced coma, administer sedatives, as ordered, and monitor vital signs. Do not give sedatives to a child with bradycardia, hypotension, or decreased respirations.

2. Encourage the parents to bring some of the child's belongings from home, such as a stuffed animal or blanket or a recording of familiar voices.

3. Encourage the parents to visit the child regularly.

4. Hold, touch, and speak soothingly to the child.

Rationales

1. Although paralytic agents can induce coma to decrease metabolic needs, they have no effect on anxiety. Sedatives can help reduce anxiety, preventing increased ICP. Because sedatives also can further suppress heart rate, blood pressure, and respiratory rate, monitoring of vital signs is warranted.

2. Familiar objects help reduce anxiety. Tape recordings are particularly helpful to adolescents; besides reducing anxiety, they also help mask environmental noises when used with earphones.

3. Regular visits maintain the parent-child relationship.

4. Such actions can help calm the child.

NURSING DIAGNOSIS

Self-esteem disturbance related to the disease or rehabilitation process (or both)

Expected outcome

The child will maintain a positive self-concept and age-appropriate development.

Interventions

1. Assess child's knowledge of the disease and his feelings about the situation.

2. Let the child to participate in his own care.

3. Provide play stimulus appropriate to the child's developmental level.

4. Provide age-appropriate explanations of all procedures and treatments.

Rationales

1. Such assessment helps determine the child's current cognitive level and emotional state (fear, anger, shame).

2. This gives the child a sense of control over his condition.

3. Play lets the child to express various emotions.

4. Such explanations help decrease anxiety.

NURSING DIAGNOSIS

Risk for altered parenting related to the child's hospital stay or lack of knowledge about the child's condition

Expected outcome

The parents will maintain appropriate interaction with the child as evidenced by visiting the child, responding to his needs, and providing support.

Interventions

1. Assess what the parents know about the child's condition.

2. Explain all procedures and nursing care measures to the parents.

Rationales

1. Such assessment serves as a basis on which to begin teaching.

2. Knowing this information eases anxiety and helps the parents feel confident about the child's care.

3. Encourage the family to assist in activities of daily living, such as baths, meals, and range-of-motion exercises.

4. Provide support to the parents by listening to their fears and concerns and referring them to auxiliary services as needed, including pastoral care and social services.

3. Helping to care for their child helps decrease the parents' anxiety.

4. Listening to the parents' fears and concerns helps decrease anxiety and stress. Auxiliary services can provide support for areas of special concern.

NURSING DIAGNOSIS

Knowledge deficit related to home care

Expected outcome

The parents will express an understanding of home care instructions.

Interventions

1. Explain to the parents the child's need for physical therapy.

2. Explain the importance of feeding the child a diet high in calories and protein (see appendix F, Guide to food values).

Rationales

1. Physical therapy helps develop wasted muscles.

2. A high-calorie, high-protein diet helps repair injured tissues.

Documentation checklist

During the hospital stay, document:
❏ child's status and assessment findings upon admission
❏ changes in the child's status
❏ pertinent laboratory and diagnostic findings
❏ fluid intake and output
❏ nutritional intake
❏ growth and development status
❏ child's neurologic status
❏ child's response to treatment
❏ child's and parents' reactions to the illness and hospital stay
❏ patient and family teaching guidelines
❏ discharge planning guidelines.

Neurologic system

Spinal cord injury

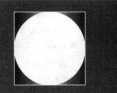

INTRODUCTION

Spinal cord injury — damage that occurs to any level of the spinal cord — can be classified according to one of three major categories: traumatic injuries (the focus of this care plan), tumors, or congenital defects.

Traumatic injuries can result from motor vehicle accidents, falls, sports injuries, or gunshot wounds. Motor vehicle accidents are the most common cause of spinal cord injury. Such injuries impair nerve impulse transmission, leading to varying degrees of dysfunction depending on the cause, the degree of transection (complete or incomplete), the location of the lesion (lower or upper motor neuron), and the level of spinal cord injury (C1 to S4). Generally, the higher the level of spinal cord damage, the more extreme the clinical manifestations.

Treatment includes preventing further trauma to the spinal cord by use of stabilization or traction. Other measures include corticosteroid administration to help decrease edema and surgery, if necessary.

This care plan focuses on the acute phase of the illness and does not fully address the rehabilitative process.

ASSESSMENT

Neurologic
- Absent voluntary motor activity
- Absence of asymmetry in sensory evaluation
- Areflexia

Respiratory
- Dyspnea
- Ineffective cough

Cardiovascular
- Bradycardia
- Hypotension

Genitourinary
- Bladder dysfunction
- Urinary tract infection (UTI)
- Urinary calculi

Gastrointestinal
- Constipation
- Impaction
- Paralytic ileum

Musculoskeletal
- Stiff neck
- Muscle spasms
- Muscle atrophy
- Contractions
- Osteoporosis

Integumentary
- Warm, dry skin
- Increased perspiration above the lesion
- Malignant hyperthermia
- Cool extremities below the lesion

NURSING DIAGNOSIS

Impaired gas exchange related to loss of use of the phrenic nerve, intercostal muscles, or abdominal muscles secondary to the spinal injury

Expected outcome

The child will exhibit adequate ventilatory effort as evidenced by clear, bilateral breath sounds and age-appropriate respiratory rate and arterial blood gas (ABG) levels.

Interventions

1. Assess the child's respiratory status every 1 to 2 hours for breath sounds, chest expansion, respiratory rate, tidal volume (if on a ventilator), and use of accessory muscles.

2. Assess the child's ability to cough every 1 to 2 hours.

3. Encourage the child to breathe deeply every 2 hours.

4. Provide gentle tracheal suctioning if the child's cough is ineffective.

5. Reposition the child every 2 hours.

6. Maintain ABG levels within normal ranges (partial pressure of arterial oxygen between 80 and 100 mm Hg and partial pressure of arterial carbon dioxide between 35 and 45 mm Hg) by adjusting oxygen flow rates or ventilator settings.

7. Administer bronchodilators or mucolytic agents, as ordered.

8. Monitor the child's temperature every 2 hours until stable.

Rationales

1. Although deterioration in respiratory function is expected, it may not develop for several days depending on the amount of spinal cord edema. Injuries above C4 are associated with partial or complete inability to breathe from loss of use of the phrenic nerve. The loss of use of intercostal muscles in low cervical or high thoracic injuries may result in the inability to breathe deeply.

2. An ineffective cough increases the risk for aspiration, infection, and atelectasis, possibly leading to respiratory failure.

3. Deep breathing helps to maintain rib cage flexibility.

4. Suctioning helps to keep the airway clear.

5. Changing position prevents the pooling of secretions.

6. Hypoxia may contribute to further degeneration of the cord injury.

7. Bronchodilators and mucolytic agents increase the diameter of the bronchioles, making breathing easier.

8. Because of the interruption of the sympathetic pathways to the hypothalamus, the child may become poikilothermic, exhibiting fluctuations in body temperature based on environment temperatures. (For each increase of 1.8° F [1° C], the brain demands about 7% more oxygen to meet metabolic demands.)

NURSING DIAGNOSIS

Decreased cardiac output related to autonomic dysfunction and immobility

Expected outcome

The child will maintain adequate cardiac output as evidenced by an age-appropriate heart rate and blood pressure.

Interventions

1. Monitor the child's heart rate, blood pressure, skin color and temperature, and capillary refill time hourly until stable.

Rationales

1. Bradycardia, hypotension, and warm, dry skin are classic signs of spinal shock as a result of the loss of sympathetic control. The higher the lesion to the spinal cord, the more severe the spinal shock will be.

Neurologic system

2. Assess for the following signs of hemorrhage from associated trauma (keeping in mind, however, that internal hemorrhage may not be detectable):
• weak, rapid, thready pulse
• tachypnea
• pallor
• tachycardia.

3. Apply antiembolism stockings or elastic bandages from the child's toes to his groin.

4. Administer vasopressors, as ordered.

5. Do not move the child or elevate the head of the bed while he has spinal shock.

6. Assess the child's extremities every 8 hours for indications of venous thrombosis, including Homans' sign, redness in the calf or thigh, and warmth.

2. Such changes in vital signs result from changes in circulatory status brought on by hemorrhage.

3. Massive vasodilatation may occur below the injury, causing pooling of venous blood in the child's abdomen, legs, and feet. Wrapping bands from the feet toward the heart promotes venous return.

4. Low-dose vasopressors can help maintain adequate cerebral and renal perfusion.

5. Position changes may cause hypotensive episodes because of loss of compensatory mechanisms with autonomic dysfunction.

6. Venous stasis or thrombosis may result from decreased blood flow and flaccid paralysis.

NURSING DIAGNOSIS

Impaired physical mobility related to spinal cord injury

Expected outcome

The child will exhibit no further injury related to impaired mobility as evidenced by absence of contractures and skin redness or breakdown.

Interventions

1. Maintain spinal alignment, as ordered, using cervical traction, a special bed, or hyperextension of the child's regular bed.

2. Reposition the child every 2 hours, and evaluate pressure points. During the acute stage, carefully position the extremities as follows:
• arms and legs extended and slightly abducted
• ankles dorsiflexed (may use high-top sneakers)
• wrist extended with metaphalangeal joints flexed about 60 to 70 degrees and interphalangeal joints flexed 35 degrees.

3. Provide passive range-of-motion exercises every 4 hours.

4. Maintain traction devices, as ordered, following the manufacturer's recommendations.

5. Assess the child for voluntary motor activity in each major muscle group during each shift.

6. Assess the child's sensory level, noting deficits and lack of symmetry. Record the sensory level by describing its location in reference to anatomic landmarks.

Rationales

1. Maintaining spinal alignment promotes healing of the lesion and prevents further injury to the spine.

2. Changing position decreases venous pooling (especially over bony prominences), which can lead to skin breakdown. Proper positioning promotes healing without producing flexor spasms or contractures.

3. Range-of-motion exercises help prevent spasms and joint contractures and maintain muscle tone.

4. Improper use of traction devices may increase the risk of improper healing.

5. Such assessment helps determine the extent of spinal cord injury and possible improvement.

6. The sensory examination helps determine the level of the spinal lesion and possible changes in neurologic status.

NURSING DIAGNOSIS

Altered urinary elimination related to interruption of neural innervation

Expected outcome

The child will maintain a urine output of 1 to 2 ml/kg/hour.

Interventions

1. Monitor the child's urine output hourly during the acute stage. Clamp the urinary catheter periodically, initially for 1 hour, then 2 hours, then gradually increasing the time.

2. After removal of the urinary catheter, assess the child's urinary function. If necessary, help the child empty his bladder by performing Credé's maneuver or by providing intermittent catheterization every 4 to 6 hours, then every 6 to 8 hours.

3. Start the child on a bladder-training program focused toward home care. Begin by clamping the catheter for increasing periods of time, then using Credé's maneuver or intermittent catheterization every 4 hours.

Rationales

1. Monitoring urine output helps evaluate fluid balance and renal function. Periodic clamping of the urinary catheter promotes development of micturition reflexes and may prevent contractions caused by either an empty bladder or prolonged distention.

2. The child may need help to empty his bladder fully after removal of the urinary catheter. Credé's maneuver and intermittent catheterization help prevent bladder distention and urinary tract infection (UTI).

3. Bladder training helps improve the bladder's muscle control and tone. Bladder control helps the child to maintain some control over his bodily functions.

NURSING DIAGNOSIS

Risk for infection related to catheterization

Expected outcome

The child will remain free from UTI as evidenced by absence of bacteria in urine and a body temperature less than 100° F (37.8° C).

Interventions

1. Monitor urinalysis results and urine culture and sensitivity tests for abnormal values.

2. Provide catheter care every 8 hours.

Rationales

1. Urinalysis and urine culture and sensitivity testing detect infection and help identify the causative organism.

2. Routine cleaning around the catheter helps decrease the risk of infection.

NURSING DIAGNOSIS

Constipation related to loss of bowel control

Expected outcome

The child will have regular bowel movements.

Interventions

1. Inspect the child's abdomen for distention, and insert a nasogastric tube for intermittent suctioning of gastric contents.

2. Monitor the child's fluid intake, and start him on an increased-fiber diet after the ileus clears.

3. Develop a bowel-training program that incorporates a digital examination at a routine time, preferably 30 minutes to 1 hour after a designated meal.

4. Administer stool softeners, as ordered.

Rationales

1. During the spinal shock stage, the child's GI system becomes atonic, possibly resulting in distention that may lead to vomiting and aspiration. Nasogastric suctioning helps prevent distention and improper bowel elimination.

2. Adequate fluid intake and increased fiber in the diet ease bowel elimination.

3. Digital examination encourages the use of the anal sphincter. Scheduling this after a designated meal enables the child to rely on normal bowel peristalsis along with digital stimulation to produce a bowel movement.

4. Stool softeners help the child pass hard, impacted stools.

NURSING DIAGNOSIS

Altered nutrition: less than body requirements related to acute injury

Expected outcome

The child will demonstrate an improved nutritional status as evidenced by minimal weight loss and no sign of skin breakdown.

Interventions

1. Administer I.V. fluids and electrolytes, as ordered, during the initial shock phase.

2. Progress from clear liquids to a normal diet, depending on the child's ability to swallow after the acute phase.

3. Carefully monitor the child's dietary intake. Increase his protein intake to one to two times the normal amount.

Rationales

1. I.V. fluids and electrolytes help ensure adequate nutrition when paralytic ileus or endotracheal intubation prevent oral or nasogastric feedings.

2. Spinal cord injury sometimes interferes with swallowing, affecting the child's ability to progress to a normal diet.

3. The child needs enough calories and protein to maintain positive nitrogen balance necessary for skin healing.

NURSING DIAGNOSIS

Body image disturbance related to physical disability

Expected outcome

The child will demonstrate a healthy self-image as evidenced by expressing an acceptance of the physical disabilities imposed by his condition.

Interventions

1. Encourage the child and parents to express their feelings about the injury.

2. Provide honest explanations about the child's expected future functioning and possible dependence.

3. Encourage the child and parents to seek counseling, if appropriate.

Rationales

1. Allowing the child and parents to express feelings helps them to overcome some of the grief brought on by the child's injury and resulting physical disabilities.

2. Honest explanations help the child and parents to face the reality of the disabilities and allow them to plan for the future.

3. Individual or family counseling may help the child and parents work through the grieving process. Peer discussions may be especially helpful, depending on the child's age.

NURSING DIAGNOSIS

Knowledge deficit related to home care

Expected outcome

The parents will express an understanding of home care instructions and demonstrate home care procedures.

Interventions

1. Assess the parents' understanding of the child's condition and prescribed treatment.

2. Explain to the parents the need for and importance of all treatments, procedures, and equipment related to home care.

3. Teach the parents the importance of encouraging the child to drink plenty of fluids.

4. Teach the parents and child the signs and symptoms of UTI — including cloudy, foul-smelling urine; fever; and burning and urgency upon urination — that can result from urinary stasis or catheterization.

5. Teach the parents and child the importance of a high-fiber diet.

6. Refer the parents and child to a physical therapist for ongoing treatment after discharge.

Rationales

1. Such assessment serves as a basis on which to begin teaching.

2. Understanding this information helps the parents recognize the importance of complying with the prescribed regimen and helps lessen their anxiety.

3. Adequate fluids dilute the child's urine, helping to prevent the buildup of bacteria. Fluids also add moisture in stools to prevent constipation.

4. Early recognition of the signs and symptoms of UTI helps prevent extensive infection.

5. Spinal cord injury increases the risk for constipation; fiber increases bulk, decreasing constipation.

6. The child needs extensive physical therapy to reach his maximum function.

Documentation checklist

During the hospital stay, document:
- ❏ child's status and assessment findings upon admission
- ❏ changes in the child's status
- ❏ pertinent laboratory and diagnostic findings
- ❏ fluid intake and output
- ❏ nutritional intake
- ❏ child's neurologic status
- ❏ child's response to treatment
- ❏ child's and parents' reactions to the injury and hospital stay
- ❏ patient and family teaching guidelines
- ❏ discharge planning guidelines.

Neurologic system

Part 4

Gastrointestinal and hepatobiliary systems

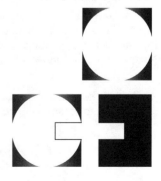

Biliary atresia

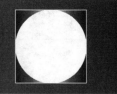

INTRODUCTION

A congenital defect, biliary atresia results from the absence or obstruction of one or more of the extrahepatic or intrahepatic bile ducts, which results in the improper drainage of bile. The accumulation of bile in the liver eventually causes cirrhosis.

Biliary atresia usually requires surgery while the child is an infant, using the Kasai procedure, in which the surgeon removes the nonfunctioning extrahepatic ducts and anastomoses a substitute duct (usually the jejunum) to the liver. This procedure does not have a high long-term success rate; as a result, liver damage tends to progress. An alternative to the Kasai procedure, liver transplantation is sometimes successful in correcting the atresia; however, it can result in several complications, including hemorrhage, organ rejection, and death.

ASSESSMENT

Gastrointestinal
- Clay-colored stools
- Distended abdomen with hepatomegaly
- Esophageal varices
- Ascites
- Anorexia
- Feeding problems (such as slowness in feeding, occasional disinterest in feeding)
- Poor nutritional status

Respiratory
- Respiratory distress

Neurologic
- Encephalopathy

Genitourinary
- Dark-colored urine

Musculoskeletal
- Lethargy
- Muscle wasting
- Failure to thrive

Eye, ear, nose, and throat
- Scleral jaundice at age 2 to 3 weeks

Hematologic
- Bleeding tendencies
- Portal hypertension

Integumentary
- Jaundice
- Dryness
- Pruritus
- Skin breakdown
- Peripheral edema

NURSING DIAGNOSIS

Fluid volume deficit related to poor absorption of nutrients

Expected outcome

The infant will maintain fluid and electrolyte balance as evidenced by a capillary refill time of 3 to 5 seconds, good skin turgor, and a urine output of 1 to 2 ml/kg/hour.

Interventions

1. Monitor the infant's fluid intake and output hourly. When measuring intake, note I.V. fluids, total parenteral nutrition, and any nasogastric or oral feedings. Weigh diapers for urine and stool content. Administer increased fluids, as ordered.

2. Weigh the infant at the same time each day, using the same scale to obtain accurate measurements.

Rationales

1. Such monitoring allows evaluation of the infant's fluid balance and the need for further intervention.

2. Changes in weight may indicate changes in the infant's fluid balance.

3. Check the pH level of the infant's stools with a reagent strip (Tes-Tape); it should be between 7 and 7.5.

4. Monitor the infant's abdominal girth, as ordered, using a consistent point of reference.

5. Observe for signs of dehydration (oliguria, dry skin, poor skin turgor, and sunken fontanels and eyes).

6. Monitor the infant's total peripheral resistance, blood pressure, electrolyte, total protein, albumin, blood urea nitrogen, and creatinine levels as well as the complete blood count (see appendix E, Normal laboratory values), as ordered. Report any abnormalities immediately.

3. Knowing the pH level of stools helps to determine the infant's absorption of fat and carbohydrates.

4. Monitoring the abdominal girth helps to detect ascites and liver enlargement.

5. Signs of dehydration indicate the need for prompt intervention to correct the child's fluid deficit.

6. Monitoring helps evaluate fluid and electrolyte balance. Uncorrected, such imbalances can lead to tachycardia, bradycardia, arrhythmias, or hypotension. Abnormal findings may indicate liver rejection or malfunction.

NURSING DIAGNOSIS

Altered growth and development related to chronic illness

Expected outcome

The infant will develop normally as evidenced by achieving developmental milestones.

Interventions

1. Institute an infant stimulation program that emphasizes the achievement of gross motor skills. Include range-of-motion exercises and positioning (sitting the infant upright). Also provide objects the infant can reach for as well as an open space for crawling.

2. Explain to the parents that their infant may not reach developmental milestones at the same rate as other, healthy infants (see appendix A, Normal growth and development). Encourage them to attend parent support group sessions or to meet with other parents of infants with biliary atresia.

3. Cluster interventions as much as possible.

Rationales

1. A planned stimulation program helps the infant achieve developmental milestones. It also helps the parents bond with their infant.

2. Parents of chronically ill infants often need special counseling about the infant's expected development. Support groups and discussions with other parents facing similar problems can help alleviate stress and fear and can provide important information on ways to stimulate development.

3. Clustering interventions allows the infant the uninterrupted rest he needs to grow and develop.

NURSING DIAGNOSIS

Knowledge deficit related to home care

Expected outcome

The parents will express an understanding of home care instructions.

Interventions

1. Teach the parents the purpose and use of all prescribed medications; include details on administration, dosages, and potential adverse reactions.

Rationales

1. Parents need this information so that they can comply with the treatment regimen. Knowing the potential adverse reactions should prompt them to seek medical help when necessary.

Gastrointestinal and hepatobiliary systems

2. Teach the parents the importance of providing the infant with auditory, visual, and tactile stimulation.

3. Explain the importance of monitoring the infant for nausea and vomiting, muscle cramps, diarrhea, and irregular heart rate and reporting such findings to the doctor.

2. Such stimulation helps the infant achieve developmental milestones.

3. These are signs and symptoms of fluid and electrolyte imbalance and may signal liver rejection or malfunctioning.

Documentation checklist

During the hospital stay, document:
- infant's status and assessment findings upon admission
- changes in the infant's status
- pertinent laboratory and diagnostic findings
- fluid intake and output
- nutritional intake
- growth and development status
- infant's response to treatment
- parents' reactions to the infant's illness and hospital stay
- family teaching guidelines
- discharge planning guidelines.

Hepatitis

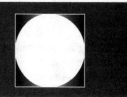

INTRODUCTION

A leading cause of illness and death in childhood, hepatitis is marked by inflammation of the liver that usually results from a viral infection. Hepatitis A and hepatitis B are the most common forms. Hepatitis A usually is transmitted by the fecal or oral route; hepatitis B, by a parenteral route or sexual contact. Vaccination can prevent hepatitis B.

Usual treatment includes isolation, bed rest, and a high-carbohydrate, low-fat diet. Although the prognosis is generally favorable, hepatitis may lead to potentially serious complications, including permanent liver damage.

ASSESSMENT

Gastrointestinal
• Gastrointestinal upset (nausea, vomiting, diarrhea)
• Anorexia
• Light-colored stools
• Right upper quadrant pain (more common in hepatitis B)

Hepatic
• Enlarged liver

Neurologic
• Mood swings
• Irritability
• Depression

Genitourinary
• Dark-colored urine

Musculoskeletal
• Lethargy, fatigue
• Arthralgia

Integumentary
• Elevated temperature
• Jaundice with pruritus
• Rash (occasionally seen early in the course of hepatitis B)
• Papular acrodermatitis (seen in young infants with hepatitis B)

NURSING DIAGNOSIS

Risk for fluid volume deficit related to vomiting, diarrhea, and bleeding

Expected outcome

The child will maintain adequate fluid volume as evidenced by moist mucous membranes, adequate skin turgor, normal electrolyte levels, normal urine output, and absence of bleeding.

Interventions

1. Weigh the child daily, and carefully monitor his fluid intake and output, including the amount and color of urine and stools. Report any output abnormalities (such as decreased urine output or diarrhea) to the doctor.

2. Assess the child's skin turgor and mucous membranes each shift. Notify the doctor of any significant changes in the child's status.

Rationales

1. Daily weighing and intake and output monitoring indicate the child's current hydration status. Children with hepatitis often have dark urine from the passage of bilirubin and urobilinogen and light-colored stools from the lack of bile pigments. Decreased urine output may indicate renal problems; diarrhea can lead to dehydration.

2. Poor skin turgor and dry mucous membranes indicate dehydration; the doctor may order increased fluid intake.

3. Monitor the child for third-space fluid shifting by:
• measuring his abdominal girth at the largest area, using the same tape measure, daily and as needed
• assessing for orthostatic hypotension at least every 4 hours
• assessing for changes in heart rate every 4 hours.

4. Monitor the child for decreased sodium levels (less than 138 mEq/L), decreased potassium levels (less than 3.4 mEq/L), and increased albumin levels. Report any abnormalities to the doctor.

5. Monitor the child for signs of bleeding, including bloody stools, bleeding from venipuncture sites, hematuria, and ecchymoses.

6. Maintain a patent I.V. access.

3. Third-space fluid shifting reflects impaired liver function. It results from edema caused by decreased albumin levels in plasma, which increases the flow of water from the capillaries to intracellular compartments.

4. Abnormal electrolyte and albumin levels indicate fluid imbalances that require prompt treatment.

5. Because of liver disease associated with hepatitis, the child's prothrombin time will be elevated, placing him at risk for increased bleeding. Bleeding can lead to decreased circulatory volume and fluid imbalances.

6. Because of anorexia and vomiting, the child may require rehydration with I.V. fluids to maintain fluid balance.

Nursing diagnosis

Pain related to inflammation of the liver

Expected outcome

The child will demonstrate increased comfort as evidenced by age-appropriate vital signs, expressions of decreased pain and itching, and relaxed body movements.

Interventions

1. Administer antipyretics, analgesics, and antihistamines, as ordered. Do not give aspirin or ibuprofen because they prolong bleeding.

2. Monitor the child's vital signs every 4 hours, as needed.

3. Encourage the use of distraction (such as toys, games, television, and books) to help decrease the child's pain. However, keep in mind that children with hepatitis should not share objects, such as toys, because of the risk of spreading infection.

4. Encourage the child to take frequent rest periods and naps.

5. If the child has a fever, give sponge baths with tepid water to reduce his temperature.

6. Use cool compresses or medicated baths (such as oatmeal, baking soda, or cornstarch baths), as desired, to decrease pruritus.

7. Each shift, assess and document the child's pain and itching along with his response to supportive measures.

Rationales

1. Analgesics may be ordered to relieve pain. Antihistamines inhibit the action of histamines on body tissues, reducing pruritus. Antipyretics reduce fever.

2. Changes in vital signs can indicate the child's current comfort level; increased blood pressure, heart rate, and respiratory rate may signify increased discomfort.

3. Distraction helps to decrease pain and discomfort by allowing the child to concentrate on objects and activities rather than on his immediate pain.

4. Rest helps combat fatigue, which can reduce the child's tolerance for pain.

5. Tepid water can help decrease the child's temperature through evaporation without causing chilling and shivering.

6. Cool compresses or baths decrease pruritus through vasoconstriction. Medicated baths have been found to decrease pruritus in some children.

7. Documentation provides data for assessing the effectiveness of nursing interventions.

NURSING DIAGNOSIS

Altered nutrition: less than body requirements related to anorexia, diarrhea, nausea, or vomiting

Expected outcome

The child will have improved nutritional intake as evidenced by stable weight and adequate caloric intake as monitored by a dietitian.

Interventions	Rationales
1. Weigh the child daily, and carefully monitor his intake and output.	**1.** Daily weighing and intake and output monitoring help determine the child's current nutritional status.
2. Consult the hospital dietitian about the child's dietary requirements.	**2.** The anorexic child requires careful dietary planning to ensure that he receives adequate nutrition.
3. Serve the child small, frequent meals that are high in carbohydrates. Make sure he has his largest meal early in the day.	**3.** Serving small, frequent meals helps ensure that the child eats most of each meal. A high-carbohydrate diet is thought to protect liver cells. The child is more likely to be well rested and hungry early in the day and can eat a larger meal.
4. Administer vitamins, as ordered.	**4.** Vitamin supplements help replenish nutrients depleted by liver disease. Improving the child's nutritional state helps the damaged liver to heal.

NURSING DIAGNOSIS

Risk for activity intolerance related to increased fatigue

Expected outcome

The child's activity level will return to normal levels without recurrence of illness.

Interventions	Rationales
1. Encourage the child to remain in bed during the acute phase of the illness.	**1.** Bed rest helps to decrease the liver's workload, helping prevent liver damage.
2. Provide a quiet environment by limiting the number of visitors and interruptions by hospital staff.	**2.** Decreasing stimuli helps to promote rest and enhance healing.
3. After the acute phase, encourage the child to increase his activities slowly, as tolerated.	**3.** Increasing activity, as tolerated, helps prevent long-term complications of bed rest (such as muscle weakness, contractures, and pressure ulcers) and promotes recovery.
4. Monitor the child's vital signs and transaminase levels (alanine aminotransferase and aspartate aminotransferase).	**4.** Changes in vital signs can indicate changes in activity tolerance. For example, increased heart and respiratory rates along with signs of respiratory distress indicate that the child needs to limit his activity level. Increased transaminase levels may result from too rapid an increase in activity, which may cause a recurrence of the illness.

Gastrointestinal and hepatobiliary systems

NURSING DIAGNOSIS

Risk for impaired skin integrity related to pruritus, frequent diarrhea, and prolonged bed rest

Expected outcome

The child will maintain skin integrity as evidenced by no signs of increased redness, irritation, or abrasions.

Interventions	Rationales
1. Keep the child's skin clean and dry at all times.	**1.** Clean, dry skin prevents skin breakdown from moisture and debris.
2. Assess the child's skin each shift for signs and symptoms of breakdown, including redness, chapping, and tenderness. If the child has any evidence of skin breakdown, change his position every 2 hours and use padding or a convoluted foam mattress.	**2.** Frequent assessments ensure the early detection and prompt treatment of skin breakdown.
3. Administer cool compresses or medicated baths (such as oatmeal, baking soda, or cornstarch baths) and antihistamines, as ordered, to help decrease pruritus.	**3.** Cool compresses or baths decrease pruritus through vasoconstriction, decreasing the risk of skin breakdown from itching. Antihistamines reduce histamine-induced pruritus.
4. Keep the child's fingernails clean and short.	**4.** Clean, short fingernails help prevent skin damage and infection from scratching.

NURSING DIAGNOSIS

Risk for infection related to spread of hepatitis virus through contact with visitors and staff members

Expected outcome

Visitors and staff members will remain free from infection as evidenced by maintaining standard precautions.

Interventions	Rationales
1. Instruct all visitors and staff members to scrub the hands thoroughly with an antimicrobial soap.	**1.** Good hand-washing technique helps reduce the spread of infection.
2. Maintain standard precautions by: • using liners for trash receptacles, according to hospital protocol • wearing and then disposing of gloves when touching soiled materials and when measuring or obtaining body fluids, such as blood, urine, or stool samples • disposing of needles in appropriate containers after use • using disposable dishes and utensils.	**2.** Standard precautions help contain any potentially contaminated specimens, needles, or containers to prevent cross-contamination and the spread of infection.

NURSING DIAGNOSIS

Social isolation related to isolation status (if the child has hepatitis B)

Expected outcome

The child will maintain social interaction with parents and significant others despite being placed in isolation.

Interventions	Rationales
1. Explain to the child and parents the purpose of isolation precautions in cases of hepatitis B (usual protocol includes the wearing of gowns and gloves when in contact with infected blood or body fluids).	**1.** Such explanations increase compliance with the isolation regimen and decrease the child's anxiety about being alone.
2. Encourage the child to maintain contact with his parents and significant others, even if only by phone.	**2.** Regular contact helps decrease feelings of isolation.
3. Encourage the child to express his feelings about the effect isolation has on his lifestyle and body perception.	**3.** Encouraging the child to express his feelings lets you assess the child's understanding of his isolation status and lets the child express any problems he may have with the lack of social interaction.
4. Encourage the parents to participate in the child's care.	**4.** Parental involvement in the child's care helps preserve some semblance of family unity and allows the child to interact with others.
5. Offer the child toys, games, books, television, and other age-appropriate materials (such as newspapers and magazines) to divert his attention from illness and isolation.	**5.** Diversional activities help decrease the trauma of isolation. Newspapers and magazines allow the child to keep up with current events, lessening his feelings of social isolation.

NURSING DIAGNOSIS

Knowledge deficit related to home care, disease, and prevention of recurrence

Expected outcome

The child and parents will express an understanding of home care instructions, the disease, and preventive measures.

Interventions	Rationales
1. Assess the child's and parents' understanding of hepatitis, including its signs and symptoms and the usual route of transmission.	**1.** Such assessment provides a basis on which to begin teaching.
2. Teach the child and parents appropriate hygiene measures to prevent the spread of infection, including: • washing hands after toileting and before eating • cleaning eating utensils with hot water and detergent • keeping the child's toothbrush, eating utensils, cups, and other personal items separate from those of other family members.	**2.** Maintaining proper hygiene practices helps prevent the spread of virus.

Gastrointestinal and hepatobiliary systems

3. If improper food storage and preparation caused the initial infection, involve the hospital dietitian in teaching sessions on how to prepare and store food properly.

4. For adolescent patients, stress the importance of avoiding alcoholic beverages while recuperating from hepatitis.

5. Instruct the parents to contact the doctor about using such over-the-counter medications as acetaminophen (Tylenol) and cold preparations; tell them not to give the child aspirin or ibuprofen.

6. Instruct the parents to monitor the child's activity level, looking for signs and symptoms of the illness' recurrence such as jaundice, pruritus, and epigastric pain.

7. Instruct family members and the child's sexual contacts (if appropriate) exposed to the virus to contact their doctor for evaluation and instruction on preventive measures.

8. Instruct the child and parents on the importance of keeping follow-up appointments.

3. The dietitian can provide detailed information on proper food storage and preparation to ensure that the virus is not transmitted through food.

4. Because alcohol has a direct toxic effect on the liver, consumption of alcoholic beverages might impair healing.

5. Many over-the-counter medications are metabolized by the liver and may cause further hepatic damage; aspirin can increase clotting time, causing further bleeding.

6. A too-rapid increase in activity level may induce a relapse or recurrence of illness.

7. Such evaluation and instruction helps prevent transmission of the disease.

8. Follow-up is necessary to evaluate the clinical progress of the disease and to prevent permanent liver damage.

Documentation checklist
During the hospital stay, document:
- ❐ child's status and assessment findings upon admission
- ❐ changes in the child's status
- ❐ pertinent laboratory and diagnostic findings
- ❐ nutritional intake
- ❐ growth and development status
- ❐ child's response to treatment
- ❐ child's and parents' reactions to the illness and hospital stay
- ❐ patient and family teaching guidelines
- ❐ discharge planning guidelines.

Hirschsprung's disease

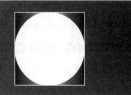

INTRODUCTION

Hirschsprung's disease, also known as aganglionic megacolon, is a congenital disease marked by the absence of parasympathetic ganglion cells in a portion of the colon (and occasionally the ileum). This aganglionosis results in lack of peristalsis in the affected bowel segment, which usually leads to obstruction and difficulty or inability to pass stool.

Hirschsprung's disease occurs more commonly in males and usually is diagnosed in infancy, although occasionally the diagnosis is made later in life. Treatment usually includes a temporary colostomy or ileostomy proximal to the affected bowel segment until corrective surgery is performed. Surgery may include resection of the affected bowel and closure of the colostomy or ileostomy.

Potential complications of this disease include bowel obstruction and dehydration. The prognosis depends on the extent of aganglionosis.

ASSESSMENT

Neonates
Gastrointestinal
- Abdominal distention
- Bilious vomitus
- No passage of meconium during the first 48 hours of life, especially if followed by diarrhea
- Lack of interest in feedings

Respiratory
- Respiratory distress

Cardiovascular
- Shock

Integumentary
- Unexplained fever

Older children
Gastrointestinal
- Constipation or ribbonlike stools
- Vomiting
- Abdominal distention
- Signs of malnutrition (weight loss, physical underdevelopment)

NURSING DIAGNOSIS

Constipation related to aganglionosis

Expected outcome

The child will have regular bowel movements as evidenced by decreased abdominal distention, decreased discomfort, and clear return of enemas or rectal irrigations.

Interventions

1. Administer enemas or rectal irrigations, as ordered.

2. Assess the child's bowel sounds and abdomen every 4 hours. Report decreased or absent bowel sounds.

3. Measure the child's abdominal girth, as ordered, using a consistent point of reference and the same tape measure each time.

Rationales

1. Bowel evacuation increases the child's comfort level and decreases the risk of bowel perforation from obstruction.

2. Such assessment is necessary to ensure proper bowel function and appropriate treatment.

3. Measuring abdominal girth helps detect distention.

NURSING DIAGNOSIS

Risk for fluid volume deficit related to decreased intake, nausea and vomiting, or increased absorptive surface of distended bowel

Expected outcome

The child will maintain fluid balance as evidenced by a urine output of 1 to 2 ml/kg/hour, capillary refill time of 3 to 5 seconds, good skin turgor, and moist mucous membranes.

Interventions

1. Weigh the child daily, and carefully monitor his fluid intake and output.

2. Administer I.V. fluids, as ordered.

3. Use saline or antibiotic solutions rather than tap water when administering enemas or rectal irrigations.

Rationales

1. Daily weighing and careful monitoring of intake and output indicate the child's fluid status.

2. The child may need I.V. fluids if he becomes dehydrated or is at risk for dehydration.

3. Tap water can cause water intoxication from the increased absorptive surface associated with bowel distention.

NURSING DIAGNOSIS

Anxiety (parent) related to lack of knowledge about the disease and prescribed treatment

Expected outcome

The parents will be less anxious as evidenced by expressing an understanding of the disease and prescribed treatment.

Interventions

1. Explain to the parents, in simple terms, the anatomy and physiology of the normal GI tract and the nature of the child's illness. Supplement the explanation with written information and diagrams or illustrations.

2. Give the parents a schedule of diagnostic studies.

3. Give the parents information about colostomy or ileostomy surgery. Provide details on the appearance and function of the colostomy or ileostomy. Use visual aids, such as an ostomy bag, if appropriate. Explain that the colostomy or ileostomy is temporary.

4. Explain to the parents the expected activities and events during the postoperative period (such as the need for I.V. fluids, nothing-by-mouth status, laboratory tests, X-rays, administration of pain medications, dressing changes, and nasogastric suctioning). Use visual aids, such as sample equipment, if available.

Rationales

1. Understanding the normal function of the GI system helps the parents to understand the seriousness of the child's condition and the need for treatment. Increased awareness of the situation should help to ease anxiety.

2. Knowing what to expect should help decrease the parents' anxieties and fears.

3. Such information helps decrease the parents' anxiety and allows them to take part in their child's care.

4. Understanding what to expect postoperatively helps alleviate the parents' anxiety by preparing them beforehand for their child's condition after surgery. Such explanations also reinforce the importance of surgical intervention and the need for parental cooperation and involvement in postoperative care.

NURSING DIAGNOSIS

Impaired skin integrity related to exposure to stool secondary to colostomy or ileostomy

Expected outcome

The child will have no signs of skin breakdown as evidenced by intact skin around the colostomy or ileostomy site that is free from redness or irritation.

Interventions

1. Use a well-fitted ostomy bag with an effective skin barrier (such as Hollihesive, Stomahesive, or Comfed) to protect the skin from coming in contact with stool.

2. Change the ostomy bag whenever it leaks or is suspected of leaking. Check the bag every 2 hours.

3. Empty the ostomy bag whenever it is one-fourth to one-third full.

4. Change the ostomy bag at least once every 24 hours until the periostomal site heals.

5. If skin breakdown occurs, administer wound treatment as ordered by the doctor, enterostomal therapist, or ostomy nurse.

Rationales

1. A properly fitting appliance and skin barrier protects the periostomal area from the caustic effects of stool. Diapering without a bag usually results in skin breakdown.

2. Leaking causes stool to come in contact with skin, increasing the risk of skin breakdown.

3. Letting the bag fill up increases the risk of leaking because the weight of stool can pull the seal away from the skin.

4. Daily changing allows for frequent monitoring of the periostomal area and ensures prompt treatment in case of improper healing (the periostomal site usually heals within 1 to 3 days).

5. Depending on the degree of skin breakdown, the child may need various treatments (such as use of a foam mattress, donut pad, skin preparations, or karaya rings).

NURSING DIAGNOSIS

Risk for infection of incision related to contamination from stool

Expected outcome

The child's incision will heal normally, as evidenced by no signs or symptoms of erythema, induration, or drainage and a body temperature less than 100° F (37.8° C).

Interventions

1. Change the ostomy bag immediately if it leaks or is suspected of leaking. This is especially important if the skin barrier or ostomy bag covers the incision.

2. If the ostomy bag covers the incision, change the ostomy bag daily until the incision heals. Note any signs of infection, including redness, purulent drainage, and swelling.

Rationales

1. Changing the ostomy bag prevents prolonged contact between the incision and stool, helping to prevent skin breakdown.

2. Changing the ostomy bag daily allows for early detection of contamination and signs of infection and promotes prompt treatment.

Gastrointestinal and hepatobiliary systems

NURSING DIAGNOSIS

Body image disturbance related to colostomy or ileostomy

Expected outcome

The child will have an improved self-concept as evidenced by age-appropriate expression about the colostomy or ileostomy and ostomy bag and showing interest in self-care. (Outcome criteria apply to children over age 5.)

Interventions

1. Promote and encourage such self-care activities as daily hygiene, grooming, feeding, and dressing.

2. Encourage the child to express his feelings about the colostomy or ileostomy.

Rationales

1. Self-care activities help the child to continue to care about himself and his appearance despite his altered body image, improving his self-esteem.

2. This allows the child to deal with his feelings without fear of rejection and helps to improve his self-image.

NURSING DIAGNOSIS

Knowledge deficit related to home care

Expected outcome

The parents will express an understanding of home care instructions and demonstrate home care procedures.

Interventions

1. Teach the parents the importance of feeding the child a high-calorie, high-fiber diet.

2. Teach the parents how to care for the child's colostomy or ileostomy (see the "Colostomy and ileostomy" plan, page 284).

Rationales

1. A high-calorie, high-fiber diet replaces lost calories and helps prevent constipation.

2. The parents need to know how to care for the colostomy or ileostomy to ensure healing and to prevent skin breakdown and other potential complications.

Documentation checklist

During the hospital stay, document:
- child's assessment findings upon admission
- changes in the child's status
- pertinent laboratory and diagnostic findings
- fluid intake and output and nutritional intake
- child's response to treatment
- child's and parents' reactions to the illness and hospital stay
- patient and family teaching guidelines
- discharge planning guidelines.

Inflammatory bowel disease

INTRODUCTION

Inflammatory bowel disease — a term used to describe ulcerative colitis and Crohn's disease — is marked by chronic inflammation of the colon. In ulcerative colitis, the mucosa and submucosa of the colon are affected. In Crohn's disease, the entire alimentary tract is involved. Crohn's disease is usually more severe and does not respond well to treatment. It is more likely to occur in school-age children and adolescents than in infants or toddlers.

Treatment for inflammatory bowel disease usually includes a high-protein, high-calorie, low-fat, low-fiber diet and anti-inflammatory medication. The prognosis for this incurable disease is not favorable; it can cause lifelong bowel problems and increases the risk of colon cancer.

ASSESSMENT

Gastrointestinal
- Abdominal pain and cramping (Crohn's disease)
- Weight loss (Crohn's disease)
- Abdominal distention
- Anorexia
- Diarrhea (ulcerative colitis)
- Steatorrhea
- Vomiting
- Bloody stools (ulcerative colitis)
- Stomatitis

Musculoskeletal
- Fatigue
- Arthralgia
- Arthritis

Endocrine
- Delayed secondary sexual development

Hematologic
- Anemia

Integumentary
- Pallor
- Dehydration
- Lesions

NURSING DIAGNOSIS

Anxiety (child and parent) related to lack of knowledge about the disease process, diagnostic studies, and expected treatment

Expected outcome

The child and parents will be less anxious as evidenced by expressing an understanding of the disease, diagnostic studies, and expected treatment.

Interventions

1. Explain to the parents and child (as appropriate) the basic anatomy and physiology of the upper and lower GI tracts. Also explain normal food passage through the GI system, paying particular attention to the nutritional aspects and functions of the small and large intestines. Use visual aids, if available, during explanations.

2. Give the parents and child a schedule of diagnostic studies, such as an upper GI series with a small-bowel follow-through, a barium enema, an upper and lower endoscopy, and biopsies.

Rationales

1. Understanding the normal function of the GI system helps the parents and child to better understand the abnormal function that occurs in inflammatory bowel disease. Visual aids help increase retention of information.

2. Knowing what to expect helps decrease anxiety and fear.

Gastrointestinal and hepatobiliary systems

3. Explain each scheduled diagnostic test to the parents and child; include information on preparing for the test, how long the test will last, and posttest care.

4. Teach the parents the importance of providing the child with a high-protein, high-calorie, low-fat, low-fiber diet to promote maximum nutritional adsorption.

5. Explain to the parents and child the purpose, use, and correct dosage of and potential adverse reactions to anti-inflammatory agents (sulfasalazine [Azulfidine], corticosteroids).

6. As indicated, provide information about the need for surgery and placement of a colostomy bag. Explain that surgery is necessary to remove the inflamed area and to create a colostomy for normal elimination. Also explain the purpose and appearance of the colostomy as well as details on the use of dressings, I.V. fluids, and pain-control medications.

7. Encourage the parents and child to express their feelings about the need for a colostomy. Refer them to a local ostomy support group, or arrange for them to meet with other parents and children with the same problem.

8. Encourage the parents and child to ask questions about the disease, diagnostic tests, or expected treatment during teaching sessions and to write down any further questions as they arise.

3. Understanding the purpose of and procedure for each test helps reduce anxiety and increases the child's cooperation. It also helps the parents to support their child while he prepares for and undergoes the test and to take part in caring for the child after the test.

4. Such a diet ensures that the child receives adequate nutrition during periods of acute illness as well as remission. A diet high in calories and protein and low in fat replaces the nutrients and blood lost through frequent diarrhea and anorexia. A diet low in fiber reduces irritation of the bowel, allowing it to heal.

5. Anti-inflammatory agents may be ordered to help reduce inflammation, allowing the bowel to rest. Teaching the parents and child about the medication regimen helps to improve compliance with therapy and with monitoring for adverse reactions.

6. This information helps the parents and child to understand and better anticipate the potential course of the disease, lessening their anxiety.

7. Because colostomy often has an effect on body image, the child and parents may have difficulty dealing with their feelings. Meeting others who share the same problem may help to reduce anxiety.

8. Asking questions during teaching sessions allows for immediate responses. Writing down questions as they occur ensures that the nurse will clarify pertinent information at a later date.

NURSING DIAGNOSIS

Altered nutrition: less than body requirements related to impaired absorption

Expected outcome

The child will have improved nutritional status as evidenced by increased intake and weight gain.

Interventions

1. Maintain the child on a high-protein, high-calorie, low-fat, low-fiber diet.

Rationales

1. Extra protein and calories help replace protein and blood lost from the ulcerated bowel and restore calories lost through diarrhea. A low-fat, low-fiber diet decreases bowel irritation that could lead to diarrhea.

2. Administer nutrition through alternative methods (such as a high-protein, high-carbohydrate, high-vitamin liquid diet; short-term, peripheral total parenteral nutrition [TPN] for 1 to 2 weeks; or long-term, central line TPN therapy) during periods of exacerbation.

2. During acute illness, the child may need an alternative feeding method to ensure adequate nutrition. An oral liquid diet replaces lost nutrients; short-term TPN replaces lost nutrients while the child's oral intake is restricted. The child may need long-term TPN if he has chronic diarrhea, fluid loss, or nutritional malabsorption.

3. Monitor the child for changes in stool consistency, melena, abdominal pain, bloating, nausea and vomiting, and fever. Monitor laboratory values (complete blood count and electrolyte, blood urea nitrogen, and glucose levels), reporting any alterations immediately.

3. These findings may signal infection, GI disturbance, or electrolyte imbalances related to nutritional imbalance.

4. Consult the hospital dietitian when planning the child's meals, and serve the child some of his favorite foods as allowed.

4. Consulting the dietitian ensures that the child receives adequately balanced meals. Serving some of the child's favorite foods helps ensure that he eats most of each meal.

NURSING DIAGNOSIS

Body image disturbance related to the disease, medication use, and the need for a colostomy

Expected outcome

The child will exhibit a positive body image as evidenced by demonstrating self-care, such as hygiene and personal grooming, and by expressing an understanding of the need for his colostomy.

Interventions

1. Instruct the child and parents to report adverse reactions to corticosteroid therapy—such as acne, rapid weight gain, and mood swings—immediately.

Rationales

1. Acne and weight gain can be devastating to a child, especially an adolescent, and mood swings can be frightening. Reporting these adverse reactions to the doctor allows for prompt treatment, decreasing their physical and emotional impact.

2. Prepare the child for the possibility of colectomy surgery and the need for a colostomy. Refer the child and parents to a local ostomy support group for ongoing counseling, if appropriate. (See the "Colostomy and ileostomy" plan, page 284.)

2. Because the need for a colostomy may have devastating psychological effects, parents and children require education, patience, support, and time to accept the condition. Local ostomy groups offer support and first-hand knowledge on ways to deal with the effects of an altered body image.

3. Encourage the child to participate regularly in an exercise program, sport, or hobby with other children his age. Also encourage participation in school, church, and community activities.

3. Such activities help distract the child's attention from the disease, helping to decrease his negative feelings about his altered body image. Interest and participation in activities with other children helps the child to maintain a healthy self-image and lifestyle.

Gastrointestinal and hepatobiliary systems

Nursing diagnosis

Knowledge deficit related to home care

Expected outcome

The parents and child will express an understanding of home care instructions and demonstrate home care procedures.

Interventions

1. Teach the parents and child the purpose and importance of proper colostomy care, including maintaining and cleaning colostomy bags, using irrigation solutions, and maintaining skin integrity (See the "Colostomy and ileostomy" plan, page 284.)

2. Explain the importance of maintaining the child on a high-protein, high-calorie, low-fat, and low-fiber diet.

3. Give the family instructions that they can give to the child's teachers, the school nurse, and any others who may care for the child.

Rationales

1. The parents and child must know how to care for the colostomy to prevent skin breakdown and infection and to ensure proper bowel function.

2. Extra calories and protein help to supplement those lost through the GI tract. Decreased levels of fat and fiber in the diet help to control diarrhea.

3. Because inflammatory bowel disease is chronic, teachers and others potential caregivers need information on what care the child may need.

Documentation checklist

During the hospital stay, document:
- ❏ child's status and assessment findings upon admission
- ❏ changes in the child's status
- ❏ pertinent laboratory and diagnostic findings
- ❏ nutritional intake
- ❏ growth and development status
- ❏ child's response to treatment
- ❏ child's and parents' reactions to the illness and hospital stay
- ❏ patient and family teaching guidelines
- ❏ discharge planning guidelines.

Liver transplantation

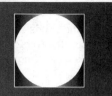

INTRODUCTION

Liver transplantation involves the surgical replacement of a nonfunctioning liver with a liver donated from a "living" donor (a brain-dead donor sustained by life support). Typically, this procedure is indicated for children with a congenital defect, such as biliary atresia. Each hospital requires that the surgery candidate meet certain criteria before being accepted for transplantation, including such compatibility factors as organ size and blood and tissue type matching.

Recovery from transplantation surgery varies, depending on the number of complications. Potential complications include hemorrhage, infection, organ rejection, and death.

ASSESSMENT

Hepatic
• Slight to moderate jaundice

Gastrointestinal
• Abdominal distention with large abdominal incision
• Malnourishment
• Poor weight gain

Respiratory
• Coarse bilateral breath sounds
• Pink, moist mucous membranes

Cardiovascular
• Pink nail beds with a capillary refill time of less than 3 seconds

Psychosocial
• Developmental delays

NURSING DIAGNOSIS

Risk for infection related to incision and immunosuppression

Expected outcome

The child will have no signs of infection as evidenced by a body temperature less than 100° F (37.8° C) and a lack of purulent drainage from the incision.

Interventions

1. Observe good hand-washing technique before caring for the child.

2. Keep the child in a private room.

3. Monitor the child's temperature every 4 hours, every 2 hours when elevated; notify the doctor of any elevation.

4. Monitor the child's vital signs every 4 hours.

5. Assess the incision for redness, edema, and drainage. Report any of these signs immediately.

6. Use sterile technique for such invasive procedures as central line care or wound care.

Rationales

1. Good hand-washing technique helps prevent nosocomial infection.

2. Keeping the child in a private room decreases the risk of exposure to patients with potentially contagious diseases.

3. A temperature higher than 100° F may indicate infection.

4. Changes in vital signs, such as elevated temperature and increased pulse rate, may indicate early infection.

5. Redness, edema, and purulent drainage are signs of wound infection.

6. Sterile technique decreases the risk of nosocomial infection.

7. Monitor the child's contact with other patients and visitors. Institute reverse isolation precautions, as ordered (see *Reverse isolation*).

7. Screening other patients and visitors for contagious diseases before they enter the child's room helps prevent infection. Reverse isolation further protects the child with further safeguards against infection.

Reverse isolation

Because immunosuppression increases the child's risk for infection, reverse (protective) isolation typically is required after surgery. Below is a list of general precautionary measures used in many hospitals.

• After locating the child in a private room, explain isolation procedures to him to help ease anxiety and promote cooperation.

• Make sure the room is cleaned and has new or scrupulously clean equipment. Because the child does not have a contagious disease, articles leaving the room require no special care after the child is discharged.

• Keep supplies, such as gowns, gloves, masks, caps, and plastic bags, in a clean, enclosed cart or in an anteroom outside the child's room. Also stock linens and head and shoe coverings for the child if he is especially susceptible to infection. Keep additional supplies, such as a thermometer, stethoscope, and blood pressure cuff, in the room to minimize trips in and out and to prevent contaminating the child with equipment used on other patients.

• Keep the door to the room closed. Post reverse isolation cards on the door.

• Put on a clean gown, mask, cap, and gloves each time you enter the child's room.

• Wash your hands with an antiseptic agent before putting on gloves to prevent bacterial growth on gloved skin; wash the gloves with an antiseptic if they become contaminated during care; wash your hands after leaving the room.

• Instruct the housekeeping staff to put on gowns, gloves, caps, and masks before entering the room; advise them not to enter the room if they are ill or infected.

• Do not allow visits by anyone known to be infected or ill. Show visitors how to put on gowns, gloves, caps, and masks, and instruct them to remove them only after they leave the room.

• Do not perform invasive procedures, such as urethral catheterization, unless absolutely necessary.

• Avoid transporting the child out of the room; if he must be moved, put a gown and mask on him first.

8. Administer antibiotics, as ordered.

8. Antibiotics are given prophylactically to prevent postoperative infection.

9. Monitor the child's complete blood count (CBC) daily.

9. An increased or decreased white blood cell count indicates infection. Shifts in the differential may also indicate infection.

10. Obtain specimens for blood and urine cultures and a chest X-ray if the child's temperature is greater than 100.4° F (38° C).

10. These tests can rule out the possibility of infection and identify the source of fever.

NURSING DIAGNOSIS

Altered cardiopulmonary tissue perfusion related to blood loss, alterations in the renin-angiotensin system, and recovering liver function

Expected outcome

The child will maintain normal tissue perfusion as evidenced by age-appropriate vital signs and CBC, capillary refill time of less than 3 seconds, and no sign of active bleeding.

Interventions

1. Assess the child's blood pressure every 4 hours. Take corrective measures, as ordered, if the pressure is increased or decreased.

Rationales

1. Decreased blood pressure may indicate active bleeding. Increased blood pressure may result from alterations in the renin-angiotensin system produced by steroid and immunosuppressant therapy.

2. Assess the child's capillary refill time, peripheral pulses, and color of skin and mucous membranes every 4 hours.

3. Assess the child for signs of active bleeding, such as bloody vomitus and tarry stools, and for color and volume of drainage. Notify the doctor immediately of any abnormal findings, and perform a type and crossmatching for blood replacement.

4. Administer antihypertensive agents (propranolol [Inderal], hydralazine [Apresoline]) or antihypotensive agents (packed red blood cells, fresh frozen plasma, or platelets), as ordered, depending on the child's blood pressure.

2. A capillary refill time greater than 5 seconds, diminished peripheral pulses, and cyanosis indicate poor peripheral perfusion and impending shock.

3. Active bleeding may indicate coagulopathies related to previous liver disease and the grafting recovery period.

4. These agents help to maintain blood pressure and hematologic values within normal limits.

Nursing diagnosis

Risk for fluid volume deficit related to high-dose steroid therapy and fluid loss

Expected outcome

The child will maintain fluid and electrolyte balance as evidenced by normal serum electrolyte levels and a urine output of 1 to 2 ml/kg/hour.

Interventions

1. Carefully monitor the child's fluid intake and output, including parenteral intake, oral intake (after the child can tolerate fluids), and urine and drainage output.

2. Weigh the child each morning using the same scale.

3. Assess for edema, weight gain, hypertension, increased ascites, gallop rhythms, and coarse breath sounds.

4. Monitor the child's serum electrolyte levels.

5. Administer diuretics, as ordered.

6. Maintain the child on a low-sodium diet.

7. When preparing I.V. medications, use the minimum amount of fluid necessary for dilution.

Rationales

1. Accurate monitoring is essential to determine the child's fluid requirements. Decreased urine output may indicate hypovolemia or acute renal failure.

2. A weight fluctuation of ± 9 oz (255 g) in a 24-hour period indicates fluid imbalance.

3. These signs of hypervolemia indicate the need for immediate treatment, such as decreased fluid intake and diuretic therapy.

4. Increased sodium levels indicate hypovolemia (usually treated with fluid volume expanders); decreased sodium levels indicate hypervolemia (usually treated with decreased fluid intake and diuretic therapy).

5. Diuretics are ordered in cases of hypervolemia to increase the excretion of excess fluids.

6. High sodium intake can cause fluid retention.

7. Using minimal fluids is especially important in small children and infants to prevent fluid overload.

Gastrointestinal and hepatobiliary systems

NURSING DIAGNOSIS

Ineffective breathing pattern related to prolonged general anesthesia and a large abdominal incision

Expected outcome

The child will maintain adequate respiratory status as evidenced by pinkish skin color, normal respiratory rate, clear breath sounds, and effective air movement.

Interventions	Rationales
1. Help the child to cough, turn, and breathe deeply every 2 hours.	**1.** Coughing helps clear mucus from the lungs; turning helps loosen secretions; deep breathing improves oxygenation.
2. Perform chest physiotherapy every 4 hours.	**2.** Chest physiotherapy helps loosen and remove secretions, making breathing easier.
3. Suction the child, as needed.	**3.** Suctioning helps to clear mucus from the airway.
4. Assess for increased respiratory rate, decreased air movements, coarse breath sounds, and changes in the color or consistency of sputum.	**4.** These signs of respiratory infection usually indicate the need for antibiotic administration.

NURSING DIAGNOSIS

Pain related to surgery

Expected outcome

The child will demonstrate increased comfort as evidenced by age-appropriate vital signs, expressions of decreased pain, and relaxed body movements.

Interventions	Rationales
1. Administer pain medication, such as meperidine hydrochloride (Demerol), morphine, or hydromorphone (Dilaudid), adjusting the dosage for the child's age and weight.	**1.** These drugs have sedative properties that help to decrease the child's pain.
2. Change the child's position every 2 hours.	**2.** Position changes help relieve pressure on bony prominences and prevent stiffness.
3. Provide diversional activities, such as toys, books, television, or games.	**3.** Such activities help to divert the child's attention from his pain.

NURSING DIAGNOSIS

Altered nutrition: less than body requirements related to chronic illness, initial postoperative nothing-by-mouth status, and anorexia

Expected outcome

The child will maintain adequate nutritional status as evidenced by adequate calorie intake and weight gain.

Interventions

1. Carefully monitor the child's intake and output.

2. Weigh the child daily.

3. When planning the child's meals, consult the hospital dietitian and consider anthropometric findings.

4. Administer nasogastric feedings or total parenteral nutrition, as ordered.

5. Serve the child some of his favorite foods, if they are within dietary limits.

Rationales

1. Intake and output monitoring provides data for assessing the child's calorie requirements.

2. Slow, steady weight gain indicates adequate nutritional intake.

3. The child needs adequate nutrition for wound healing. Anthropometric findings help to determine the child's current nutritional status and calorie requirements.

4. The child may need supplemental nutrition when his oral intake does not meet calorie needs.

5. Offering some of the child's favorite foods helps ensure that he will eat more of each meal.

NURSING DIAGNOSIS

Anxiety (child and parent) related to the extended hospital stay and chronic illness

Expected outcome

The child and parents will be less anxious as evidenced by expressing their fears and demonstrating a realistic problem-solving approach to coping with those fears.

Interventions

1. Assume the role of the primary nurse to establish a trusting relationship with the child and parents.

2. Explain all procedures to the child and parents in appropriate terms.

3. Develop a daily schedule of all activities and treatments for the staff and family to use.

4. Answer all questions honestly, consulting appropriate resources as needed.

5. Allow the child and parents to express their fears and frustrations.

6. Allow the child and parents to make choices concerning the child's care (such as bathing and feeding), when possible.

7. Integrate the services of a social worker, child-life worker, and spiritual counselor, as needed, in the child's care.

Rationales

1. Generally, the primary nurse establishes consistent nursing care and serves as advocate for the patient and family, which helps ease anxiety.

2. Such explanations help to reduce anxiety by preparing the child and parents for upcoming events.

3. A daily schedule provides a sense of consistency and structure, which can help reduce anxiety.

4. Answering all questions enhances the parents' and child's knowledge and understanding of the disease, decreasing anxiety.

5. Expression of feelings promotes trust and open communication, helping to decrease anxiety.

6. This helps to ease anxiety by fostering a sense of control and allowing for active participation in the child's care.

7. Offering ancillary support helps to ease anxiety during particularly stressful times.

Gastrointestinal and hepatobiliary systems

NURSING DIAGNOSIS

Altered growth and development related to the chronic illness and extended hospital stay.

Expected outcome

The child will achieve his appropriate developmental level as evidenced by demonstrating age-appropriate developmental tasks.

Interventions

1. Provide the child with age-appropriate toys and activities.

2. Use the Denver Developmental Screening Test (DDST) to assess the child's current developmental level (up to age 6).

3. Provide for routine psychological evaluation of the child's coping skills and support systems.

Rationales

1. Providing such toys and activities encourages normal development.

2. The DDST is widely accepted as a measure of a child's current developmental level.

3. Such evaluation provides information on the child's developmental progress and ability to cope with the illness.

NURSING DIAGNOSIS

Altered parenting related to chronic life-threatening disease

Expected outcome

The parents will interact appropriately with the child as evidenced by visiting regularly, talking with the child, and providing support.

Interventions

1. Encourage the parents to visit or stay with child (if permitted).

2. Explain all treatments and procedures to the parents.

3. Encourage the parents to attend support group meetings.

Rationales

1. Regular visits or rooming-in allows for continued parent-child contact.

2. Such explanations help decrease fear and anxiety, which can lead to stress and alterations in the parent-child relationship.

3. Attending support group meetings allows the parents to interact with other parents of children with chronic illnesses, which encourages improved parenting skills.

NURSING DIAGNOSIS

Knowledge deficit related to home care

Expected outcome

The parents will express an understanding of home care instructions.

Interventions

1. Teach the parents:
• the signs and symptoms of infection, such as elevated temperature and purulent drainage from the incision
• the signs and symptoms of organ rejection, such as elevated temperature, pain at the graft site, swelling and tenderness, jaundice, and decreased hemoglobin and hematocrit values.

2. Teach the parents about all ordered medications; include details on proper administration and potential adverse reactions. Explain that long-term steroid use can cause Cushing's syndrome, excessive hair growth, growth retardation, and infertility.

3. Explain to the parents the child's immunosuppressed state and the need for certain precautions, such as avoiding persons with known infection and avoiding large crowds, to protect the child from infection.

4. Instruct the parents to monitor the child's temperature twice daily.

5. Explain the importance of keeping regular laboratory appointments when the child is receiving cyclosporine (Sandimmune) or other immunosuppressant therapy. Discuss the adverse effects of the drug, which include nausea, vomiting, tremors, headache, hepatotoxicity, and nephrotoxicity.

Rationales

1. Knowing the signs and symptoms of infection and organ rejection should prompt the parents to seek medical help when necessary.

2. Such teaching helps ensure that the parents administer medications accurately and comply with the medication regimen. Knowing the potential adverse reactions should prompt parents to seek medical help when necessary. Understanding the effects of long-term steroid use can help the parents respond effectively if they occur.

3. Because of the child's immunosuppressed state, he is at risk for infection, which may have life-threatening implications.

4. Frequent monitoring ensures early recognition of rejection or infection and allows for prompt treatment.

5. Regular laboratory visits ensure accurate blood level measurements and help to determine when medication adjustments are necessary. The parents need to recognize adverse effects so they can seek medical help when necessary.

NURSING DIAGNOSIS

Body image disturbance related to effects of steroid therapy

Expected outcome

The child will have an improved self-concept as evidenced by verbalizing acceptance of his body.

Interventions

1. Listen attentively to the child's feelings and concerns about his body. Do not negate the feelings.

2. Help the child focus on his assets and positive features.

3. Encourage the child to attend support group meetings, such as those designed for transplant patients in his age-group.

4. Encourage the child's siblings and peers to visit.

Rationales

1. Listening provides emotional support and allows the nurse to assess the child's acceptance of his appearance.

2. Focusing on assets and positive features helps de-emphasize the negative aspects of the child's condition.

3. Support groups help decrease the child's feelings of isolation by introducing him to other children with similar problems. Such groups also allow the child to see how others cope with an altered body image.

4. Visits from siblings and peers enable the child to maintain contact with others outside the hospital, thereby fostering a sense of normalcy.

Gastrointestinal and hepatobiliary systems

NURSING DIAGNOSIS

Noncompliance with drug regimen related to drug effects

Expected outcome

The child and parents will comply with the prescribed drug regimen.

Interventions

1. Instruct the child and parents on potential adverse reactions to immunosuppressive drug therapy, including acne, weight gain, and cushingoid appearance. Explain that these effects should decrease as the dosage is decreased.

2. Instruct the child and parents on how to control weight gain and acne. Teach the importance of performing proper skin care, monitoring daily fluid intake, and following the prescribed diet.

Rationales

1. Knowing this information should decrease the child's and parents' anxiety and encourage them to comply with the medication regimen.

2. Knowing that they can control some of the negative aspects of drug therapy should encourage the child and parents to comply with the medication regimen.

Documentation checklist

During the hospital stay, document:
- ❒ child's status and assessment findings upon admission
- ❒ changes in the child's status
- ❒ pertinent laboratory and diagnostic findings
- ❒ fluid intake and output
- ❒ nutritional intake
- ❒ growth and development status
- ❒ child's response to treatment
- ❒ child's and parents' reactions to the illness and hospital stay
- ❒ patient and family teaching guidelines
- ❒ discharge planning guidelines.

Pyloric stenosis

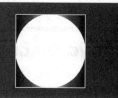

INTRODUCTION

Pyloric stenosis—a narrowing of the passageway that leads from the stomach to the small intestine—is characterized by hypertrophy of the pyloric sphincter. Apparent soon after birth (usually within 6 weeks), this disorder is marked by severe projectile vomiting, dehydration, and weight loss or poor weight gain.

The prognosis for pyloric stenosis is favorable. Usual treatment includes pyloromyotomy and rehydration. Potential complications include aspiration pneumonia and infection.

ASSESSMENT

Gastrointestinal
- Projectile vomiting
- Weight loss
- Palpable mass in the upper abdomen
- Distended abdomen
- Visible peristaltic waves
- Prolonged stomach emptying
- Decreased volume and number of stools

Integumentary
- Dry skin and poor skin turgor

NURSING DIAGNOSIS

Anxiety (parent) related to lack of understanding about the disease, diagnostic studies, and treatment

Expected outcome

The parents will be less anxious as evidenced by expressing an understanding of the disorder and the need for diagnostic testing and treatment.

Interventions

1. Explain to the parents the anatomy and the process of food passage through the normal upper GI tract. Use visual aids, if available.

2. Give the parents a schedule of the ordered diagnostic tests.

3. Teach the parents about each diagnostic test (upper GI series, ultrasonography, and laboratory testing); include information on preparing for the test, how long the test will last, and posttest care.

4. Provide the parents with information on preoperative and postoperative events. Include details on withholding oral feedings, laboratory workups, X-rays, pain medication, the feeding plan, how to hold the infant, and nasogastric intubation.

5. Encourage the parents to write down any questions that arise about the infant's care. Answer their questions simply and honestly.

Rationales

1. Understanding the GI system helps parents to better understand the disorder and the need for testing and treatment.

2. Having a schedule of diagnostic tests helps the parents to anticipate upcoming events.

3. Knowing this information should help to decrease the parents' anxiety and increase their cooperation, support, and involvement in diagnostic testing and posttest care.

4. Knowing what to expect helps decrease the parents' anxiety and fear and increases their involvement in the infant's care.

5. Encouraging the parents to write down questions can be reassuring and helps to lessen anxiety.

NURSING DIAGNOSIS

Altered nutrition: less than body requirements related to frequent projectile vomiting

Expected outcome

The infant will maintain adequate nutritional status as evidenced by retained feedings and decreased vomiting.

Interventions

1. Feed the infant in upright position, burping him after every ½ to 1 oz (15 to 30 ml). Maintain a quiet, relaxed environment. Before surgery, the infant should receive nothing by mouth for 3 to 4 hours, depending on the infant's age and the doctor's order.

2. Offer small, frequent feedings every 1 to 2 hours. Feed again after each vomiting episode.

3. Offer oral feedings of an electrolyte solution (such as Pedialyte or Ricelyte) during diagnostic workups.

4. Assess the infant for signs of worsening dehydration, including decreased urine output, dry skin, poor skin turgor, and sunken fontanels and eyes. Report these signs immediately.

5. Position the infant upright after each feeding.

Rationales

1. Feeding and burping the infant in this manner prevents aerophagia and ensures optimal retention of feeding.

2. Small, frequent feedings decrease the total fluid volume in the stomach at one time, which decreases the risk for vomiting and provides optimal hydration until I.V. therapy is initiated.

3. Electrolyte solutions replace electrolytes lost through repeated vomiting.

4. The doctor may order I.V. fluids to replace fluids and prevent shock.

5. The upright position helps prevent aspiration.

NURSING DIAGNOSIS

Fluid volume deficit related to dehydration or shock (or both)

Expected outcome

The infant will maintain normal fluid and electrolyte balance as evidenced by a normal urine output (11 to 18 ml/hour for a neonate; 17 to 25 ml/hour for an older infant), a capillary refill time of 3 to 5 seconds, good skin turgor, and age-appropriate potassium levels and vital signs.

Interventions

1. Rehydrate the infant, as indicated, with an oral electrolyte solution or I.V. fluids.

2. Monitor laboratory test results for complete blood count, specific gravity, and electrolyte, blood urea nitrogen, and arterial blood gas levels.

3. Monitor the infant every 2 to 4 hours for signs of shock, including increased heart and respiratory rates, decreased blood pressure, and pallor.

Rationales

1. Oral electrolyte solutions and I.V. fluids replace fluids and electrolytes lost through vomiting and dehydration.

2. Dehydration causes increases in the hemoglobin and hematocrit values. Vomiting causes decreased potassium and sodium levels, increased specific gravity, increased partial pressure of arterial carbon dioxide levels, and decreased pH.

3. Frequent monitoring allows for early detection and treatment of shock, which can occur with vomiting and postoperative hypervolemia. Treatment may include the administration of fluids and electrolytes (sodium and potassium) or a plasma volume expander (albumin).

4. Assess the infant's skin for signs of dehydration, including grayish color, dryness, poor turgor, and depressed fontanels.

5. Weigh the infant daily, and monitor his fluid intake and output hourly, including the amount of I.V. and oral intake, vomitus, nasogastric drainage, urine, and stool. Be sure to weigh diapers.

4. These signs indicate the need for increased fluid intake.

5. Daily weighing and frequent monitoring of intake and output ensure continual assessment of the infant's fluid status.

NURSING DIAGNOSIS

Risk for infection related to surgery

Expected outcome

The infant's surgical incision will remain free from infection after surgery as evidenced by decreased swelling and redness around the incision site and a lack of foul-smelling odor and purulent discharge.

Interventions

1. Monitor the incisional dressing and site for signs of infection (erythema, purulent drainage, edema, increased tenderness, wound dehiscence, elevated core temperature) every 2 hours. Administer antibiotics, as ordered.

2. Use sterile technique when in contact with the incision site until it completely heals; wash hands before any skin contact, keep dressings sterile, and clean the wound thoroughly.

Rationales

1. Frequent monitoring allows for early detection and prompt treatment of infection.

2. Sterile technique helps prevent bacterial infection.

NURSING DIAGNOSIS

Pain related to surgical incision

Expected outcome

The infant will have minimal pain as evidenced by decreased irritability, fussing, and crying.

Interventions

1. Administer analgesics regularly during the first 24 hours after surgery. Document the medication's effectiveness.

2. Change the infant's position (from side to back to abdomen) every 2 hours, when possible.

3. Show the parents the proper holding technique; encourage them to hold and cuddle the infant.

4. Monitor the infant for abdominal distention, peristaltic waves, absent or decreased bowel sounds, and signs of obstruction (such as bilious vomitus) every 4 hours. Report these abnormalities immediately.

Rationales

1. The infant usually receives analgesics after surgery to relieve pain. Documenting the medications' effectiveness helps to determine the infant's comfort level.

2. Position changes increase mobility, comfort, and muscle relaxation and decrease guarding of the incision.

3. Demonstrating the proper technique ensures that the parents will not cause the infant any discomfort. Holding promotes bonding, increasing the infant's sense of security, love, and support.

4. Such abnormalities are signs of postoperative complications, such as bowel obstruction or paralytic ileus, and require prompt treatment.

Gastrointestinal and hepatobiliary systems

NURSING DIAGNOSIS

Knowledge deficit related to home care

Expected outcome

The parents will express an understanding of home care instructions.

Interventions

1. Teach the parents about feeding the infant; include details on specific formulas to use, preparation methods, feeding volume, and feeding technique.

2. Teach the parents how to care for the surgical wound; include details on dressing changes, cleaning techniques, and signs of infection.

3. Teach the parents the purpose and use of medications (such as bethanechol chloride [Duvoid]); include details on administration, dosages, and potential adverse reactions.

Rationales

1. Such teaching should help the parents to comply with the feeding regimen, ensuring that the infant receives adequate nutrition.

2. Such teaching should help the parents to provide adequate care and recognize and report signs of infection.

3. Such teaching promotes compliance with the medication regimen. Knowing the signs potential adverse reactions should prompt parents to seek medical help when necessary.

Documentation checklist

During the hospital stay, document:
- ❏ infant's status and assessment findings upon admission
- ❏ changes in the infant's status
- ❏ pertinent laboratory and diagnostic findings
- ❏ fluid intake and output
- ❏ nutritional intake
- ❏ growth and development status
- ❏ infant's response to treatment
- ❏ parents' reactions to the infant's illness and hospital stay
- ❏ family teaching guidelines
- ❏ discharge planning guidelines.

Tracheoesophageal fistula

INTRODUCTION

A congenital malformation of the trachea and esophagus, a tracheoesophageal fistula is an abnormal opening between the trachea and esophagus. The abnormality commonly results in obstruction of the infant's normal swallowing route. It may occur as a blind pouch that terminates at the proximal end of the esophagus and connects to a fistula extending from the trachea at the distal end; as a fistula between the trachea and esophagus; or as some other abnormality.

Usual treatment includes anastomosis of the esophagus and closure of the fistula. Potential complications include aspiration pneumonia and bowel obstruction. The prognosis usually is favorable.

ASSESSMENT

Gastrointestinal
- Excessive mucus around the mouth
- Frothy saliva around the mouth and nose
- Abdominal distention

Respiratory
- Triad of choking, coughing, and cyanosis with first feeding
- Sneezing
- Apnea
- Pneumonia
- Rhonchi and crackles

NURSING DIAGNOSIS

Ineffective breathing pattern related to choking, coughing, and cyanosis during feeding

Expected outcome

The infant will have decreased respiratory distress as evidenced by quiet, relaxed breathing during feedings.

Interventions

1. Keep the head of the infant's crib elevated 45 degrees until the defect is corrected.

2. Observe the infant's behavior before, during, and after feedings. Notify the doctor immediately if the infant shows signs of choking, increased respiratory rate, vomiting, and cyanosis.

3. Carefully suction the infant's oropharynx; do not suction past the pharynx.

4. Prepare the infant for diagnostic X-ray studies, according to hospital protocol.

Rationales

1. Elevating the head of the crib helps prevent aspiration of secretions.

2. Observing the infant's behavior ensures early detection and prompt treatment of complications.

3. Careful suctioning helps decrease the risk for aspiration. Suctioning past the pharynx may accidentally perforate the esophagus.

4. Diagnostic X-rays identify the specific abnormality and define the appropriate intervention.

NURSING DIAGNOSIS

Anxiety (parent) related to lack of knowledge about the disorder, diagnostic testing, and treatment

Expected outcome

The parents will be less anxious as evidenced by expressing an understanding of the disorder and the need for diagnostic testing and treatment.

Interventions

1. Explain to the parents the basic anatomy and physiology of the normal upper GI tract and the passage of food through this section of the GI system. Use visual aids, if available, in your explanation.

2. Give the parents a schedule of the ordered diagnostic tests.

3. Explain that the infant may need a gastrostomy tube until he is mature enough to undergo temporary or permanent repair of the abnormality.

4. Explain what will happen preoperatively and postoperatively. Include details on withholding oral fluids, I.V. lines, laboratory workups, X-rays, pain medication, feeding plans, and how to hold the infant. Explain that the child may need surgery or esophageal dilation in the future.

5. Encourage the parents to write down any further questions as they arise. Answer their questions honestly and simply.

Rationales

1. Understanding the normal function of the GI system helps parents understand the abnormal functioning that results from the disorder and the need for diagnostic testing and treatment.

2. A schedule helps the parents anticipate upcoming events, reducing their anxiety and fear.

3. Understanding that the infant may need a gastrostomy tube for feedings helps the parents comply with the treatment.

4. Knowing what to expect preoperatively and postoperatively helps decrease the parents' anxiety and increases their involvement in the infant's care.

5. Parents often have many questions after meeting with the nurse. Encouraging them to write down questions can be reassuring and helps to lessen anxiety.

NURSING DIAGNOSIS

Ineffective breathing pattern related to aspiration of secretions or feedings or both

Expected outcome

The infant will have improved respiratory status as evidenced by stable respirations and no signs of respiratory distress.

Interventions

1. To maintain the infant's respiratory status and help prevent pneumonia:
• Position the nasal catheter in the esophageal pouch when providing gentle suctioning.
• Elevate the infant's head and chest 20 degrees.
• Suction the infant, as needed.
• Maintain a patent airway

2. Administer antibiotics, as ordered.

Rationales

1. These measures ensure that the infant receives adequate oxygenation at all times.
• Maintaining the catheter in this position helps drain secretions and prevent aspiration.
• Elevation helps prevent aspiration.
• Suctioning clears the airway of secretions.
• A patent airway promotes adequate oxygenation.

2. The infant may need antibiotics to treat pneumonia.

NURSING DIAGNOSIS

Altered growth and development related to the hospital stay and deprivation of normal parent-infant interactions and environmental stimulation

Expected outcome

The infant will grow and develop normally as evidenced by achieving optimal growth and developmental milestones.

Interventions

1. Provide the infant with appropriate auditory, visual, and tactile stimulation (such as music, bright colors, mirrors, and different shaped objects).

2. Show the parents how to hold the infant and encourage them to hold and cuddle the infant frequently.

3. Help the parents to understand and distinguish among the infant's behavioral cues, such as crying, grimacing, and fussing.

4. Teach the parents to perform range-of-motion (ROM) exercises or to use appropriate play when the infant is not confined by I.V. setups or dialysis.

5. Encourage the parents to talk to and establish eye contact with the infant.

Rationales

1. Consistent auditory, visual, and tactile stimulation help the infant achieve optimal growth and development.

2. Holding and cuddling help promote infant-parent bonding, which the infant needs for normal growth and development.

3. Parents of an infant who requires emergency care may have difficulty understanding their infant's needs. Helping them to differentiate behavioral cues allows them to respond appropriately, promoting normal growth and development.

4. ROM exercises and play techniques increase infant stimulation and parental bonding, which promote normal growth and development.

5. Such contact increases bonding and helps to stimulate the infant.

NURSING DIAGNOSIS

Knowledge deficit related to home care

Expected outcome

The parents will express an understanding of home care instructions.

Interventions

1. Teach the parents how to recognize the signs of aspiration, including respiratory distress, vomiting of bright red blood, elevated temperature, and choking. Make sure they receive proper training in cardiopulmonary resuscitation and abdominal thrust technique before the infant is discharged from the hospital.

2. Teach the parents to keep the infant's head elevated during feedings and to place the infant on his side after feedings.

3. Explain the need for follow-up care, including surgery or dilation of the esophagus.

Rationales

1. Parents need to know the signs of aspiration so that they can provide emergency treatment when necessary.

2. These positions help prevent the aspiration of food.

3. The infant may require surgery at a later date if he was too unstable to undergo corrective surgery during the initial hospital stay.

Documentation checklist

During the hospital stay, document:
- ❏ infant's status and assessment findings upon admission
- ❏ changes in the infant's status
- ❏ pertinent laboratory and diagnostic findings
- ❏ nutritional status
- ❏ growth and development status
- ❏ infant's response to treatment
- ❏ parents' reactions to the infant's illness and hospital stay
- ❏ family teaching guidelines
- ❏ discharge planning guidelines.

Gastrointestinal and hepatobiliary systems

Vomiting and diarrhea

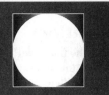

INTRODUCTION

Vomiting may result from several disorders, such as pyloric stenosis, intestinal obstruction, increased intracranial pressure, gastroesophageal reflux, appendicitis, and viral or bacterial infection. Vomiting depletes water and electrolytes. Initially, vomiting can cause metabolic alkalosis with increased pH and bicarbonate (HCO_3^-). Prolonged vomiting may result in the loss of base, and metabolic acidosis can occur.

Diarrhea, the passage of numerous watery stools, also occurs in many disorders, including bacterial and viral infection, inflammatory bowel disease, gastroenteritis, malabsorption syndrome, and food allergies. Diarrhea can cause metabolic acidosis with decreased pH and HCO_3^-. Young children are at particular risk for dehydration from vomiting and diarrhea because water makes up a higher percentage of their total body weight than it does of adults.

ASSESSMENT

Vomiting
Gastrointestinal
• Nausea
Respiratory
• Decreased respiratory rate
Cardiovascular
• Increased heart rate
• Arrhythmias
Neurologic
• Fatigue
• Lethargy
Hematologic
• pH greater than 7.45
• HCO_3^- above 26 mEq/L
• Increased partial pressure of carbon dioxide ($Paco_2$) levels
• Hypokalemia
Genitourinary
• Decreased urine output
Integumentary
• Poor skin turgor
• Sunken fontanels

Diarrhea
Gastrointestinal
• Loose, watery stools
• Blood and mucus in stools
• Abdominal cramping
Respiratory
• Hyperventilation
• Kussmaul's respirations
• Fruity breath odor
Cardiovascular
• Increased heart rate
Neurologic
• Headache
• Weakness
• Fatigue or lethargy
• Coma
Hematologic
• pH less than 7.35
• HCO_3^- below 22 mEq/L
• Decreased $Paco_2$ levels
• Hypokalemia
Integumentary
• Poor skin turgor
• Sunken fontanels

NURSING DIAGNOSIS

Fluid volume deficit related to vomiting or diarrhea

Expected outcome

The child will maintain adequate fluid volume as evidenced by moist mucous membranes, adequate skin turgor, age-appropriate electrolyte levels, and a urine output of 1 to 2 ml/kg/hour.

Interventions

1. Monitor the child's fluid intake and output.

Rationales

1. Fluid intake and output determine the child's hydration status and guide fluid replacement therapy.

2. Weigh the child daily.

3. Assess the child's skin color, skin turgor, fontanels (in an infant), level of consciousness, capillary refill time, and mucous membranes each shift. Notify the doctor immediately of any significant changes in the child's status.

4. Monitor the child for fever.

5. Monitor the child's serum electrolyte levels.

6. Administer an oral electrolyte solution (such as Pedialyte), as ordered.

7. Maintain a patent I.V. access and administer I.V. fluids, as ordered.

2. Weight directly measures hydration status.

3. Paleness, poor skin turgor, sunken fontanels, decreased level of consciousness, increased capillary refill time, and dry mucous membranes indicate dehydration.

4. Fever increases dehydration and can signal infection.

5. Abnormal serum electrolyte levels indicate fluid imbalances that require prompt treatment.

6. Oral electrolyte solutions replace fluids and electrolytes lost through vomiting and diarrhea.

7. The child may need I.V. fluids if he becomes dehydrated or is at risk for dehydration. However, too-rapid infusion may cause fluid overload.

NURSING DIAGNOSIS

Altered nutrition: less than body requirements related to vomiting or diarrhea

Expected outcome

The child will maintain adequate nutritional intake as evidenced by stable weight.

Interventions

1. Weigh the child daily, and carefully monitor intake and output.

2. Consult the hospital dietitian about the child's dietary requirements.

3. Allow the child nothing by mouth until vomiting subsides; then slowly introduce clear liquids.

4. Add carbohydrate-rich foods to the diet, such as plain rice, noodles, and potatoes. As an alternative, introduce the BRAT diet (B = bananas, R = rice or rice cereal, A = applesauce, T = tea and toast) to relieve diarrhea.

Rationales

1. Monitoring daily weight and intake and output determine the child's nutritional status.

2. The child requires careful dietary planning to ensure that he receives adequate nutrition despite vomiting or diarrhea.

3. Nothing-by-mouth status allows the GI system to rest and reduces vomiting. Clear liquids are less irritating to the GI tract than solid foods and help to replace lost fluids.

4. A high-carbohydrate diet thickens stool. The BRAT diet helps counteract the effects of diarrhea. Bananas replace potassium, rice and applesauce improve stool consistency, tea replaces lost fluid and decreases inflammation, and toast relieves irritation.

NURSING DIAGNOSIS

Knowledge deficit related to home care

Expected outcome

The parents will express an understanding of home care instructions.

(Text continues on page 140.)

Gastrointestinal and hepatobiliary systems

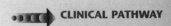

Diarrhea, vomiting, and dehydration

	Day 1
Consults	
Tests	• Lab work as ordered • Stool specimen as ordered
Treatments	• Enteric precautions • I.V. • Strict intake and output (I & O) • Vital signs (VS) q 4 hr with blood pressure • Daily weight • Developmental appropriate interventions provided
Medication	
Diet	• Age specific, as ordered
Activity	• Age specific, as ordered
Nursing process	• Patient history/assessment admission form • Systems assessment • Growth curve by doctor—within 12 hr • Assess for signs of dehydration—tears, mucous membranes, fontanels, blood pressure, turgor, and capillary refill.
Teaching C = class H = handout R = reference V = video	• Orient to unit routine. • Review signs/symptoms of dehydration. • Review diet and restrictions. • Teach about enteric precautions. • Save diapers for nursing, and monitor frequency. • Review plan of care.
Discharge planning	• Assess support network. • Reinforce length of stay.
Needs and outcomes	• Patient does not exhibit further signs of dehydration. • Patient is free from harm. • Patient maintains developmental level. • Parent verbalizes understanding of unit routine and policies. • Parent verbalizes an understanding of enteric precautions. • Parent verbalizes understanding of plan of care.

Day 2	Day 3
• Child life	• Child life
• Enteric precautions • I.V. • Strict I & O • VS q 4 hr with blood pressure • Daily weight	• Enteric precautions • I.V. • Strict I & O • VS q 4 hr with blood pressure • Daily weight
• Antipyretics as needed	• Antipyretics as needed
• Age specific, as ordered	• Age specific, as ordered
• Age specific, as ordered	• Age specific, as ordered
• Systems assessment • Assess for signs of dehydration — tears, mucous membranes, fontanels, blood pressure, turgor, and capillary refill.	• Systems assesment • Assess for signs of dehydration — tears, mucous membranes, fontanels, blood pressure, turgor, and capillary refill.
• Review diet and restrictions. • Save diapers and monitor frequency. • Hand-washing techniques	• Review diet and restrictions. • Save diapers and monitor frequency.
• 24-hour written discharge notice given	• Discharge by 11 a.m. • Written discharge instructions • Follow-up appointment with doctor
• Patient's lab values are within acceptable parameters. • Patient is no longer vomiting (if applicable). • Patient has a decrease frequency of stools (if applicable). • Parent displays confidence in self-care of child. • Patient/parent utilizes appropriate developmental supportive services. • Parent demonstrates proper hand-washing techniques.	• Patient is tolerating diet. • Parent verbalizes understanding of discharge instructions.

Adapted with permission from Northshore University Hospital, Manhasset, N.Y. (Revised 6/95).

Gastrointestinal and hepatobiliary systems

Interventions

1. Teach the parents the purpose and use of any pre-scribed medications (such as antiemetics or antidiar-rheals); include details on administration, dosages, and potential adverse reactions.

2. Explain the importance of monitoring the child for continued nausea, vomiting or diarrhea, muscle cramps, and irregular heart rate. Tell them to report such signs and symptoms to the doctor immediately.

3. Teach the parents how to manage vomiting and diarrhea at home.

Rationales

1. Such instruction promotes compliance with the medication regimen. Knowing potential adverse reactions should prompt the parents to seek medical help when necessary.

2. These are signs and symptoms of fluid and electrolyte imbalances.

3. Knowing how to manage vomiting and diarrhea at home allows the parents to intervene before the child needs hospitalization.

Documentation checklist

During the hospital stay, document:
- ❏ child's status and assessment findings upon admission
- ❏ changes in the child's status
- ❏ pertinent laboratory and diagnostic findings
- ❏ fluid intake and output
- ❏ nutritional intake and daily weight
- ❏ growth and development status
- ❏ child's response to treatment
- ❏ child's and parents' reactions to the illness and hospital stay
- ❏ patient and family teaching guidelines
- ❏ discharge planning guidelines.

Part 5

Genitourinary system

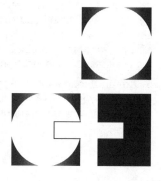

Acute glomerulonephritis

INTRODUCTION

The most common noninfectious renal disease of childhood, acute glomerulonephritis affects the glomeruli and filtration rate of the kidneys, resulting in water and sodium retention and hypertension. Usually caused by a reaction to streptococcal infection, this disease seldom has any long-term effects on the renal system.

Acute glomerulonephritis affects boys more commonly than girls and usually occurs at about age 6. Treatment typically includes the administration of antibiotics, antihypertensives, and diuretics as well as dietary restrictions. Potential complications include hypertension, congestive heart failure, and end-stage renal disease.

ASSESSMENT

Genitourinary
- Cloudy, smoky brown urine
- Proteinuria
- Elevated urine specific gravity
- Decreased urine output
- Hematuria

Cardiovascular
- Mild hypertension

Neurologic
- Lethargy
- Irritability
- Seizures

Gastrointestinal
- Anorexia
- Vomiting
- Diarrhea

EENT
- Moderate periorbital edema

Hematologic
- Transient anemia
- Azotemia
- Hyperkalemia

Integumentary
- Pallor
- Generalized edema

NURSING DIAGNOSIS

Altered cerebral tissue perfusion related to water retention and hypernatremia

Expected outcome

The child has normal tissue perfusion as evidenced by normal blood pressure, reduced water retention, and no signs of hypernatremia.

Interventions

1. Monitor and document the child's blood pressure every 1 to 2 hours during the acute phase.

2. Institute the following seizure precautions:
- Keep an oral airway and suction equipment at the child's bedside.
- Post signs above the child's bed and on his door alerting health care personnel to the child's seizure status.

3. Administer an antihypertensive agent, such as hydralazine hydroxide (Apresoline), as ordered. Monitor the child for adverse reactions.

Rationales

1. Frequent monitoring allows for early detection and prompt treatment of changes in the child's blood pressure.

2. Instituting seizure precautions helps prevent injury during a seizure episode. Although uncommon in acute glomerulonephritis, seizures can result from lack of oxygen perfusion to the brain.

3. Antihypertensives may be ordered because uncontrolled hypertension can cause kidney damage. Although the exact reason for hypertension is unknown, it may be related to fluid overload in the circulatory system.

4. Monitor the child's fluid volume status every 1 to 2 hours. Monitor urine output; it should be 1 to 2 ml/kg per hour.

5. Assess the child's neurologic status (level of consciousness, reflexes, and pupillary response) every 8 hours. Notify the doctor immediately of any significant changes in the child's status.

6. Administer diuretics, such as hydrochlorothiazide (Esidrix) or furosemide (Lasix), as ordered.

4. Monitoring is essential because volume expansion further increases blood pressure.

5. Frequent assessments allow for early detection and prompt treatment of any changes in the child's neurologic status.

6. Diuretics promote excretion of fluid.

Nursing diagnosis

Fluid volume excess related to oliguria

Expected outcome

The child maintains normal fluid volume as evidenced by a urine output of approximately 1 to 2 ml/kg/hour.

Interventions

1. Weigh the child daily, and monitor his urine output every 4 hours.

2. Assess the child for edema, measure abdominal girth every 8 hours, and (for boys) check for scrotal swelling.

3. Monitor the child closely for adverse reactions to diuretic therapy, especially when using hydrochlorothiazide or furosemide.

4. Monitor and record the child's fluid intake.

5. Assess the color, consistency, and specific gravity of the child's urine.

6. Monitor the results of all ordered laboratory tests.

Rationales

1. Daily weighing and frequent monitoring of urine output allow for early detection and prompt treatment of changes in the child's fluid status. Rapid weight gain indicates fluid retention. Decreased urine output may indicate impending renal failure.

2. Frequent assessments and measurements allow for early detection and prompt treatment of any changes in the child's condition. Increased abdominal girth and scrotal swelling usually indicate ascites.

3. These diuretics can cause hypokalemia, which requires the administration of I.V. potassium supplements.

4. The child may need his fluid intake restricted because of fluid retention and decreased glomerular filtration rate; he may also need sodium intake restricted.

5. Frothy urine indicates increased protein depletion, a sign of impaired kidney function.

6. Elevated blood urea nitrogen and creatinine levels may indicate impaired kidney function.

Nursing diagnosis

Altered nutrition: less than body requirements related to anorexia

Expected outcome

The child has improved nutritional intake as evidenced by eating at least 80% of each meal.

Interventions

1. Provide a high-carbohydrate diet.

2. Serve small, frequent meals that include some of the child's favorite foods.

3. Restrict the child's sodium and protein intake, as ordered.

Rationales

1. A high-carbohydrate diet is usually more palatable to a child and provides essential calories.

2. Serving smaller quantities of food at one meal seems less overwhelming to a child, encouraging him to eat more at each sitting. Serving some the child's favorite foods helps ensure that he eats more of each meal.

3. Because sodium causes fluid retention, it is usually restricted in children with this disorder. In severe cases, the kidneys cannot metabolize protein, necessitating protein restrictions.

Nursing diagnosis

Activity intolerance related to fatigue

Expected outcome

The child has increased activity tolerance as evidenced by the ability to play for increasing periods of time.

Interventions

1. Schedule rest periods to follow each activity.

2. Provide quiet, challenging, age-appropriate games.

3. Cluster the child's nursing care to allow for periods of uninterrupted sleep at night.

Rationales

1. Frequent rest periods conserve energy and decrease the production of metabolic wastes, which can further stress the kidney.

2. Such games conserve energy while preventing boredom.

3. Clustering care helps the child get needed sleep.

Nursing diagnosis

Risk for impaired skin integrity related to immobility and edema

Expected outcome

The child maintains normal skin integrity as evidenced by pinkish skin color and the absence of redness, edema, and skin breakdown.

Interventions

1. Provide a convoluted foam mattress for the child's bed.

2. Help the child change position every 2 hours.

3. Bathe the child daily using a high-fat soap.

Rationales

1. A convoluted foam mattress pads bony prominences, decreasing the risk of skin breakdown.

2. Frequent position changes reduce pressure on the capillary beds and improve circulation, decreasing the risk of skin breakdown.

3. Deodorant or perfumed soaps dry the skin, contributing to skin breakdown.

4. Support and elevate edematous extremities.

5. If the child is a boy, place padding around the scrotum.

4. Supporting and elevating extremities promotes venous return and helps decrease swelling.

5. Padding helps prevent skin breakdown.

NURSING DIAGNOSIS

Anxiety (parent) related to the child's hospital stay

Expected outcome

The parents are less anxious as evidenced by expressing their fears and an understanding of the child's condition.

Interventions

1. Listen to the parents' concerns.

2. Explain all procedures to the parents and involve them in discussions about the child's care.

3. Refer the parents to an appropriate support group, if needed.

Rationales

1. Listening provides support during stress.

2. Keeping the parents informed and involving them in discussions about the child's care fosters a sense of control that helps to decrease anxiety.

3. A support group provides parents with an outlet for expressing their feelings and concerns.

NURSING DIAGNOSIS

Knowledge deficit related to home care

Expected outcome

The parents express an understanding of home care instructions.

Interventions

1. Explain to the parents the pathophysiology of the disease.

2. Reassure the parents that the disease rarely causes long-term effects.

3. Explain to the parents the need to maintain the child on a sodium-restricted diet until his edema subsides and the kidneys resume normal function.

4. Instruct the parents to limit the child's activity until the doctor approves a return to normal activity level.

5. Teach the parents the signs and symptoms of upper respiratory infection, such as elevated temperature, sore throat, and cough; also teach them signs of renal failure, such as decreased urine output, weight gain, and edema.

Rationales

1. Such explanations help the parents understand the disease and the need to continue treatment at home.

2. Parents usually are worried about the effects of the disease, especially if the child has received dialysis during the acute stage of the disease.

3. A sodium-restricted diet is necessary because excessive sodium intake limits water excretion.

4. Activity restrictions are necessary to prevent stress on the kidneys, which could cause a relapse of the disease.

5. Knowing the signs and symptoms of recurring infection and renal failure should prompt parents to seek medical help when necessary.

6. Advise the parents of the importance of keeping all follow-up appointments.

6. Follow-up visits are essential to determine resolution of disease and detect any complications.

Documentation checklist

During the hospital stay, document:
- ❏ child's status and assessment findings upon admission
- ❏ changes in the child's status
- ❏ pertinent laboratory and diagnostic findings
- ❏ fluid intake and output
- ❏ nutritional intake
- ❏ child's response to treatment
- ❏ child's and parents' reactions to the illness and hospital stay
- ❏ patient and family teaching guidelines
- ❏ discharge planning guidelines.

Hypospadias and epispadias

INTRODUCTION

Congenital defects that are detectable at or shortly after birth, hypospadias and epispadias involve abnormalities of the male urethral opening. In hypospadias, the more common defect, the urethral opening usually appears along the ventral side of the penile shaft. Often, although not always, the defect is associated with a chordee, a downward bowing of the penis. In epispadias, the urethral opening appears on the dorsal side of the penis.

Treatment for hypospadias or epispadias involves surgery to restore the appearance and normal function of the penis. Surgery usually is not scheduled until age 1 to 2, when the penis is of a more operable size. Potential complications include infection and urethral obstruction.

ASSESSMENT

Preoperative
Genitourinary
- Absence of ventral foreskin
- Dimple or groove at tip of penis
- Spade-shaped glans penis
- Possible chordee (bowing) with or without an erection
- Urethral opening on the ventral (hypospadias) or dorsal (epispadias) side of penis

Postoperative
Genitourinary
- Penile swelling
- Bleeding at surgical site
- Dysuria

Neurologic
- Irritability
- Restlessness

NURSING DIAGNOSIS

Anxiety (child and parent) related to surgical procedure (urethroplasty)

Expected outcome

The child and parents are less anxious as evidenced by expressing an understanding of the surgical procedure.

Interventions

1. Explain to the child and parents the surgical procedure and expected postoperative care. Use pictures and dolls when explaining procedures to the child. Explain that surgery involves correcting the placement of the urethral opening. Also explain that an indwelling urinary catheter will be in place and that the child may need restraints to prevent him from disturbing the catheter. Advise them that the child may be discharged with the catheter in place.

2. Allow the child to act out fears and fantasies with puppets and dolls.

Rationales

1. Explaining the surgery and postoperative care helps alleviate anxiety and fear by allowing the child and parents to anticipate and prepare for the upcoming events. Using pictures and dolls to explain procedures helps the child understand complicated concepts.

2. Acting out allows the child to vent his fears and allows you to assess the child's cognitive level and ability to understand the condition and need for surgery.

NURSING DIAGNOSIS

Risk for infection (urinary tract) related to placement of indwelling catheter

Expected outcome

The child remains free from infection as evidenced by normal urinalysis results and a body temperature less than 100° F (37.8° C).

Interventions

1. Keep the catheter drainage bag below the child's bladder level, making sure the tubing is free from kinks and loops.

2. Use aseptic technique when emptying the catheter bag.

3. Monitor the child's urine for cloudiness or sedimentation. Also check surgical dressings every 4 hours for foul odor or purulent drainage; promptly report such signs to the doctor.

4. Encourage the child to drink at least 2 oz (60 ml) of fluid per hour.

5. Administer prophylactic antibiotics, as ordered, to help prevent infection. Monitor the child for therapeutic effects and adverse reactions.

Rationales

1. Maintaining the drainage bag in this position prevents infection by preventing nonsterile urine from flowing back into the bladder.

2. Aseptic technique prevents contaminants from entering the urinary tract.

3. These signs may indicate infection.

4. Increased fluid intake dilutes urine and encourages voiding.

5. Such monitoring helps determine the efficacy of as well as the child's tolerance to antibiotics.

NURSING DIAGNOSIS

Pain related to surgery

Expected outcome

The child exhibits increased comfort as evidenced by decreased crying, restlessness, and expression of pain.

Interventions

1. Administer analgesics, as ordered.

2. Make sure the child's catheter is correctly positioned and free of kinks.

Rationales

1. Analgesics may be ordered to provide pain relief.

2. Improper catheter positioning may cause pain from inadequate drainage or friction resulting from tension on the inflated balloon.

NURSING DIAGNOSIS

Risk for injury related to dislodged urinary catheter or urinary catheter removal

Expected outcome

The child remains free from injury as evidenced by maintaining correct urinary catheter placement until removal by the nurse or doctor.

Interventions

1. Secure the catheter to the child's penis with bandages and tape.

2. Place restraints on the child's arms when he is unsupervised or asleep.

3. Use a bed cradle to keep linens from contacting the catheter and penis.

Rationales

1. A secure dressing helps decrease the chance of accidental removal.

2. Restraints prevent the child from pulling out or dislodging the catheter.

3. Keeping bed linens from contact with the catheter and penis helps prevent accidental dislodgment.

NURSING DIAGNOSIS

Anxiety (parent) related to the appearance of the child's penis after surgery

Expected outcome

The parents are less anxious as evidenced by expressing their feelings about the child's defect.

Interventions

1. Encourage the parents to express their feelings and concerns about the child's imperfection. Focus on questions of sexuality and reproduction.

2. Help the parents through the normal grieving process.

3. Refer the parents to an appropriate support group, if needed.

4. If appropriate, explain the need for multiple surgeries and answer any questions the parents may have.

Rationales

1. Allowing the parents to express feelings and concerns provides support and understanding, reducing their anxiety. They are likely to be most concerned with the effects of the defect on sexuality and reproduction.

2. Grieving allows the parents to work through their anxiety and distress.

3. A support group can help the parents to cope with the child's imperfection.

4. Surgical repair may need to take place in stages. Discussing this with the parents and allowing them to express their feelings may help lessen their anxiety.

NURSING DIAGNOSIS

Knowledge deficit related to home care

Expected outcome

The parents express an understanding of home care instructions and demonstrate home care procedures.

Interventions

1. Teach the parents the signs and symptoms of urinary tract or incisional infection, including increased temperature, cloudy urine, and purulent drainage from the incision.

2. Teach the parents how to care for the catheter and penis, including cleaning around the catheter, emptying the drainage bag, and securing the catheter; explain the importance of monitoring the color and clarity of urine.

Rationales

1. Knowing the signs and symptoms of infection should prompt parents to seek medical help when needed.

2. Such information promotes increased compliance with the home care regimen and helps prevent catheter dislodgment and infection.

3. Tell the parents to keep the child from straddling a bicycle or rocking horse.

4. As appropriate, teach the parents the purpose and use of antibiotics and medication for bladder spasms (meperidine hydrochloride [Demerol], acetaminophen [Tylenol]); include details on administration, dosages, and potential adverse effects.

3. Straddling could cause the catheter to dislodge and damage the operative site.

4. Analgesics help control pain. Bladder spasms may occur from bladder irritation. Knowing the potential adverse effects should prompt parents to seek medical help when necessary.

Documentation checklist

During the hospital stay, document:
- ❏ child's status and assessment findings upon admission
- ❏ changes in the child's status
- ❏ pertinent laboratory and diagnostic findings
- ❏ fluid intake and output
- ❏ nutritional intake
- ❏ child's response to treatment
- ❏ child's and parents' reactions to the surgery and hospital stay
- ❏ family teaching guidelines
- ❏ discharge planning guidelines.

Kidney transplantation

INTRODUCTION

Kidney transplantation may be indicated for a child whose kidneys no longer function because of infection, end-stage renal disease, or cancer. The procedure involves the replacement of the nonfunctioning kidney with a fully functioning kidney taken from a living donor or a cadaver. The nonfunctioning kidney is usually left in place and the new kidney is attached to the iliac artery and hypogastric vein. A child awaiting kidney transplantation must meet certain hospital criteria before being put on a waiting list.

Potential complications include hemorrhage, infection, organ rejection, and death. The survival rate usually is above 50%.

ASSESSMENT

Postoperative complications
Genitourinary
• Increased urine output
Cardiovascular
• Hypertension

Neurologic
• Restlessness
• Irritability
Gastrointestinal
• Increased appetite
• Gastric distress
Eye, ear, nose, and throat
• Periorbital edema

Transplant rejection
Genitourinary
• Tenderness and swelling at graft site
• Decreased urine creatinine levels
• Proteinuria
• Hematuria
• Decreased urine output
Cardiovascular
• Hypertension
Hematologic
• Increased white blood cell count
• Increased serum creatinine levels
Musculoskeletal
• General malaise
Integumentary
• Fever

NURSING DIAGNOSIS

Fluid volume excess related to function of transplanted kidney

Expected outcome

The child maintains appropriate fluid volume status as evidenced by good skin turgor, moist mucous membranes, lack of periorbital edema, and urine output of 1 to 2 ml/kg/hour.

Interventions

1. Weigh the child at same time each day, with the child in the same clothes, using the same scale.

2. Monitor the child's fluid intake and output hourly for the first 48 to 72 hours, then every 4 hours until stable, and then every 8 hours.

3. Monitor the child's blood pressure hourly until stable, then every 4 hours.

4. Monitor the child for hematuria, which should clear within 2 to 4 days of surgery.

Rationales

1. Daily weighing helps determine the child's fluid status.

2. Frequent monitoring provides information on the child's fluid status and kidney function.

3. Monitoring is essential because blood pressure changes with fluid shifts and degree of shock.

4. Increased bleeding may signal transplant rejection or hemorrhage.

5. Assess the child's skin turgor and mucous membranes every 8 hours.

6. Closely monitor serum electrolyte and creatinine levels.

7. Maintain the child on a sodium-restricted diet.

5. Poor skin turgor and dry mucous membranes indicate dehydration.

6. Electrolyte and creatinine levels should return to normal with normal kidney function.

7. A sodium-restricted diet helps decrease fluid retention.

Nursing diagnosis

Risk for infection related to immunosuppression

Expected outcome

The child remains free from infection as evidenced by maintaining a temperature less than 100° F (37.8° C), clear lungs, and normal urinalysis results.

Interventions

1. Monitor the child for fever and for swelling, redness, warmth, or drainage at the surgical site.

2. Assess the child's pulmonary status (respiratory rate, depth, and rhythm) every 4 hours. Notify the doctor immediately of any significant changes in the child's status.

3. Have the child turn, cough, and breathe deeply every 2 hours. Splint the incision before having the child cough.

4. Assess the child's urine for cloudiness or increased sediment.

5. Use sterile technique during all dressing changes.

6. Clean the incision with hydrogen peroxide or sterile saline solution.

7. Provide appropriate catheter care, including cleaning around the catheter and urinary meatus with an antimicrobial agent.

Rationales

1. These signs indicate possible infection and the need for appropriate interventions, such as the administration of antibiotics.

2. Such assessment allows for early detection and prompt treatment of infection.

3. Turning, coughing, and deep breathing help mobilize secretions, helping to prevent infection. Splinting supports the incision during coughing.

4. These signs indicate possible infection and require prompt treatment with antibiotics.

5. Sterile technique helps prevent the introduction of bacteria into the wound.

6. Cleaning decreases crusting and bacterial buildup.

7. Keeping the catheter clean helps prevent entry of bacteria into the urinary tract.

Nursing diagnosis

Altered nutrition: potential for more than body requirements related to increased appetite secondary to use of immunosuppressant agents

Expected outcome

The child maintains appropriate nutrition as evidenced by ingesting a balanced diet.

Interventions

1. Monitor the child's daily weight and dietary intake.

Rationales

1. Such monitoring provides data for assessing the child's nutritional status and detecting changes that require intervention.

2. Discuss dietary modifications, such as sodium and potassium restrictions, with the child and parents.

3. Inform the child and parents that the child's appetite should decrease in 2 to 4 months, when the immunosuppressant drug dosage is decreased.

4. Incorporate some of the child's favorite foods, as allowed, into the diet.

2. Understanding the reasons for dietary modifications should promote compliance. Sodium increases fluid retention; potassium excretion stresses the kidneys.

3. Immunosuppressant drugs increase appetite. Knowing this should help the child and parents comply with the prescribed diet.

4. Serving some of the child's favorite foods helps the child to comply with the prescribed diet by increasing his sense of control.

NURSING DIAGNOSIS

Pain related to frequent invasive procedures and surgery

Expected outcome

The child exhibits increased comfort as evidenced by relaxed facial features, active involvement in play, and expression of comfort.

Interventions

1. Such explanations help to decrease anxiety, fear, and feelings of loss of control.

2. Assess the child for the severity and location of any pain or discomfort, using pediatric pain assessment tools (such as a face interval or number line pain-rating scale).

3. Place the child in a comfortable position while maintaining proper body alignment and supporting pressure points.

4. Allow the child to have familiar objects from home, such as toys and blankets.

5. Administer an analgesic, as ordered.

6. Provide diversional activities, such as toys, games, television, or books.

Rationales

1. Before any invasive procedure, explain to the child and parents what will occur.

2. Knowing the severity and location of the child's pain helps to determine appropriate pain-control measures. Interventions might include medication, positioning, diversion, imagery, relaxation, and breathing techniques.

3. Such positioning avoids the development of contractures, cramping, and putting pressure on one part of the body for extended periods.

4. Familiar objects help increase feelings of security and decrease anxiety, which can affect the child's comfort level.

5. Analgesics provide pain relief, increasing the child's comfort level.

6. Diversional activities distract the child from pain.

NURSING DIAGNOSIS

Ineffective individual coping related to sensory overload

Expected outcome

The child demonstrates effective coping skills as evidenced by age-appropriate responses and behavior.

Interventions	Rationales
1. Allow the child to make small decisions about his care, such as scheduling baths and meals. Let him have some input into medication and treatment choices; for example, ask him if he wants his medication now or in 10 minutes.	**1.** Allowing the child some control helps him to cope with his situation by increasing feelings of self-control.
2. Set limits for the child to help him maintain acceptable behavior. Encourage the parents to maintain discipline as they would at home.	**2.** Establishing reasonable behavioral limits and providing consistent discipline increase feelings of security and normalcy, helping the child to cope with his situation.
3. Take the child to a treatment room for any invasive procedure.	**3.** Performing invasive procedures in a treatment room allows the child to feel secure in his own hospital room, which fosters a sense of normalcy and helps the child cope.
4. Schedule periods of quiet time for the child.	**4.** Quiet time gives the child a chance to block out sensory stimuli that may hinder his ability to cope.

Nursing diagnosis

Body image disturbance related to effects of steroid therapy

Expected outcome

The child has an improved self-concept as evidenced by expressing acceptance of his body.

Interventions	Rationales
1. Listen attentively and nonjudgmentally to the child's feelings and concerns about his body.	**1.** Listening provides emotional support and lets you assess how well the child accepts his appearance.
2. Help the child focus on his assets and positive features.	**2.** Focusing on assets and positive features helps to de-emphasize the negative aspects of the child's condition.
3. Encourage the child to attend support group meetings, such as those designed for transplant patients in his age-group.	**3.** A support group helps decrease the child's feelings of isolation by introducing him to other children with similar problems. Such a group also allows the child to see how others cope with an altered body image.
4. Encourage the child's siblings and peers to visit.	**4.** Visits from siblings and peers help the child maintain contact with others outside the hospital, fostering a sense of normalcy.

Nursing diagnosis

Noncompliance with drug regimen related to drug effects

Expected outcome

The child and parents comply with the prescribed drug regimen.

Interventions

1. Teach the child and parents the potential adverse effects of immunosuppressive drug therapy, including acne, weight gain, and cushingoid appearance. Explain that these effects should decrease as the dosage is decreased.

2. Teach the child and parents how to control weight gain and acne. Teach the importance of proper skin care, monitoring daily fluid intake, and following the prescribed diet.

Rationales

1. Knowing this information should decrease the child's and parents' anxiety and encourage them to comply with the medication regimen.

2. Knowing that they can control some of the negative aspects of drug therapy should encourage the child and parents to comply with the medication regimen.

NURSING DIAGNOSIS

Knowledge deficit related to home care

Expected outcome

The parents and child express an understanding of home care instructions and demonstrate home care procedures.

Interventions

1. Teach the parents and child the signs and symptoms of transplant rejection (see the "Assessment" section at the beginning of this plan). Tell them to report these signs immediately to the doctor should they occur.

2. Teach the parents and child the purpose of laboratory tests (creatinine, blood urea nitrogen, calcium, and phosphorus levels; white blood cell count; and glomerular filtration rate).

3. Teach the parents how to take the child's blood pressure and how and when to administer antihypertensive medications. Explain the importance of monitoring for adverse reactions and the need to notify the doctor if they occur.

4. Teach the parents the purpose and use of steroids; include details on administration, dosages, and potential adverse effects (nausea and vomiting, GI bleeding, increased susceptibility to infection, fluid retention, and growth retardation).

5. Teach the parents the purpose and use of cyclosporine (Sandimmune); include details on administration, dosages, and potential adverse effects (hypertension, accelerated hair growth, nephrotoxicity, and diarrhea).

6. Teach the parents and child the signs and symptoms of infection, including fever and increased pain; tell them to report such signs and symptoms at once.

7. Emphasize the need for the child to limit his exercise level and to avoid contact sports and long-distance running.

Rationales

1. Early recognition of transplant rejection ensures prompt medical intervention.

2. The parents and child should have a basic understanding of these tests so they know what the values mean when the child receives such tests as an outpatient.

3. Knowing this information helps promote compliance with the medication regimen. Knowing the potential adverse reactions (hypotension, bradycardia, faintness, and dizziness) should prompt the parents to seek medical help when necessary.

4. Knowing this information helps the parents comply with the medication regimen. Knowing the potential adverse effects should prompt the parents to seek medical help when necessary. The parents and child may need support and counseling if steroid use affects the child's growth.

5. Knowing this information helps promote compliance with the medication regimen. Knowing the potential adverse effects should prompt the parents to seek medical help when necessary.

6. Recognizing and reporting indications of infection ensures prompt treatment to prevent complications.

7. The child needs to limit his activities because heavy exercise may cause dehydration; contact sports and long-distance running may result in trauma to the kidney.

8. Encourage the child and parents to join one or more support groups, such as a hospital transplantation support group or one sponsored by the National Association on Hemodialysis and Transplantation.

8. Such groups offer support by allowing the parents and child to meet with others undergoing similar problems.

Documentation checklist

During the hospital stay, document:
- [ ] child's status and assessment findings upon admission
- [ ] changes in the child's status
- [ ] pertinent laboratory and diagnostic findings
- [ ] fluid intake and output
- [ ] nutritional intake
- [ ] child's response to treatment
- [ ] child's and parents' reactions to the illness, surgery, and hospital stay
- [ ] patient and family teaching guidelines
- [ ] discharge planning guidelines.

Nephrotic syndrome

INTRODUCTION

A manifestation of many glomerular disorders, nephrotic syndrome is marked by proteinuria, hypoalbuminemia, and edema and sometimes hematuria, hypertension, and a decreased glomerular filtration rate. Nephrotic syndrome is classified as either primary or secondary: primary nephrotic syndrome is limited to renal injury; secondary nephrotic syndrome is associated with systemic illness. Usually of unknown etiology, nephrotic syndrome affects more boys than girls, usually between ages 2 and 7.

Typical treatment includes dialysis and the administration of antihypertensives, diuretics, and steroids. A child may have several relapses throughout treatment. Potential complications include renal disease, renal failure, and heart failure.

ASSESSMENT

Genitourinary
- Oliguria
- Proteinuria
- Hematuria

Cardiovascular
- Hypertension (sometimes)

Integumentary
- Edema of face (in the morning)
- Generalized edema of the extremities and abdomen (as the day progresses)
- Pallor

NURSING DIAGNOSIS

Risk for impaired skin integrity related to edema and immobility

Expected outcome

The child has no signs or symptoms of skin breakdown as evidenced by absence of redness, irritation, and muscle wasting.

Interventions

1. Help the child change position every 2 hours.

2. Provide proper skin care, including daily baths with moisturizing soap, massages, position changes, and changing soiled linens and clothing.

3. Assess the child's skin for evidence of irritation and breakdown, such as redness, edema, and abrasions, every 4 to 8 hours.

4. Support or elevate edematous areas, such as the arms, legs, and scrotum, with pillows or bed linens. Use powder on these areas.

5. Increase the child's activity level as edema subsides.

Rationales

1. Frequent position changes help to prevent skin breakdown by alleviating pressure on body surfaces.

2. Proper skin care helps keep the skin free from irritating substances and helps prevent skin breakdown.

3. Frequent assessments allow for early detection and prompt intervention, when necessary.

4. Elevating or supporting edematous areas helps to decrease edema. Using powder decreases the moisture and friction that often occur when body surfaces rub together.

5. Increased activity helps prevent skin breakdown from prolonged bed rest.

NURSING DIAGNOSIS

Risk for infection related to immunosuppression

Expected outcome

The child remains free from infection as evidenced by a body temperature less than 100° F (37.8° C) and an absence of purulent drainage, cough, and sore throat.

Interventions

1. Do not allow anyone with an acute infection to visit the child.

2. Administer antibiotics, as ordered.

3. Monitor the child daily for signs and symptoms of infection, including cough, fever, runny nose, purulent drainage, and sore throat.

Rationales

1. Immunosuppression makes the child vulnerable to infection.

2. The immunosuppressed child usually receives prophylactic antibiotics to help prevent infection.

3. Monitoring ensures early recognition and prompt treatment of infection.

NURSING DIAGNOSIS

Altered peripheral tissue perfusion related to hypertension

Expected outcome

The child maintains normal tissue perfusion as evidenced by age-appropriate blood pressure, the absence of headaches and seizures, and a capillary refill time of 3 to 5 seconds.

Interventions

1. Monitor the child's blood pressure every 4 hours.

2. Institute the following seizure precautions:
• Keep an oral airway and suction equipment near the child's bedside.
• Post a sign above the child's bed and on his door alerting all health care personnel to the child's seizure status.
• Document the child's seizure status on his chart.

3. Administer antihypertensive medications, as ordered.

Rationales

1. Monitoring ensures early recognition and prompt treatment of hypertension.

2. Severe hypertension and cerebral hypoxia increase the risk for seizures.

3. The child may need antihypertensives to decrease his blood pressure and reduce the risk of complications, including seizures, cerebrovascular accident, heart failure, and headaches.

NURSING DIAGNOSIS

Altered nutrition: less than body requirements related to disease

Expected outcome

The child has an improved nutritional intake as evidenced by eating at least 80% of each meal.

Interventions

1. Offer the child small, frequent meals.

2. Serve the child some of his favorite foods within dietary restrictions.

Rationales

1. A child with this disease typically has a decreased appetite. Eating small, frequent meals rather than a few large meals prevents the child from becoming tired and too full and ensures that he eats more at each sitting.

2. The child is more likely to eat more of each meal if he is served some of his favorite foods.

NURSING DIAGNOSIS

Fluid volume excess related to disease

Expected outcome

The child has no signs of fluid volume excess as evidenced by decreased edema and a urine output of 1 to 2 ml/kg/hour.

Interventions

1. Weigh the child at the same time each day, using the same scale and with the child wearing the same clothes.

2. Carefully monitor the child's fluid intake and output.

3. Place the child on a sodium-restricted diet during the edematous phase of the disease.

4. Administer diuretics, as ordered.

5. Monitor the child for decreased urine specific gravity.

6. Assess skin integrity and provide skin care.

Rationales

1. Daily weighing helps determine fluctuations in the child's fluid status.

2. Monitoring helps determine the child's fluid status.

3. A sodium-restricted diet helps prevent fluid retention.

4. Diuretics help eliminate fluid from the child's body. However, they are sometimes ineffective in children with nephrosis.

5. Decreased urine specific gravity indicates diuresis.

6. Edema from fluid volume excess may increase the risk of skin breakdown.

NURSING DIAGNOSIS

Knowledge deficit related to home care

Expected outcome

The parents express an understanding of home care instructions.

Interventions

1. Assess the parents' and child's understanding of the disease and prescribed treatment.

2. Teach the parents the importance of maintaining the child on a sodium-restricted diet.

3. Advise the parents that the child might have mood swings and increased irritability. Make sure that they understand that this is normal, but advise them not to let the child become manipulative.

Rationales

1. Such assessment serves as a basis on which to begin teaching.

2. Reducing the child's sodium intake prevents fluid retention.

3. Mood swings and irritability commonly result from a hospital stay and medication use.

4. Instruct the parents not to limit the child's activity level unless the child becomes overtired.

5. Teach the parents how to test the child's urine for protein.

4. Children with nephrotic syndrome usually can tolerate increased activity after the edematous phase has passed.

5. An increase in protein in the urine may indicate the need for a change in medication.

Documentation checklist

During the hospital stay, document:
- ❏ child's status and assessment findings upon admission
- ❏ changes in the child's status
- ❏ pertinent laboratory and diagnostic findings
- ❏ fluid intake and output
- ❏ nutritional intake
- ❏ child's response to treatment
- ❏ child's and parents' reactions to the illness and hospital stay
- ❏ patient and family teaching guidelines
- ❏ discharge planning guidelines.

Part 6

Musculoskeletal system

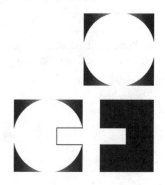

Congenital hip dysplasia

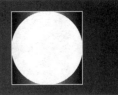

INTRODUCTION

One of the most common congenital malformations, congenital hip dysplasia refers to displacement of the head of the femur out of the acetabulum, or hip socket. This defect can be categorized into one of three types: acetabular dysplasia, subluxation, or dislocation.

Although the exact etiology is unknown, congenital hip dysplasia may result from fetal malpositioning within the uterus. It is more common in girls and occurs in approximately 1 of every 750 live births.

Usually, the defect can be treated without surgical intervention. Treatment typically includes maintaining abduction of the affected hip using a double or triple diapering technique, Pavlik harness, braces, or a spica cast.

The degree of success in correcting this deformity depends on the age at which the deformity is detected (generally, the earlier the deformity is detected, the more successful the treatment will be). Potential complications include shortening of the leg, limping, muscle contractures, and permanent damage to the femur and acetabulum.

ASSESSMENT

Musculoskeletal
- Immobility of affected hip and leg
- Clicking of hip (felt on examination)
- Unequal skin folds on buttocks

NURSING DIAGNOSIS

Risk for impaired skin integrity related to immobility, traction, or spica cast

Expected outcome

The child maintains skin integrity as evidenced by warm, pink, intact skin and no signs of skin breakdown.

Interventions

1. Inspect the child's skin, especially around bony prominences and cast openings, at least once every 4 hours.

2. If the child is in a spica cast, place him in a tilted position on his back or abdomen and turn him every 2 hours. When lying the child on his abdomen, position his face so that he can breathe.

3. Bathe the child daily. Massage his skin during baths and every 4 to 6 hours.

4. Pad the cast with plastic wrap around the child's perianal area.

5. Petal the cast after it dries. Use strips of waterproof tape or an occlusive dressing to overlap the cast edges.

Rationales

1. Frequent inspection allows for early detection of reddened skin and prompt treatment to prevent skin breakdown.

2. Turning helps restore circulation to pressure areas.

3. Cleanliness helps prevent skin breakdown. Massage promotes good circulation.

4. Plastic wrap helps keep the cast clean and prevents body fluids from contacting the skin, helping to prevent skin breakdown.

5. Petaling the cast helps keep it dry and prevents skin irritation.

NURSING DIAGNOSIS

Constipation related to immobility

Expected outcome

The child has normal bowel elimination as evidenced by regular bowel movements; soft, formed stools; and bowel sounds in all four quadrants.

Interventions

1. Obtain a history of the child's normal bowel habits.

2. Maintain a bowel record, including the times of bowel movements, stool consistency and pH, and results of any stool testing.

3. Encourage the child to drink plenty of fluids, especially fruit juices; monitor for diarrhea.

4. Administer stool softeners or suppositories, as ordered.

Rationales

1. Knowing the child's normal bowel habits helps to assess the child's current elimination pattern and the need for intervention.

2. Such a record helps identify the cause of constipation.

3. Increased fluid intake helps prevent constipation. Fruit juices may act as a cathartic; too much juice can cause diarrhea.

4. These agents stimulate fecal elimination by moisturizing and lubricating the feces to help ease their expulsion.

NURSING DIAGNOSIS

Risk for infection related to break in skin integrity secondary to traction (if pins are used)

Expected outcome

The child remains free from infection as evidenced by pink skin around pin sites, lack of purulent drainage, and no signs of edema.

Interventions

1. Assess the child's skin around pin sites every shift for signs of infection (redness, warmth, edema, and purulent drainage).

2. Clean the skin around the pin sites according to hospital policy or at least every 8 hours. (Hydrogen peroxide or saline solution typically is used for cleaning.)

3. Use aseptic technique for pin care.

Rationales

1. Frequent assessments allow for early detection and prompt treatment of infection.

2. Routine cleaning around the pin sites helps prevent infection.

3. Aseptic technique helps prevents infection when caring for a break in skin integrity.

NURSING DIAGNOSIS

Risk for injury related to possible mechanical malfunctioning of traction or circulatory compromise

Expected outcome

The child suffers no injuries resulting from mechanical malfunctioning or circulatory compromise as evidenced by a capillary refill time of 3 to 5 seconds, strong pedal pulses, warm extremities, and pink skin.

Musculoskeletal system

Interventions

1. Maintain the traction apparatus by checking the ropes for fraying and making sure the knots are secure. Tighten all bolts, and make sure the weights are hanging freely off the bed.

2. Assess the child's peripheral circulation every 2 hours, noting warmth, movement, capillary refill time, sensation in extremities, and pulse rate. Report any indications of pain, paresthesia, or paralysis.

Rationales

1. The traction apparatus should be set up according to hospital policy; routine checking helps ensure the patient's safety.

2. The traction device or spica cast may interfere with circulation, causing such complications as tissue necrosis or compartment syndrome. Increasing pain, paresthesia, or paralysis may indicate compartment syndrome.

NURSING DIAGNOSIS

Diversional activity deficit related to immobility secondary to traction or spica cast

Expected outcome

The child engages in diversional activities despite his immobility.

Interventions

1. Provide the child with environmental stimulation by placing his bed near a window, occasionally moving the bed outside of the room, placing brightly colored objects on the walls and bed, and putting toys within the child's reach.

2. Provide the child with age-appropriate activities and stimulation.

3. Provide for increased socialization by encouraging family members to visit or stay with the child, arranging for a volunteer to stay with him when possible, and encouraging interaction with other children when appropriate.

Rationales

1. Varying the child's physical environment helps decrease boredom from immobility.

2. Age-appropriate activities and stimulation decrease boredom and promote normal development.

3. Increased socialization helps prevent feelings of isolation and loneliness.

NURSING DIAGNOSIS

Knowledge deficit related to home care

Expected outcome

The parents express an understanding of home care instructions and demonstrate any home care procedures.

Interventions

1. Teach the parents routine cast care as follows:
• Inspect the skin for redness (especially around bony prominences and cast openings) at least once every 4 hours. If irritation develops, keep the skin clean and dry and apply a protective ointment to the site.
• Turn the child every 2 hours if he is in a spica cast.

• Bathe the child daily. Massage his skin during baths and every 4 to 6 hours.

• Pad the cast with plastic wrap around the child's perianal area.

• If the cast edges become soiled, petal the cast by overlapping the edges with strips of waterproof tape or an occlusive dressing.

2. Explain to the parents the importance of maintaining the child on a diet that is high in calories, calcium, and protein. Also explain the benefits of fruits, juices, and high-fiber cereals.

3. Instruct the parents to provide environmental and developmental stimulation by:
• placing the child's bed near a window, if possible
• occasionally moving the child's bed outside of his room
• placing brightly colored objects on the walls and bed
• putting toys within the child's reach
• providing age-appropriate activities.

Rationales

1. Routine cast care helps prevent skin breakdown.
• Frequent skin inspection allows for early detection and prompt treatment of irritation that could lead to breakdown.

• Regular turning restores circulation to pressure areas, helping to prevent skin breakdown.
• Daily bathing cleans the skin thoroughly and helps prevent skin breakdown. Massage promotes good circulation.
• Plastic wrap keeps the cast clean and prevents body fluids from contacting skin surfaces, helping to prevent skin breakdown.
• Petaling the cast helps keep it dry and prevents skin irritation.

2. A diet high in calories, calcium, and protein promotes healing and bone development. Fruits, juices, and high-fiber cereals prevent constipation from immobility.

3. Varying the child's physical environment helps decrease boredom from prolonged bed rest and immobility; age-appropriate activities promote normal development.

Musculoskeletal system

Documentation checklist

During the hospital stay, document:
❏ child's status and assessment findings upon admission
❏ changes in the child's status
❏ pertinent laboratory and diagnostic findings
❏ nutritional intake
❏ growth and development status
❏ child's response to treatment
❏ child's and parents' reactions to the illness and hospital stay
❏ patient and family teaching guidelines
❏ discharge planning guidelines.

Craniosynostosis

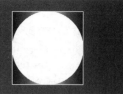

INTRODUCTION

Caused by premature closure of one or more of the skull sutures (commonly the sagittal sutures), craniosynostosis results in abnormal skull development and possible brain damage or mental retardation. Abnormalities usually result from continued brain growth where sutures remain open.

Treatment involves surgical separation of the sutures, usually at age 2 to 3 months. The prognosis is usually favorable when the surgery is performed as early as possible. Potential complications include increased intracranial pressure, brain damage, and death.

ASSESSMENT

Musculoskeletal
• Abnormal shape and symmetry of head
• Premature closure of skull sutures

Neurologic
• Signs and symptoms of increased intracranial pressure (ICP), including papilledema, nausea and vomiting, irritability, blindness, and mental retardation

NURSING DIAGNOSIS

Anxiety (parent) related to lack of knowledge about the infant's condition and need for surgery

Expected outcome

The parents are less anxious as evidenced by expressing an understanding of the infant's condition and need for surgery and by participating in the infant's care.

Interventions

1. Assess the parents' understanding of the infant's condition and need for surgery. Explain the condition and surgical procedure in simple terms.

2. Explain to the parents the events surrounding the surgery, including details on shaving the infant's head, preparing and caring for the incision site, the expected degree of swelling and pain, and the expected length of stay in the intensive care unit (ICU).

3. Allow the parents to visit the ICU before surgery.

4. Encourage the parents to ask questions and to express their fears and expectations about the infant's condition and surgery.

Rationales

1. Explaining the infant's condition and surgical procedure should help to clear up any misconceptions, easing the parents' anxiety.

2. Such explanations should help the parents adjust to the infant's need for surgery and ease their anxieties by allowing them to anticipate events surrounding the surgery.

3. Visiting the ICU should help to prepare the parents for the infant's postoperative environment, reducing their anxiety.

4. Encouraging the parents to ask questions and express fears and expectations allows you to clarify any misconceptions and offer reassurance, reducing the parents' anxiety.

NURSING DIAGNOSIS

Altered cerebral tissue perfusion related to cerebral edema and increased ICP

Expected outcome

The infant has no indications of cerebral edema or increased ICP as evidenced by age-appropriate vital signs, alertness, flat fontanels, and no signs of nausea.

Interventions

1. Keep the infant's head elevated at all times by raising the head of the crib 30 degrees.

2. Monitor the infant's vital signs hourly, reporting any significant changes (such as hyperthermia, decreased respiratory rate, bradycardia, and hypertension with a widening pulse pressure) immediately.

3. Monitor the infant's neurologic status every 2 hours, reporting any significant changes (such as decreased level of consciousness, unilateral or bilateral dilated pupils with decreased response to light, vomiting, irritability, and restlessness) immediately.

4. Carefully monitor the infant's fluid intake and output.

5. Turn the infant every 2 hours. If the child is older, encourage him to perform deep-breathing and coughing exercises to maintain respiratory function.

6. If possible, do not subject the infant to:
• painful stimuli
• respiratory procedures (especially suctioning and percussion)
• procedures that involve head rotation or neck flexion and extension
• application of pressure to neck veins
• Trendelenburg's position.

Rationales

1. This position promotes venous drainage and decreases swelling.

2. Such changes in vital signs indicate increased ICP, which requires prompt intervention.

3. Such changes in neurologic status indicate increased ICP, which requires prompt intervention.

4. Careful monitoring helps prevent fluid overload and cerebral edema.

5. The child must maintain respiratory function to prevent hypercapnia or hypoxia.

6. These positions and procedures may increase ICP.

NURSING DIAGNOSIS

Risk for infection related to surgical incision

Expected outcome

The infant remains free from infection as evidenced by closed sutures, body temperature less than 100° F (37.8° C), and no signs of purulent drainage and edema.

Interventions

1. Monitor the infant's temperature every 4 hours, and notify the doctor of any elevation.

Rationales

1. Increased temperature may indicate infection, which requires administration of antibiotics and antipyretics.

Musculoskeletal system

2. Observe the infant for signs of cerebrospinal fluid (CSF) leakage (usually from the eyes or nose). Check for glucose in the discharge using a reagent strip, and report positive findings immediately.

3. Keep the incision clean and dry, and apply antibiotic ointment (as ordered) to the suture line. Immediately report any signs of redness, swelling, or drainage.

2. A dural tear during surgery can result in CSF leakage, a potential source of meningeal infection. A positive glucose test indicates CSF drainage.

3. Skin or tissue infection can occur at the incision and usually requires the administration of antibiotics.

NURSING DIAGNOSIS

Risk for injury related to unstable bone fragments at the surgical site

Expected outcome

The infant suffers no injuries to the surgical site.

Interventions

1. Do not apply pressure anterior to the incision, down to and including the eye orbits and bridge of the nose.

2. Pad the crib side rails.

3. Support the back of the infant's head when lifting him.

Rationales

1. Pressure on the surgical site may disrupt normal healing.

2. Padding the crib side rails provides a cushion in case the infant accidentally bumps his head.

3. Supporting the head minimizes pressure at the surgical site, reducing the risk of injury.

NURSING DIAGNOSIS

Altered nutrition: less than body requirements related to postoperative diet

Expected outcome

The infant maintains an adequate nutritional status as evidenced by stable weight and consuming at least 80% of each feeding.

Interventions

1. Weigh the infant daily, using the same scale. Carefully monitor the infant's intake and output.

2. Administer I.V. fluids until the infant can tolerate oral fluids, usually 12 hours after surgery.

3. Introduce solids slowly, as tolerated.

Rationales

1. Daily weighing and careful monitoring of intake and output provide an accurate measure of the infant's nutritional status.

2. I.V. fluids help maintain the infant's nutritional status during the immediate postoperative period.

3. Rapid introduction of solids may cause nausea.

NURSING DIAGNOSIS

Fluid volume excess related to surgery and possible syndrome of inappropriate antidiuretic hormone secretion (SIADH)

Expected outcome

The infant maintains normal fluid volume as evidenced by the absence of edema and ascites, normal ICP, and no signs of headache or heart failure.

Interventions

1. While the infant is in the ICU, monitor his fluid intake and output hourly.

2. Monitor the infant for decreased serum sodium concentration, high urine osmolality, low urine volume, irritability, and lethargy. Report any of these findings immediately.

Rationales

1. Frequent monitoring allows for early detection and prompt treatment of any fluid status problems.

2. These signs may indicate SIADH, a common occurrence after neurosurgical procedures that involves intracranial manipulation.

NURSING DIAGNOSIS

Pain related to surgical procedure

Expected outcome

The infant exhibits decreased crying and irritability.

Interventions

1. Observe the infant for crying, restlessness, loss of appetite, flushing, and increased sweating.

2. Provide appropriate comfort measures (such as positioning, distraction, and massage), and administer pain medication, as needed.

Rationales

1. Such behavioral changes and physiologic responses indicate pain.

2. Comfort measures and pain medications can effectively control the infant's pain.

NURSING DIAGNOSIS

Sensory alteration (visual) related to postoperative orbital edema

Expected outcome

The infant exhibits decreased orbital edema.

Interventions

1. Prepare the parents for expected orbital and facial edema and bruising (the infant's eyes may be swollen shut for the first few days after surgery but should gradually reopen by the 5th day). Offer reassurance during times of peak swelling.

2. Elevate the head of the crib 30 degrees, and apply warm compresses to the orbital area every 4 hours.

3. Help orient the older child to his immediate surroundings. Give him with a call light and put up the bed's side rails.

Rationales

1. Swelling and bruising may prevent the infant from seeing for a few days. This can be particularly frightening for the parents, who may need continual reassurance.

2. Elevating the head of the crib and applying warm compresses help reduce swelling.

3. The unfamiliar environment and sounds of the ICU can frighten a child with impaired vision, compromising his safety.

NURSING DIAGNOSIS

Knowledge deficit related to home care

Expected outcome

The parents express an understanding of home care instructions and demonstrate home care procedures.

Musculoskeletal system

Interventions

1. Teach the parents the importance of:

• keeping the incision clean (with one-half strength hydrogen peroxide) and dry (with dressings) until sutures are removed and watching for indications of infection (purulent drainage or swelling at the site, fever, and signs of headache and malaise)
• elevating the head of the crib or bed 30 degrees

• maintaining safety precautions in the home, such as using side rails or bumper pads, placing the infant on a rug or thick blanket when on the floor, and prohibiting the older child from roughhousing and running.

2. Emphasize the need to keep follow-up appointments, as scheduled.

Rationales

1. The parents need to be informed of the importance of home care.
• Routine incision care helps decrease the risk of serious complications, such as infection.

• Elevating the head of the crib or bed helps reduce orbital edema.
• Maintaining safety helps prevent accidental bumping of the head, which could impair healing.

2. Follow-up appointments allow monitoring of growth or changes in the infant's or child's head shape and evaluation of the effectiveness of surgery.

Documentation checklist

During the hospital stay, document:
❐ infant's status and assessment findings upon admission
❐ changes in the infant's status
❐ pertinent laboratory and diagnostic findings
❐ fluid intake and output
❐ nutritional intake
❐ growth and development status
❐ infant's response to treatment
❐ parents' reactions to the infant's surgery and hospital stay
❐ family teaching guidelines
❐ discharge planning guidelines.

Fractures

INTRODUCTION

Usually the result of childhood accidents (such as falls or motor vehicle accidents), fractures can be classified as follows:

• In a *complete fracture*, the bone breaks entirely across, resulting in a break in the continuity of bone (such a fracture may be further classified as transverse, oblique, spiral, or torsion).

• In an *incomplete fracture*, the break extends only partially through the bone, and the bone remains continuous.

• In a *closed (simple) fracture*, the break does not puncture the skin surface.

• In an *open (compound) fracture*, the break punctures through the skin surface.

Common fracture sites include the arm, clavicle, knee, and femur. Treatment includes reduction and immobilization of the fracture and may involve traction, casting, or surgery. The outcome usually depends on the severity of the fracture and the treatment provided. Potential complications include the development of fat emboli, improper bone growth, compartment syndrome, and infection.

ASSESSMENT

Musculoskeletal
• Skeletal deformity
• Muscle spasm
• Pain or tenderness
• Bony crepitus

Neurologic
• Loss of motor function
• Impaired sensation
• Paresthesia
• Paralysis

Integumentary
• Swelling
• Bruising

NURSING DIAGNOSIS

Pain related to muscle spasm, swelling, or bleeding

Expected outcome

The child has no signs of pain as evidenced by relaxed facial expressions, expression of comfort, ability to sleep, decreased need for analgesics, decreased agitation, and low scores on pain assessment scales.

Interventions

1. Assess the degree and level of the child's pain using pediatric assessment tools (such as a face interval or line number pain-rating scale).

2. Institute the following comfort measures:
• Keep the child in proper body alignment.

• Provide support above and below the fracture site when moving the child. Move the child carefully, and avoid jarring the bed.
• Monitor for any pressure areas caused by traction, the child's cast, or bedclothes.
• Elevate the fracture above the level of the heart.

• Apply ice to the fracture, as ordered.

Rationales

1. Assessing the child's pain allows you to determine the specific area of pain, monitor for changes in the degree of pain before and after interventions, and monitor for complications, such as impaired circulation.

2. Promoting comfort helps relieve the child's pain.
• Maintaining proper body alignment decreases joint strain and prevents contractures.
• Any movement may increase pain, so supporting the child above and below the fracture site and avoiding sudden, jerking motions help promote comfort.
• Prolonged pressure may cause ischemia, which results in pain.
• Elevating the fracture above the level of the heart promotes venous return and decreases edema, which can exert pressure on nerve endings and cause pain.
• Ice causes vasoconstriction, which inhibits edema and pain.

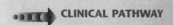 **CLINICAL PATHWAY**

Closed reduction-femur fracture-spica cast application

Plan	ED phase/Clinic outpatient surgery	Admit from ED/OR
Goals	• Initial social work assessment • Skeletal survey completed (if performed or related to abuse workup) • Caregiver/child prepared for procedure	• Initial cast teaching complete • Patient comfortable with oral pain medications
Treatments	• Spica cast application	• Petal cast with pink tape and mole skin when cast dry.
Activity	• Bed rest/caregiver may hold after casted • Turn q 2 hr.	• May be held by caregiver, out of bed (OOB) to wagon, wheelchair, stroller
Diet	• Nothing by mouth until casted • Regular diet for age after casted	• Nothing by mouth until casted • Regular diet for age after casted
Tests	• X-ray-femur-AP/Lateral • Skeletal survey before spica cast application if abuse is differential diagnosis	• Post cast X-ray in ED or OR
Medications/I.V.	• Conscious sedation (ED) • General anesthesia (OR)	• Pain medications and diazepam (Valium) by mouth
Consults	• Social services/Pediatrics if ED questions abuse • Child life for procedure preparation	• Social work • Case manager • Child life • Pediatrics
Teaching/Discharge planning	• Spica cast application information to family • Social services — for initial family assessment	• Cast care booklet • Demonstrate neurovascular checks, positioning, turning, and hygiene measures. • Caregiver assists with neurovascular checks, turning, hygiene measures, and positioning.
Patient flow	• ED to X-ray to ED • Clinic outpatient surgery (closed reduction with casting)	• Admit to patient care unit. • Admit to postanesthesia care unit. • If indicated, admit to hospital overnight.
Equipment and supplies	• I.V. fluids and supplies • Medications for sedation • Pulse oximeter • Handheld resuscitation bag and mask at bedside for conscious sedation • Casting materials • Spica table	• Moleskin — 1 can • Pink tape — 4 rolls • Diapers • Sanitary pads

Adapted with permission from Vanderbilt Children's Hospital, Nashville, Tennessee.

Day 1 (Femur fracture, closed reduction and casting, extended recovery)

• Social services assessment is complete.
• Staff is aware of who the child may be discharged to in abuse cases.
• Caregiver accurately verbalizes/demonstrates how to care for patient at home and has necessary equipment.
• Patient is comfortable with oral pain medications.

• May be held by caregiver, OOB to wagon, wheelchair, stroller
• Turn q 2 hr.

• Nothing by mouth until casted
• Regular diet for age after casted

• Pain medications and Valium by mouth

• Social services/Case manager, Child life, Pediatrics

• Caregiver demonstrates all skills: neurovascular checks, hygiene and diapering, positioning/turning, setting up Bradford frame and its use, and skin care.
• Discussed with caregiver and he accurately verbalizes understanding of troubleshooting, problem solving, clothing and transportation requirements, behavioral management needs; when to call doctor; use of stroller, wagon, and wheelchair; and how to adapt activities.
• Clinical nurse specialist/Case manager follows up by phone after discharge.

• Discharge; return to clinic 1 week after discharge.

• Assess need for wagon/stroller/wheelchair for home use.

3. Administer analgesics or muscle relaxants or both, as ordered. Give medications promptly, especially when the child indicates by complaints, facial expressions, irritability, or body positioning that he is in pain.

3. Analgesics help relieve pain; muscle relaxants help reduce muscle spasms. Giving medications promptly helps ensure that the child's pain remains controllable.

NURSING DIAGNOSIS

Altered peripheral tissue perfusion related to bleeding, swelling, the cast, or traction

Expected outcome

The child maintains adequate peripheral tissue perfusion as evidenced by decreasing pain; strong pulses; pinkish, warm skin; a capillary refill time of 3 to 5 seconds; normal sensation; and pain-free movement in the extremity distal to the fracture.

Interventions

1. Assess the rate and volume of the pulse distal to the fracture every 2 to 4 hours.

2. Assess the color, temperature, and capillary refill time of the affected extremity; compare findings with those of the unaffected extremity.

3. Assess the child's sensation distal to the fracture (using touch, pressure, or the pin prick method) every 15 minutes for the first hour, then hourly for the next 24 hours, and then every 4 hours.

4. Assess movement distal to the fracture site every 2 to 4 hours.

5. Assess the degree and level of the child's pain using pediatric assessment tools (such as a face interval or line number pain-rating scale).

6. Notify the doctor immediately of abnormal signs or symptoms, including decreased sensation, pallor, cool temperature at the fracture, and decreased peripheral pulses.

Rationales

1. Such assessment can indicate impeded blood flow to the distal extremity, requiring replacement of the cast or readjustment of the traction device.

2. Comparing the two extremities helps determine whether the affected extremity is adequately perfused.

3. Such assessment determines whether perfusion to the nerves is intact.

4. Such assessment helps determine whether the fracture has impaired the child's movement, which could result in neurologic damage.

5. Such assessment helps to determine the specific area of pain, detect any changes in pain before and after intervention, and identify complications, such as impaired circulation.

6. Early detection ensures prompt treatment to prevent impaired circulation from causing tissue necrosis and nerve damage, which could lead to permanent damage and possible amputation.

NURSING DIAGNOSIS

Risk for impaired skin integrity related to immobility from cast or traction

Expected outcome

The child maintains skin integrity as evidenced by the absence of irritation, redness, and breaks in the skin.

Interventions

1. Assess the child's skin for redness or irritation, especially around pressure points. If you note redness or irritation, massage pressure points at least once every 4 hours. Also check to see whether the cast needs trimming or the traction device needs padding to relieve pressure.

2. Turn and reposition the child at least once every 2 hours.

3. Provide the child with sheepskin padding, elbow and heel pads, a convoluted foam mattress, and an overbed trapeze.

4. Keep the child's skin dry and free from irritants by taking the following measures:
• Tuck plastic-backed disposable diapers or plastic wrap around the cast in the perianal region to protect the cast from moisture or soiling.
• Instruct the child not to insert any object between the cast and skin.
• Petal the edges of the cast.

Rationales

1. Redness or irritation may signal impending skin breakdown. Massaging and relieving pressure points promptly should prevent skin breakdown.

2. Turning and repositioning help relieve pressure, preventing skin breakdown.

3. Sheepskin padding and elbow and heel pads can help reduce skin abrasion. A convoluted foam mattress helps reduce pressure by distributing body weight evenly on the bed surface. An overbed trapeze allows the child to lift himself without abrading the skin.

4. Moisture and irritation may skin breakdown in children with fractures.
• Protecting the cast from moisture prevents bacterial growth that could lead to infection and skin breakdown.
• Inserting any object between the cast and skin may break the skin and cause infection.
• Petaling the cast decreases the likelihood that loose plaster might fall into the cast and irritate the skin.

NURSING DIAGNOSIS

Impaired gas exchange related to complications secondary to the fracture and immobility

Expected outcome

The child does not develop signs of impaired gas exchange as evidenced by age-appropriate vital signs, unlabored respirations, and normal level of consciousness.

Interventions

1. Assess the child's vital signs and neurologic status, noting any wheezing, cyanosis, sluggish pupil response, and lethargy. Report any of these abnormalities immediately to the doctor.

2. Instruct the child to turn, cough, and breathe deeply every 2 hours.

3. Monitor the child's hematocrit and hemoglobin values.

Rationales

1. Such assessment may indicate complications, such as hypovolemia secondary to hemorrhage or pulmonary embolus, altered level of consciousness secondary to pulmonary embolus or hypovolemia, or respiratory distress secondary to lung secretions or pulmonary embolus.

2. Turning, coughing, and deep breathing help clear secretions and expand the lungs fully.

3. These values directly measure the oxygen-carrying capacity of the blood. Low levels may indicate the need for the administration of packed red blood cells.

Musculoskeletal system

NURSING DIAGNOSIS

Constipation related to immobility

Expected outcome

The child maintains normal bowel elimination as evidenced by having regular bowel movements and passing soft, formed stools.

Interventions

1. Check and record all bowel movements, noting the frequency and consistency of all stools.

2. Increase the child's fluid and dietary fiber intake, as necessary. Encourage the child to drink plenty of fluids and to eat whole-grain cereals, fruits, and vegetables.

3. Administer stool softeners, as ordered.

Rationales

1. Monitoring the child's bowel movements helps determine the need for intervention.

2. Fluid helps move food along the digestive tract. Fiber increases the bulk of feces.

3. Stool softeners help water penetrate fecal material, making it easier for the child to pass stool.

NURSING DIAGNOSIS

Risk for activity intolerance related to immobility from cast or traction

Expected outcome

The child participates in self-care and social activities as evidenced by performing activities of daily living (ADLs), exercising, and engaging in age-appropriate activities.

Interventions

1. Encourage the child to perform ADLs (as tolerated) and to participate in decisions about his care.

2. Involve the child in a regular exercise program, as ordered. Exercises may include:
• active range-of-motion (ROM) exercises on all unaffected joints every 4 hours
• isometric exercises (flexing and extending extremity, and tightening and relaxing muscles) involving the affected area every 2 to 4 hours
• limb-strengthening exercises, if appropriate.

3. Encourage the child to socialize by providing him with a wheelchair or crutches for easy ambulation. If the child cannot ambulate on his own, move him around on a stretcher or move his bed into the playroom.

4. Provide the child with age-appropriate activities, such as toys, games, television, and reading materials.

5. Encourage the parents to bring in the child's school assignments (and a tutor, if necessary) and to arrange for siblings and peers to visit (if appropriate).

Rationales

1. Allowing the child to participate in his care promotes independence and feelings of self-control.

2. Regular exercise helps maintain muscle tone and joint mobility and, if the child will need crutches, helps prepare him for crutch walking.

3. Ambulation promotes feelings of independence and increases the likelihood that the child will socialize and engage in age-appropriate activities.

4. Such activities promote normal development.

5. School work and visits from siblings and peers encourage the child to maintain contact with outside interests.

Nursing diagnosis

Knowledge deficit related to home care

Expected outcome

The parents express an understanding of home care instructions and demonstrate home care procedures.

Interventions

1. Explain to the parents the normal healing of a fracture. Also explain the importance of routine cast care, including:
• protecting the cast from moisture and soil with a plastic-backed diaper or plastic wrap
• petaling the cast to prevent loose plaster from falling into the cast
• notifying the doctor if the cast breaks or becomes loose.

2. Instruct the parents to assess the child's neurovascular status by noting the child's skin color and temperature (it should be warm and dry) and capillary refill time (it should be 3 to 5 seconds) and by checking for impaired sensation or movement, pain, and swelling.

3. Teach the parents how to care for their child's skin, especially on his buttocks and back. Tell them to clean the skin using a moisturizing lotion and powder and to check for redness and irritation. Also instruct them to keep the child from inserting objects into the cast.

4. Teach the parents the importance of regular exercise, such as active ROM exercises, isometric exercises, and physical therapy (if needed for crutch walking).

5. Help the parents assess their home environment to determine the child's special needs. Ask about the location of the child's bed, the bathroom, and stairs and whether the child will need any special equipment, such as an overbed trapeze, bedpan, urinal, side rails, shower stool, crutches, or wheelchair. Also ask about the child's school needs, such as an alternative means of transportation, special clothing, and tutoring.

6. Instruct the parents to encourage the child to drink plenty of fluids and to increase his dietary fiber intake.

7. Offer suggestions for age-appropriate activities.

Rationales

1. Understanding the normal healing of a fracture and the importance of cast care should promote compliance with home care.

2. Such assessments identify possible complications that require immediate medical attention.

3. Proper skin care decreases the risk of infection or trauma to the skin.

4. Regular exercise helps prevent muscle stiffness and contractures.

5. Helping to assess the child's home environment helps the parents anticipate and prepare for the child's needs.

6. Increased fluid and dietary fiber intake help prevent constipation, a common complication of immobility.

7. Age-appropriate activities promote normal development and help divert the child's attention from his immobility.

Documentation checklist

During the hospital stay, document:
❏ child's status and assessment findings upon admission
❏ changes in the child's status
❏ pertinent laboratory and diagnostic findings
❏ nutritional intake
❏ growth and developmental status
❏ child's response to treatment
❏ child's and parents' reactions to the injury and hospital stay
❏ patient and family teaching guidelines
❏ discharge planning guidelines.

Musculoskeletal system

Osteomyelitis

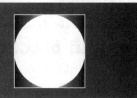

INTRODUCTION

An infection of the bone and marrow, osteomyelitis is caused by septicemia (usually from a *Staphylococcus* infection in older children and a *Haemophilus* infection in younger children) resulting from a wound, fracture, surgery, or burn injury. This disease occurs most commonly in children ages 5 to 15, with a higher incidence among boys.

Treatment usually involves administering antibiotics I.V. and immobilizing the infected bone. Surgery may be necessary to drain subperiosteal or subcutaneous abscess. The prognosis generally depends on the severity of the infection and the response to antibiotic therapy. Potential complications include hematologic, hepatic, or renal damage related to high doses of antibiotics; joint or bone damage; abscesses; and amputation.

ASSESSMENT

Musculoskeletal
- Localized tenderness (usually over a bone or joint)
- Limited range of motion
- Guarding of extremity
- Restlessness

Cardiovascular
- Increased pulse rate

Neurologic
- Generalized malaise
- Irritability

Hematologic
- Increased white blood cell (WBC) count
- Increased erythrocyte sedimentation rate

Integumentary
- Elevated temperature
- Increased warmth with edema at affected site

NURSING DIAGNOSIS

Risk for infection related to wound contamination

Expected outcome

The child remains free from further infection as evidenced by decreases in edema, fever, erythema, warmth at the infection site, WBC count, and sedimentation rate.

Interventions

1. Use good hand-washing technique before treating the child.

2. Assess the infection site each shift and document any signs of exudate, edema, erythema, or warmth.

3. Monitor the child's vital signs every 4 hours for increases in temperature, heart rate, and respiratory rate.

4. Monitor the child's WBC count, erythrocyte sedimentation rate, and blood cultures. Notify the doctor of any significant changes.

5. Administer antibiotics (cephalosporins and penicillinase-resistant agents are the drugs of choice) and antipyretics, as ordered. Monitor the child for drug compatibility and adverse reactions.

Rationales

1. Good hand washing decreases the spread of nosocomial infection.

2. Exudate, edema, erythema, and warmth indicate ongoing infection, which may signal the need for medication adjustment.

3. Such changes in vital signs indicate ongoing infection, which may signal the need for medication adjustment.

4. Elevated WBC count and erythrocyte sedimentation rate indicate ongoing infection. Blood cultures (positive in 60% of children with osteomyelitis) indicate an ongoing systemic infection.

5. Antibiotics help fight bacterial infections. Antipyretics help decrease fever.

6. Maintain a patent drainage system, as indicated.

7. Maintain universal precautions when handling infective material.

8. Use sterile technique for all dressing changes.

6. Proper drainage prevents tissue damage from the accumulation of purulent exudate or clots.

7. Such precautions help prevent the risk of contamination.

8. Sterile technique helps prevent the introduction of bacteria into the wound.

Nursing diagnosis

Impaired skin integrity related to infection

Expected outcome

The child has no signs of skin breakdown as evidenced by decreased edema and new skin growth at the surgical site.

Interventions

1. Elevate the affected extremity 30 degrees.

2. Assess peripheral pulses, skin color, and sensation in the affected extremity every 4 hours. Also check capillary refill time in the extremity distal to the splint or cast every 4 hours.

3. Monitor the amount of drainage, especially bloody drainage, around the cast or splint every 4 hours. Notify the doctor if the drainage soaks through the cast.

4. Use sterile technique when changing dressings.

5. Provide the following cast or splint care, as needed:

• Petal the child's cast.

• Keep the cast or splint dry.
• Instruct the child not to put objects into the cast or splint.

Rationales

1. Elevation ensures venous return, decreasing edema and the risk of skin breakdown.

2. In edematous or splinted extremities, frequent assessment of pulses, skin color, and sensation help ensure adequate circulation and prevent nerve impairment. Capillary refill time should be 3 to 5 seconds.

3. Monitoring allows the determination of the amount of wound drainage. Excessive bloody drainage may indicate hemorrhage or infection.

4. Sterile technique decreases the risk of contamination and possible skin breakdown. Frequent dressing changes keep the wound clean and dry and allow you to evaluate the wound.

5. Proper care of the cast or splint helps prevent breaks in the child's skin integrity.
• Petaling the cast helps to prevent loose plaster from falling into the cast, which could cause irritation and possible skin breakdown.
• Moisture can lead to skin breakdown.
• Putting objects, such as food or toys, into the cast or splint can injure or irritate the skin.

Nursing diagnosis

Pain related to inflammation and infection

Expected outcome

The child has increased comfort as evidenced by decreased irritability and agitation, expression of decreased pain, and relaxed behavior when interacting with others.

Interventions

1. Assess and document characteristics of the child's pain, including location, type, duration, and pattern. To determine the severity of pain, use a face interval or number line pain-rating scale.

2. Administer analgesics, as ordered or needed. Document the child's response.

3. Elevate the affected extremity 30 degrees.

4. Move the affected extremity smoothly and gently.

5. Use distraction techniques, such as television, music, or games, to comfort the child.

6. Provide periods of quiet and rest.

7. Document the most effective strategy for pain relief in the child's record.

Rationales

1. Frequent assessment and documentation help determine the need for intervention and evaluate the effectiveness of previous interventions.

2. Analgesics help relieve pain.

3. Elevating the affected extremity decreases edema and pain by promoting venous return.

4. Any sudden or abrupt movements may increase the child's pain.

5. Distraction diverts the child's attention from his pain and helps him focus on other activities.

6. Fatigue can lessen the child's tolerance for pain.

7. Documentation helps ensure that all team members follow consistent pain-relief measures.

NURSING DIAGNOSIS

Impaired physical mobility related to infection

Expected outcome

The child demonstrates optimal mobility (as allowed or tolerated) as evidenced by performing passive range-of-motion (ROM) exercises and moving his extremities.

Interventions

1. Keep the affected extremity immobile with a splint or cast, as ordered.

2. Assess the skin color, sensation, and movement of the affected extremity every 4 hours.

3. Consult a physical therapist or occupational therapist, as necessary, to develop an effective exercise program that includes ROM and isometric exercises.

Rationales

1. Immobilization with a splint or cast helps maintain proper bone alignment, helping ensuring proper healing and optimal mobility.

2. Such assessment helps prevent circulatory or nerve impairment and allows evaluation of the effectiveness of the splint or cast.

3. An effective exercise program maintains muscle strength, ensures optimal recovery, and prevents potential complications from immobility, such as contractures, limb shortening, and limping.

NURSING DIAGNOSIS

Altered nutrition: less than body requirements related to increased metabolic needs for wound healing

Expected outcome

The child has an improved nutritional intake as evidenced by maintaining a stable weight and consuming at least 80% of each meal.

Interventions

1. Assess the child's nutritional and emotional status, noting any sign of apathy, irritability, pallor, edema, or cachexia (a long-term complication).

2. Monitor the child's fluid intake and output, reporting a urine output of less than 1 ml/kg/hour.

3. Document and evaluate the child's food intake every shift.

4. Serve the child small, frequent, high-calorie meals and drinks. Consult the hospital dietitian, as necessary, to ensure that the child receives a well-balanced diet and enough calories.

5. Serve some of the child's favorite foods, if they meet dietary guidelines.

Rationales

1. Such findings may indicate bowel obstruction or constipation, possibly contributing to the child's unstable weight.

2. Oliguria, a sign of dehydration, commonly occurs in osteomyelitis.

3. Knowing the child's food intake helps determine whether he is getting the nutrition he needs for wound healing.

4. Eating small, frequent meals allows the child to eat more of each meal without feeling too full. A high-calorie diet promotes healing.

5. Serving the child some of his favorite foods helps ensure compliance with the prescribed diet.

NURSING DIAGNOSIS

Ineffective family coping: compromised related to prolonged hospital stay

Expected outcome

The child and family members demonstrate appropriate coping and support mechanisms as evidenced by maintaining communication among family members and significant others.

Interventions

1. Encourage the parents and other family members to take part in the child's daily activities. Designate at least two activities each day for the family to do with the child.

2. Arrange for a foster grandparent or volunteer to stay with the child when the parents are away from the child's hospital room.

3. Perform any invasive procedure in the treatment room.

4. Encourage the parents to bring in the child's school assignments and arrange for a tutor, if necessary.

5. Provide the parents with daily updates on the child's status.

Rationales

1. Family involvement in the child's activities helps foster a sense of family unity, helping family members to cope during the child's hospital stay.

2. The parents may need time away from the child to rest and attend to other family matters. Arranging for someone to stay with the child provides a means of support in the parents' absence.

3. Performing invasive procedures in a treatment room allows the child to feel secure in his own hospital room, helping him to cope with the hospital stay.

4. Continuing with school work allows the child to maintain a sense of normalcy.

5. Daily updates help the parents to cope by decreasing anxiety and fostering trust in the health care team.

NURSING DIAGNOSIS

Knowledge deficit related to home care

Expected outcome

The parents express an understanding of home care instructions and demonstrate home care procedures.

Musculoskeletal system

Interventions

1. Explain to the parents the basic etiology and pathophysiology of osteomyelitis.

2. Review with the parents the signs and symptoms of recurring infection (see the "Assessment" section at the beginning of this plan).

3. Teach the parents the purpose and use of antibiotics; include details on administration, dosage, and potential adverse effects.

4. Teach the parents the importance of providing a well-balanced diet.

5. Teach the parents the importance of cast or splint care, including details on:
• petaling the cast edges
• keeping the cast or splint dry
• instructing the child not to place objects in the cast or splint.

6. Explain the importance of keeping all follow-up appointments.

7. Refer the parents to the school nurse or a home health nurse, as necessary.

Rationales

1. Such explanations help the parents to take measures to prevent a recurrence of the infection.

2. Knowing the signs and symptoms of infection promotes early detection and prompt treatment, which decreases the risk of complications.

3. This promotes compliance with the medication regimen and allows the parents to recognize the need for medical help when necessary.

4. A well-balanced diet provides essential vitamins, calories, protein, and calcium to promote healing.

5. Proper cast or splint care helps prevent complications of the skin or affected extremities.

6. Follow-up appointments are necessary to evaluate healing and to help prevent reinfection.

7. A school nurse or home health nurse can monitor the child's progress and compliance with treatment.

Documentation checklist

During the hospital stay, document:
❐ child's status and assessment findings upon admission
❐ changes in the child's status
❐ pertinent laboratory and diagnostic findings
❐ nutritional intake
❐ growth and development status
❐ child's response to treatment
❐ child's and parents' reactions to the illness and hospital stay
❐ patient and family teaching guidelines
❐ discharge planning guidelines.

Rheumatoid arthritis

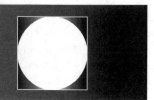

INTRODUCTION

Juvenile rheumatoid arthritis—characterized by joint inflammation that results in decreased mobility, pain, and swelling—is classified as polyarticular, pauciarticular, or systemic.

Polyarticular arthritis, which involves many joints (particularly the small joints of the hands), and *pauciarticular* arthritis, which primarily affects only a few joints (such as the knees, ankles, and elbows), occur more frequently in girls. *Systemic* arthritis, which characteristically causes a high fever, rheumatoid rash, and polyarthritis, affects boys and girls equally.

Although the exact cause of rheumatoid arthritis remains unknown, it seems to be linked with certain immunodeficiencies. Peak onset occurs from ages 2 to 5 and again from ages 9 to 12.

Treatment may include the administration of corticosteroids, nonsteroidal anti-inflammatory agents, aspirin, gold salts, and penicillamine (Cuprimine) as well as physical therapy and joint replacement surgery. Potential complications include joint deformity and adverse reactions resulting from medication use, including bleeding, GI distress, ulcers, blindness, and death. Although the prognosis usually depends on the severity of the disease, many children have some form of joint disability.

ASSESSMENT

Musculoskeletal
- Joint pain
- Joint swelling
- Decreased mobility
- Joint inflammation
- Morning stiffness
- Delayed growth

Hematologic
- Elevated erythrocyte sedimentation rate
- Positive rheumatoid factor titer

NURSING DIAGNOSIS

Pain related to inflamed joints, joint immobility, and gastric irritation secondary to aspirin use

Expected outcome

The child has increased comfort as evidenced by the ability to perform range-of-motion (ROM) exercises, expression of decreased pain, and absence of gastric irritation.

Interventions

1. Assess the intensity and location of the child's pain as well as the relationship of the pain to the time of day and activities performed. Use pediatric pain assessment tools, such as a face interval or line number pain-rating scale, in your evaluation.

2. Provide a warm bath or shower (approximately 100° F [37.8° C]) each morning for 10 to 12 minutes.

3. Administer analgesics and anti-inflammatory medications, as ordered (most commonly enteric-coated aspirin four times daily). To prevent stomach irritation or pain, administer aspirin with food, milk, or an antacid about half an hour before the child rises in the morning.

Rationales

1. Such an assessment helps determine the type and amount of pain medication needed.

2. Heat helps relieve pain and joint stiffness. A morning shower provides the most relief because joint stiffness usually is worse in the morning.

3. Aspirin provides pain relief and decreases the joint inflammation associated with arthritis. Administering aspirin with food, milk, or an antacid decreases the risk of gastric irritation; giving it in the early morning provides the most relief because joint stiffness is usually the worst upon rising.

4. Monitor the child for signs and symptoms of aspirin toxicity, including ringing in the ears, decreased hearing, drowsiness, nausea, vomiting, irritability, unusual behavior, and rapid, deep breathing.

4. These signs and symptoms may signal the need for a dosage reduction or discontinuation of aspirin therapy.

5. Help the child perform active and passive ROM exercises after consulting with the physical therapist. Encourage ambulation during play activities.

5. Moving the joints helps relieve joint stiffness; however, excessive exercise may worsen pain. The physical therapist can help plan an individualized program for the child.

6. Maintain proper body alignment by propping the child with pillows when he is in bed.

6. Proper body alignment helps ease pain and prevents contractures.

7. Consult the physical therapist about the use of splints. Set up a schedule for application and removal of splints.

7. The child may need splints to help prevent contractures. They should be removed at regular intervals to ease pain and prevent skin breakdown.

NURSING DIAGNOSIS

Self-care deficit related to pain, immobility, and joint contractures

Expected outcome

The child has no self-care deficits as evidenced by his ability to perform age-appropriate activities of daily living (ADLs).

Interventions

1. Assess the child's current level of self-care.

2. Work with the child to establish a self-care program based on mutual goals and expectations. Consult the occupational and physical therapists before completing the plan.

3. Encourage the child to perform ADLs himself, but help when necessary.

Rationales

1. Such an assessment establishes a baseline that can be used to evaluate his progress.

2. Helping to design his own self-care plan fosters the child's sense of control and encourages participation and compliance. An occupational therapist can provide advice about the child's ADLs and the need for adaptive devices, such as bathroom and bedside support bars, tongs (to lift and reach objects), and fasteners (to help buckle and button clothing). A physical therapist can individualize an exercise program designed to maintain ROM of the affected joints.

3. The child's ability to perform ADLs himself may vary depending on the severity of pain.

NURSING DIAGNOSIS

Body image disturbance related to the effects of the chronic illness and the disabling nature of the disease

Expected outcome

The child has no disturbance in self-concept as evidenced by expressing an acceptance of his altered body image and interacting positively with others.

Interventions

1. Establish a therapeutic relationship with the child, and encourage him to express his feelings about his body.

2. Correct any misconceptions the child may have about his condition and build on his positive feelings and coping skills.

3. Encourage the child to interact with his peers, family, and the hospital staff.

4. Consult social services, a child-life worker, or a psychologist, as needed.

5. Provide time for the child and parents to express their feelings about the crippling effects of the disease.

6. Help the child prepare to deal with his peers at school; enlist school counselors and the child's teachers to help the child and his classmates understand and accept each other.

Rationales

1. Establishing a therapeutic relationship helps the child to develop trust, which improves communication. Encouraging him to express his feelings lets you determine his current cognitive and emotional level.

2. The child may feel overwhelmed and need help separating facts from misconceptions and coping with his negative feelings.

3. Interaction with and acceptance by others helps build a positive self-concept.

4. Such professionals can help identify the child's needs and improve his self-concept by using play therapy and teaching appropriate coping skills.

5. The child and parents must express their feelings about the disabling nature of the disease before they can begin to cope effectively.

6. A chronically ill child may have trouble dealing with his peers, resulting in anger and depression; classmate may also have misunderstandings and biases about the illness. Helping the child prepare to deal with classmates and heading off classmates' misunderstandings make it easier for the child to function at school.

Nursing diagnosis

Ineffective family coping: compromised related to the effects of the child's chronic illness

Expected outcome

The family exhibits effective coping skills as evidenced by expressing their feelings about the child's chronic illness and by stating what resources are available to them.

Interventions

1. Assess the family's dynamics and interactions, including role expectations and boundaries.

2. Assess the family's knowledge and current use of support systems.

3. Encourage family members to express their feelings, and help them deal with such feelings as guilt, anger, hopelessness, grief, and anxiety.

4. Help family members recognize ineffective coping patterns and find other ways to deal with their problems.

5. Refer the family to available resources within the hospital and the community, such as to a social services department and the American Juvenile Arthritis Organization, 1330 West Peachtree Street, Atlanta, GA 30309.

Rationales

1. Such assessment may reveal ineffective family communication patterns and unrealistic expectations.

2. Support systems, such as extended family, friends, and church and community resources, help the family remain healthy and intact. Understanding how the family uses these resources allows you to suggest appropriate alternative coping and support systems.

3. The family members of a chronically ill child often harbor negative feelings; expressing such feelings allows them to receive emotional support.

4. Identifying ineffective behaviors is the first step toward change. Teaching problem-solving skills encourages family members to discover alternative solutions.

5. The family needs to know what resources are available.

Musculoskeletal system

NURSING DIAGNOSIS

Knowledge deficit related to home care

Expected outcome

The parents express an understanding of home care instructions.

Interventions

1. Explain to the parents the purpose and use of pain medications; include details on administration, dosages, and potential adverse effects.

2. Explain to the parents the importance of regular exercise, including active and passive ROM exercises.

3. Tell the parents to encourage the child to care for himself as much as possible, based on his degree of pain.

4. Teach the parents and child how to use adaptive devices, such as fasteners and tongs.

5. Refer the parents to appropriate community resources, such as the Juvenile Arthritis Foundation.

Rationales

1. Understanding the purpose and use of pain medications helps the parents comply with the medication regimen. Knowing the potential adverse effects should prompt them to seek medical help when necessary.

2. Regular exercise helps relieve joint stiffness and prevent contractures.

3. Self-care promotes self-esteem.

4. Using such devices promotes independence and improves self-esteem.

5. Community resources provide information and support to families of chronically ill children.

Documentation checklist

During the hospital stay, document:
- ❏ child's status and assessment findings upon admission
- ❏ changes in the child's status
- ❏ pertinent laboratory and diagnostic findings
- ❏ nutritional intake
- ❏ growth and development status
- ❏ child's response to treatment
- ❏ child's and parents' reactions to the illness and hospital stay
- ❏ patient and family teaching guidelines
- ❏ discharge planning guidelines.

Part 7

Eye, ear, nose, and throat

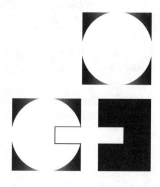

Cleft lip and cleft palate

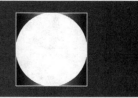

INTRODUCTION

Congenital defects of the lip and palate, cleft lip and cleft palate may occur separately or together. Caused by the failure or incomplete union of embryonic facial structures, these defects tend to be hereditary but may result from nongenetic factors. They may be associated with other anomalies as well. The incidence of these defects is 1 in 750 live births.

Cleft lip, more common in boys, may range from a slight indentation to an open cleft. Treatment involves surgical repair to correct the child's appearance, usually between ages 1 and 3 months. Cleft palate, more common in girls, may involve only the soft palate or may extend to the hard palate and nose. Treatment for this defect also involves surgical repair, usually between ages 1 and 2, before the child's speech is well developed.

Potential complications include infection, otitis media, hearing loss, and lack of parental attachment. The expected outcome for these defects is generally favorable; however, children with cleft palate may have speech and dental problems.

ASSESSMENT

Eye, ear, nose, and throat
• Abnormal separation of the upper lip or palate (or both)
• Separation of the upper gum
• Impaired dentition
• Impaired speech
• Easy choking
• Increased otitis
Respiratory
• Respiratory distress with aspiration
• Possible dyspnea
Musculoskeletal
• Failure to thrive
Gastrointestinal
• Difficulty feeding
Psychosocial
• Impaired parent-infant bonding¯
• Impaired body image

NURSING DIAGNOSIS

Altered nutrition: less than body requirements related to impaired feeding (preoperative)

Expected outcome

The infant maintains adequate nutritional status as evidenced by appropriate monthly weight gain (1 to 2 lb [0.5 to 1 kg]).

Interventions

1. Use an appropriate nipple and bottle (soft, cross-cut nipple; regular or squeeze bottle; a bottle especially designed for premature infants) to feed the infant.

2. Place the nipple in the infant's mouth on the side opposite the cleft, toward the back of the tongue.

3. Place the infant in a relaxed upright or semisitting position during feeding.

Rationales

1. Because of his inability to create a vacuum, an infant with cleft palate may have an ineffective sucking reflex. Use of an appropriate nipple and bottle eases the flow of liquid, promoting feeding. The specific nipple used depends on the severity of the cleft.

2. Placing the nipple in this manner stimulates the infant's "stripping" action (pressing the nipple against the tongue and the roof of the mouth to expel milk).

3. This position prevents nasal regurgitation and choking.

4. Burp the infant after every ½ to 1 oz (15 to 30 ml), but do not remove the nipple too frequently during feedings.

5. Try to keep each feeding to 45 minutes or less.

6. If the infant cannot feed without choking or aspirating, place him in an upright position and feed him with a syringe and soft rubber tubing.

4. The infant needs frequent burping because the defect may cause him to swallow more air, causing discomfort. Removing the nipple too frequently may tire and frustrate the infant, resulting in incomplete feedings.

5. Longer feedings may tire the infant, resulting in poor weight gain.

6. The upright position reduces the risk for aspiration; using a syringe and soft rubber tubing deposits liquid in the back of the infant's mouth, reducing aspiration through the cleft.

NURSING DIAGNOSIS

Risk for infection related to the defect (preoperative)

Expected outcome

The infant has no signs of infection as evidenced by a body temperature of less than 100° F (37.8° C) and no signs of ear drainage, coughing, wheezing, crackles in the lung field, or irritability.

Interventions

1. Offer the infant ⅛ to ⅜ oz (5 to 10 ml) of water after each feeding.

2. Remove crusted formula or milk with a moist cotton-tipped applicator.

3. After each feeding, place the infant in an infant seat or position him in his crib on his right side with the head of the bed elevated 30 degrees.

4. Assess the infant for signs of infection, including ear drainage, odor, and fever. Administer antibiotics, as ordered.

Rationales

1. Water cleans the nasal passages and palate and prevents milk from collecting in the eustachian tubes, which in turn prevents the growth of bacteria that could lead to infection.

2. Loosening and removing crusted material helps keep the cleft clean and free from bacteria, decreasing the risk of infection.

3. Positioning the infant in this manner helps prevent aspiration that could lead to pneumonia.

4. Recurring otitis media, resulting from an abnormal eustachian tube, is associated with cleft lip and cleft palate.

NURSING DIAGNOSIS

Risk for altered parenting related to the stress of hospitalization (preoperative)

Expected outcome

The parents ask appropriate questions about the infant's condition, incorporate the infant's care into their normal lifestyle, and express their feelings about the infant's appearance.

Interventions

1. Provide opportunities for the parents to hold and cuddle the infant and to practice caregiving tasks before discharge.

Rationales

1. Such opportunities promote bonding and prepare the parents to care for the infant at home.

Eye, ear, nose, and throat

2. Encourage the parents to prepare family members, including siblings and other relatives, for the infant's arrival home. Advise them to explain to the family the infant's appearance in simple terms, to show them pictures, and to have them visit the infant in the hospital.

3. Encourage the parents to treat the infant as a normal family member and to incorporate his care into their daily routine.

4. Encourage the parents to seek help from other family members or friends in feeding and caring for the infant.

5. Refer the parents to an appropriate support group and craniofacial center, if available.

2. Preparing family members for the infant's arrival allows them to adjust to the infant's appearance and allows the parents to focus on the infant's immediate needs.

3. The parents need to think of their infant as a normal child with a cleft lip or cleft palate—not as a sick child—to provide adequate home care and to preserve family unity.

4. Having others help in the infant's care and feeding gives the parents a chance to rest and focus on their own needs.

5. A support group gives the parents a chance to share their feelings and experiences with other parents in similar situations, decreasing anxiety and enhancing coping and problem-solving skills. A craniofacial center has experience in providing care for children with cleft lip or palate.

NURSING DIAGNOSIS

Anxiety (parent) related to surgery

Expected outcome

The parents are less anxious as evidenced by expressing an understanding of the need for surgery and by participating in the infant's or child's preoperative and postoperative care.

Interventions

1. Assess the parents' understanding of the defect and the need for surgery.

2. Explain to the parents the procedures surrounding the surgery, including the surgical procedure itself, the length of surgery, and the infant's or child's expected postoperative appearance.

3. Demonstrate to the parents the proper feeding technique to use after surgery (placing a tube on the buccal mucosa and squirting small amounts of liquid through a syringe); have them practice the technique. Also demonstrate the proper use of arm restraints, which prevent the infant or child from touching and disturbing the incision.

Rationales

1. Such assessment serves as a basis for teaching.

2. Such explanations prepare the parents for the perioperative events and the expected outcome, helping to relieve anxiety.

3. Demonstrating the proper feeding technique and use of arm restraints familiarizes the parents with postoperative care, helping to decrease their anxiety.

NURSING DIAGNOSIS

Ineffective airway clearance related to the effects of anesthesia, postoperative edema, and excessive mucus production

Expected outcome

The infant or child remains free from respiratory complications as evidenced by maintaining clear, regular respirations.

Interventions

1. Assess the infant's or child's respiratory status every 4 hours for abnormal breath sounds, cyanosis, retractions, grunting, or nasal flaring.

2. Reposition the infant or child every 2 hours. After cleft lip surgery, the infant or child may be placed as appropriate in an infant seat or on his back or side with his head elevated; after cleft palate surgery, he may be placed in a prone position.

3. Place the infant or child in a mist tent, as ordered. Keep the infant covered, and change the sheets regularly.

4. Keep the infant or child in an upright position during feeding.

Rationales

1. These signs of respiratory distress may indicate pneumonia, which requires antibiotic therapy.

2. Frequent repositioning promotes drainage of lung secretions.

3. Cool, humidified air helps to liquefy secretions, which helps the infant or child to breathe easier. Covers prevent chills.

4. The upright position decreases the risk of choking and aspiration.

Nursing diagnosis

Altered nutrition: less than body requirements related to new feeding technique and postoperative dietary changes

Expected outcome

The infant or child maintains adequate nutrition as evidenced by adapting to the new diet and feeding methods and continuing to gain weight.

Interventions

1. If the infant or child has undergone cleft lip repair, feed him through a syringe and soft rubber tubing placed inside the cheek and away from the suture line. Also use a syringe and tubing to feed the infant who has undergone cleft palate repair. Do not use a nipple. For an older child who has undergone cleft palate repair, use a regular drinking cup, not a straw, for liquid feedings. As the child progresses from a full liquid diet, use a spoon for feeding, not a fork.

2. Encourage small, frequent feedings at first; then progress to age-appropriate fluid intake.

3. If the child has undergone cleft palate repair, instruct the parents to feed him a full liquid diet (such as high-calorie drinks) for the first 3 weeks after surgery.

Rationales

1. Sucking on a nipple causes too much pressure on the suture line; a fork or straw can damage suture lines.

2. The infant or child may require smaller feedings while adapting to the new feeding method.

3. A full liquid diet during the first 3 weeks prevents damage to the suture line.

Eye, ear, nose, and throat

Nursing diagnosis

Impaired skin integrity related to surgical incision

Expected outcome

The infant or child suffers no break in skin integrity as evidenced by an intact incision, no signs of infection, and signs of healing.

Interventions

1. Provide the following suture line care after feedings and as needed:
• Clean the suture line with saline solution and a cotton-tipped applicator.
• Apply an antibiotic ointment, as ordered, to moisturize the mouth and prevent separation of the sutures.
• Monitor for signs and symptoms of infection.
• Offer small amounts of water after feedings to rinse the mouth of any milk residue that could lead to bacterial growth.

2. Apply arm restraints, as ordered. Evaluate circulation and perform range-of-motion (ROM) exercises every 2 hours.

3. After cleft lip surgery, position the infant or child as appropriate in an infant seat or on his side or back— not stomach—keeping the head of the bed elevated; after cleft palate surgery, place the infant or child in a prone position.

4. Anticipate the child's needs to decrease his crying.

Rationales

1. Proper suture line care ensures cleanliness, prevents separation of sutures, decreases the risk of infection, and reduces the amount of crusted material around the suture line that might result in an enlarged scar.

2. Arm restraints prevent the infant or child from rubbing the suture line or placing objects in his mouth until the incision heals. Evaluation ensures adequate circulation, and ROM exercises prevent muscle stiffness and contractures.

3. Sitting in an infant seat or lying on his side or back after cleft lip surgery prevents the child from rubbing his lip on the bed linens, reducing the risk of rupture; lying prone after cleft palate surgery prevents pressure on the suture line.

4. Crying causes tension on the suture line, which could lead to rupture.

NURSING DIAGNOSIS

Pain related to surgery

Expected outcome

The infant or child maintains a degree of comfort as evidenced by decreased crying and irritability.

Interventions

1. Assess the infant or child for irritability, loss of appetite, and restlessness every 2 hours after surgery.

2. Administer analgesics, as ordered.

3. Provide diversional activities, such as games, cards, videotapes, and reading materials, for the older child.

Rationales

1. The infant or child may be too young to express discomfort with words; behavioral cues are the only indication of pain.

2. Analgesics help decrease pain.

3. Diversional activities refocus the child's attention, reducing his perception of pain.

NURSING DIAGNOSIS

Knowledge deficit related to home care

Expected outcome 1

The parents express an understanding of preoperative home care instructions, and demonstrate home care procedures.

Interventions

1. Explain to the parents the nature of the defect and the need for follow-up care.

2. Teach the parents of an infant with cleft lip or palate the following feeding techniques:
• Feed the infant with an appropriate nipple and bottle (a soft, cross-cut nipple or one specially designed for premature infants; a regular or squeeze bottle).
• Position the nipple in the infant's mouth opposite the cleft and toward the back of the tongue.

• Keep the infant in an upright or semisitting position.

• Burp the infant after every ½ to 1 oz (15 to 30 ml).

• Clean the cleft immediately after feedings.

3. Explain to the parents the purpose and use of an apnea monitor, if one is prescribed for home use.

Rationales

1. Such explanations help decrease anxiety and increase compliance with the prescribed treatment and upcoming surgery.

2. Because of the defect, the parents need to pay particular attention to the infant's feeding.
• Because of the infant's defect, he may have an ineffective sucking reflex. Using an appropriate feeding device helps ensure that he consumes each feeding.
• Placing the nipple in this manner stimulates the "stripping" action the infant uses to draw liquid from the bottle.
• Positioning the infant upright or semisitting prevents nasal regurgitation and choking.
• Frequent burping reduces the amount of air swallowed during feeding, reducing the infant's discomfort.
• Cleaning the cleft immediately after feedings decreases the risk of infection.

3. The infant may need an apnea monitor to detect apneic episodes related to respiratory difficulty from aspiration of feedings.

Expected outcome 2

The parents express an understanding of postoperative home care instructions and demonstrate home care procedures.

Interventions

1. Teach the parents the following feeding techniques:
• Use a spoon, not a fork, to feed the child solid foods and a rubber-tipped syringe or a cup (if appropriate) to feed the infant or child fluids.
• Do not allow the child to use a straw.

2. Teach the parents how to care for the suture line:
• Use saline solution and a cotton-tipped applicator to clean the suture line.
• Apply antibiotic ointment, as ordered, to cover the incision.
• Check the incision for signs of infection, such as redness, swelling, and purulent drainage, and report such findings to the doctor.
• Offer small amounts of water after feedings to rinse away any milk residue that could lead to bacterial growth and infection.

3. Tell the parents they must keep the infant's or child's arms restrained. Explain that they should remove the restraints periodically, keeping the infant or child under supervision.

Rationales

1. Using a spoon for solid foods and a rubber-tipped syringe for fluids reduces the risk of trauma to the suture line. Using a straw can damage the suture line.

2. Proper suture line care ensures cleanliness, reduces the risk of infection, and reduces crust formation that may result in an enlarged scar; infection requires medical intervention.

3. Arm restraints prevent the infant or child from rubbing the suture line or placing objects in his mouth. Removing the restraints allows full range of motion and prevents neurovascular compromise.

Eye, ear, nose, and throat

4. After cleft lip surgery, instruct the parents to position the infant or child in an infant seat or on his side or back—never on his stomach—with the head of the bed elevated; after cleft palate surgery, instruct the parents to place him in a prone position.

5. Advise the parents to anticipate the infant's or child's needs to decrease his crying.

6. Explain to the parents the importance of follow-up care, including the need for ear inspections and hearing evaluations every 2 to 4 months and routine checkups and immunizations.

7. Discuss the possibility of further follow-up care—at a regional craniofacial center, if possible—including speech therapy, orthodontic care, and surgery.

4. Positioning the infant or child in this manner prevents him from rubbing his lip on the bed linens.

5. Prolonged crying causes tension on the suture line.

6. Frequent ear inspections and hearing evaluations are necessary because abnormal eustachian tube development predisposes the infant or child to frequent attacks of otitis media, which may lead to hearing loss. Routine checkups and immunizations help maintain optimal health.

7. Children with cleft palate may have speech impediments and dental problems that require surgery. Depending on the severity of the defect, the child may need extensive care.

Documentation checklist

During the hospital stay, document:
- ❐ infant's or child's status and assessment findings upon admission
- ❐ changes in the infant's or child's status
- ❐ pertinent laboratory and diagnostic findings
- ❐ nutritional intake
- ❐ growth and development status
- ❐ infant's or child's response to treatment
- ❐ child's and parents' reactions to the surgery and hospital stay
- ❐ patient and family teaching guidelines
- ❐ discharge planning guidelines.

Myringotomy

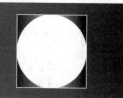

INTRODUCTION

Myringotomy is the surgical incision of the inferior portion of the tympanic membrane to drain fluid from the middle ear. The insertion of myringotomy (tympanostomy) tubes allows fluid to drain continuously and encourages pressure in the middle ear to equalize.

Surgery, which is usually indicated for children who have recurring ear infections (common in children under age 3), can be performed on an outpatient basis. The expected outcome depends on the effectiveness of the myringotomy tubes in preventing infections from recurring. Potential complications include hearing loss and infection.

ASSESSMENT

Eye, ear, nose, and throat
- Chronic ear infections (usually at least four per year)
- Ear pain
- Yellowish-green drainage from the ear
- Pain upon swallowing

Integumentary
- Fever

Psychosocial
- Irritability

NURSING DIAGNOSIS

Risk for injury (hemorrhage) related to surgery

Expected outcome

The child has no signs of hemorrhage resulting from surgery as evidenced by lack of bleeding, age-appropriate hemoglobin and hematocrit values, and pink mucous membranes.

Interventions

1. Monitor the amount of ear drainage during the postoperative period. Immediately report to the surgeon heavy bleeding or bleeding that occurs more than 3 days after surgery.

2. Administer antihistamines and decongestants, as ordered.

3. Monitor hemoglobin and hematocrit values.

Rationales

1. A small amount of reddish drainage is normal during the first few days after surgery. Heavy bleeding or bleeding that occurs more than 3 days after surgery is abnormal.

2. These agents constrict vessels, reducing the amount of bleeding.

3. Abnormally low values may indicate hemorrhage.

NURSING DIAGNOSIS

Anxiety (child and parent) related to the surgical procedure and perioperative events

Expected outcome

The child and parents are less anxious as evidenced by expressing an understanding of the surgical procedure and the events surrounding surgery.

Interventions

1. Explain the surgical procedure to the child and parents in simple terms. If the child undergoes local anesthesia, explain that he will be awake during the procedure so that the surgeon can test his hearing. Answer any questions simply and honestly.

2. Explain that, depending on the time of surgery, the child may not be given anything to eat or drink after midnight on the day of surgery to prevent vomiting and aspiration during surgery.

3. Explain to the parents that surgery may not be performed if the child has signs and symptoms of an acute infection, including elevated temperature, runny nose, and ear pain, on the day of surgery.

4. Inform the parents about the expected length of surgery and where they may wait during the procedure and recovery period. Make sure they know who will contact them when the procedure is over.

5. Explain to the child and parents the expected postoperative events, including expected ear drainage, hearing loss, and pain.

Rationales

1. Such information helps to decrease fear and anxiety by preparing the child and parents for the anticipated surgical events.

2. The child may become frightened if he cannot have food or drink throughout the night or on the morning of surgery. Explaining this to him beforehand should help to lessen his anxiety and fear.

3. Surgery cannot be performed under these circumstances because of the risk of septicemia or rampant infection.

4. Not knowing how long the surgery may last may make the parents unduly anxious during surgery. Knowing how long the surgery should last and who will talk with them after the procedure should lessen their fear and apprehension.

5. Understanding what to expect after the procedure should reduce anxiety.

NURSING DIAGNOSIS

Knowledge deficit related to home care

Expected outcome

The parents express an understanding of home care instructions.

Interventions

1. Instruct the parents to report to the doctor immediately any evidence of fever, increased bloody drainage, or increased pain.

2. Tell the parents to keep water out of the child's ears. Suggest they place cotton balls or earplugs in the child's ears during baths and shampoos until the tubes fall out or the doctor tells them otherwise. Also suggest they not allow the child to swim during this time.

3. Instruct the parents to cover the child's ears when he goes out in cold, windy weather.

4. Tell the parents to face the child when talking to him and to speak more clearly and slightly more loudly.

5. Teach the parents the purpose and use of antibiotics and analgesics; include detail on administration, dosages, and adverse effects. Warn them not to give the child aspirin.

Rationales

1. These may indicate infection or hemorrhage.

2. Tube placement allows water to enter the middle ear easily, increasing the risk of infection.

3. Cold may cause ear pain.

4. The child may have some hearing loss during the first few weeks after surgery.

5. The child may need antibiotics to reduce the risk of postoperative infection and analgesics to help control pain. Aspirin may cause bleeding.

Documentation checklist

During the hospital stay, document:
❐ child's status and assessment findings upon admission
❐ changes in the child's status
❐ pertinent laboratory and diagnostic findings
❐ nutritional intake
❐ child's response to treatment
❐ child's and parents' reactions to the surgery and hospital stay
❐ patient and family teaching guidelines
❐ discharge planning guidelines.

Tympanoplasty

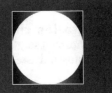

INTRODUCTION

Tympanoplasty, the surgical reconstruction of the hearing mechanism of the middle ear, repairs eardrums ruptured by frequent ear infections. The expected outcome is generally favorable; however, some children experience permanent hearing loss.

ASSESSMENT

Eye, ear, nose, and throat
• Chronic ear infections (usually more than four per year)
• Hearing loss
• Ear pain
• Drainage from ears
Integumentary
• Elevated temperature

NURSING DIAGNOSIS

Anxiety (child and parent) related to surgical procedure and perioperative events

Expected outcome

The child and parents are less anxious as evidenced by expressing an understanding of the surgical procedure and the events surrounding the surgery.

Interventions

1. Explain the surgical procedure to the child and parents and answer any questions honestly and simply. If the child is to undergo local anesthesia, he will be awake during surgery so that the surgeon can test his hearing but he will feel no pain.

2. Explain that, depending on the time of surgery, the child may not be permitted to eat or drink anything after midnight on the day of surgery to prevent the risk of vomiting and aspiration.

3. Explain to the parents that surgery may not be performed if the child has signs and symptoms of an acute infection, including elevated temperature, runny nose, and ear pain.

4. Inform the parents about the expected length of surgery and where they should wait during the procedure and recovery period. Make sure they know who will contact them when the procedure is over.

5. Explain to the child and parents the usual postoperative events, including details on expected pain, bleeding, and hearing loss. Explain that the child can expect some pain, which is usually controlled with analgesics, and that he may have a minimal amount of bleeding, probably in the form of bloody drainage. Also explain that the child's hearing may decrease initially but that it will improve in time.

Rationales

1. Explaining the surgical procedure and answering questions should promote a sense of security, helping to lessen anxiety and fear.

2. The child may become frightened if he is denied food or drink during the night or on the morning of surgery. Explaining this to him beforehand should help lessen his fear and anxiety.

3. The parents may become alarmed if the surgery is suddenly postponed.

4. Not knowing how long the surgery may last may make the parents unduly anxious during surgery. Knowing how long the surgery should last and who will talk with them after the procedure should lessen their fear and apprehension.

5. Understanding what to expect prepares the child and parents for what will happen after surgery, helping to relieve their anxiety and fear.

NURSING DIAGNOSIS

Risk for injury (hemorrhage) related to surgery

Expected outcome

The child has no signs of bleeding as evidenced by a lack of drainage and age-appropriate hemoglobin and hematocrit values.

Interventions

1. Check the child's dressing every 1 to 2 hours for signs of excessive bleeding. Draw a circle around the outer edge of drainage each time.

2. Elevate the head of the bed 30 degrees.

3. Apply a pressure dressing for the first 24 hours after surgery.

4. Instruct the child to cough and sneeze with an open mouth, avoid blowing his nose, and avoid exposure to loud noises or music.

Rationales

1. A minimal amount of bleeding sometimes occurs after surgery. However, excessive bleeding may indicate hemorrhage and should be reported immediately to the doctor. Marking the dressing shows the progression or resolution of drainage.

2. Raising the head of the bed reduces intracranial pressure, decreasing the risk of bleeding.

3. Pressure dressings help decrease postoperative bleeding and swelling.

4. Coughing or sneezing with a closed mouth, nose blowing, and exposure to loud sounds increase pressure in the ears and may cause bleeding.

NURSING DIAGNOSIS

Knowledge deficit related to home care

Expected outcome

The parents express an understanding of home care instructions.

Interventions

1. Instruct the parents to monitor the child for fever, increased bloody drainage, and increased pain.

2. Tell the parents to keep water out of the child's ears. Tell them not to wash his hair for 1 week after surgery, to place cotton balls or earplugs in his ears during baths or showers, and to prohibit him from swimming until the doctor approves.

3. Instruct the parents to give the child mild analgesics (not aspirin) for pain.

4. Advise the parents that they may need to speak more slowly and loudly to the child and turn up the volume on the radio or television.

5. Advise the parents to instruct the child to avoid elevator rides of more than eight floors. If he must go more than eight floors, he should get out of the elevator after eight floors, wait for his equilibrium to return, and than get back on.

Rationales

1. These may indicate infection or hemorrhage and require immediate medical attention.

2. Water in the ear may cause the absorbable packing to be absorbed prematurely or to break down. It also can be painful and lead to infection.

3. Analgesics help control pain; aspirin increases the risk of bleeding.

4. The child may have impaired hearing in the affected ear for 3 to 6 weeks after surgery.

5. High altitudes increase pressure in the eustachian tube and inner ear, possibly resulting in dislodgment of the tympanic membrane graft.

Eye, ear, nose, and throat

Documentation checklist

During the hospital stay, document:

- ❏ child's status and assessment findings upon admission
- ❏ changes in the child's status
- ❏ pertinent laboratory and diagnostic findings
- ❏ nutritional intake
- ❏ child's response to treatment
- ❏ child's and parents' reactions to the surgery and hospital stay
- ❏ patient and family teaching guidelines
- ❏ discharge planning guidelines.

Part 8

Hematologic and immunologic systems

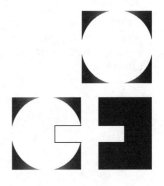

Acquired immunodeficiency syndrome

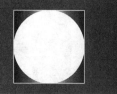

INTRODUCTION

Acquired immunodeficiency syndrome (AIDS), caused by human immunodeficiency virus (HIV), weakens the child's immunity to several opportunistic infections, including *Pneumocystis carinii* pneumonia, cytomegalovirus, herpesvirus, toxoplasmosis, and Kaposi's sarcoma. The virus may be transmitted through sexual contact with an infected person, contact with an infected person's body fluids, sharing I.V. needles and syringes with an infected person, or the transfusion of contaminated blood products. AIDS also may be contracted congenitally from an HIV-positive mother through placental transfer or breast milk.

To help prevent the spread of HIV, the Centers for Disease Control and Prevention has published *Guidelines for Prevention of Transmission of HIV and HBV to Health-Care and Public-Safety Workers* and recommends that all hospital caregivers follow standard precautions when handling blood or body fluids.

AIDS has a high mortality rate and, as of this time, no cure. Treatment usually includes measures to control signs and symptoms, such as the administration of antibiotics, antifungal agents, and pain medications. Various combinations of drugs are currently being used to lower viral counts.

ASSESSMENT

Immunologic
- Lymphadenopathy
- Decreased number of T cells

Hematologic
- Anemia

Respiratory
- Respiratory distress
- *P. carinii* pneumonia

Gastrointestinal
- Hepatomegaly
- Hepatitis (fungal)

Musculoskeletal
- Malaise

Eye, ear, nose, and throat
- Parotitis

Integumentary
- Elevated temperature

NURSING DIAGNOSIS

Risk for infection related to immunosuppressive state

Expected outcome

The child has no sign of infection as evidenced by a body temperature less than 100° F (37.8° C) and lack of pain or purulent drainage.

Interventions

1. Assess the child for fever, rash, cough, purulent drainage, and behavior changes, such as tiredness and irritability.

2. Institute reverse isolation precautions, as necessary, to prevent exposing the child to further infection. Do not allow anyone with a known infection to enter the child's room.

Rationales

1. These signs may indicate infection, which requires the administration of antibiotics.

2. Such precautions may be needed to help protect the child, whose immunosuppressive state makes him highly susceptible to infections.

NURSING DIAGNOSIS

Self-esteem disturbance related to stigma of disease and isolation

Expected outcome

The child has improved self-esteem as evidenced by expressing positive feelings about himself to his parents and significant others.

Interventions

1. Explain to the child, in appropriate terms, the nature of the disease and the need for reverse isolation (if applicable).

2. If the child is not in reverse isolation and poses no risk to other children on the unit, allow him to leave his room.

3. Allow the child to participate in his care, if appropriate.

4. Explain all procedures to the child.

5. Encourage the child to express his feelings.

Rationales

1. The child may not understand the seriousness of his disease and the need to protect him from further infection. Such explanations should help to increase his awareness of the condition and promote increased self-esteem.

2. Isolation usually is necessary only when the child is at risk for infection or when he poses a risk to others. Allowing the child to interact with others promotes normal growth and development and helps improve self-esteem.

3. Performing self-care helps increase the child's self-esteem by fostering a sense of control over the situation.

4. Explaining the reason for and steps involved in procedures helps alleviate fear and fosters a sense of control.

5. Such encouragement helps the child to vent his anxieties, frustrations, and fears — emotions that may interfere with self-esteem.

NURSING DIAGNOSIS

Fear (child and parent) related to life-threatening implications of the child's disease

Expected outcome

The child and parents exhibit less fear as evidenced by appearing less anxious and by asking appropriate questions about the child's condition.

Interventions

1. Explain to the parents and child, in appropriate terms, the nature of the child's illness and the need for medical care. Answer all questions simply and honestly.

Rationales

1. The parents and child need to understand the reason for hospitalization and the seriousness of the child's condition. However, they also need reassurance that the child is receiving the best care possible and that researchers are constantly searching for new treatments and a cure.

Hematologic and immunologic systems

2. Encourage the parents and child to express their feelings.

2. Allowing the parents and child to vent their fears, anxieties, and frustrations helps them face the seriousness of the child's illness and develop new ways of coping. The parents may feel an overwhelming sense of guilt, especially if the child contracted the disease congenitally, and may need special counseling. Both the parents and child may need help to deal with others' misconceptions and biases about the disease.

3. Explain all procedures to the parents and child.

3. Explaining the reason for and steps involved in procedures helps to lessen fear and apprehension about the child's care.

4. Encourage the parents and child to join a local AIDS support group. Offer referrals, as needed.

4. Support groups allow the parents and child to interact with other families facing similar circumstances. Knowing that they are not alone and can turn to others for emotional support should help to lessen their fear.

Nursing diagnosis

Knowledge deficit related to home care

Expected outcome

The parents express an understanding of home care instructions.

Interventions

1. Explain to the parents the importance of keeping the child away from persons with known infections.

2. Instruct the parents to provide a diet high in calories and protein.

3. Advise the parents to encourage the child to interact socially with other children and to return to school (if applicable). Give the parents information to pass on to the school to help educate students and teachers about the disease.

Rationales

1. Avoiding exposure to infection is essential because the child's immunosuppression makes him highly susceptible to infection.

2. A diet high in calories and protein replenishes the child's diminished reserves and helps him fight infection.

3. Social interaction and education are important aspects of normal development. As long as the child poses no risk to other children, he should be encouraged to return to normal activities. Learning about the disease can help decrease fear and correct any misconceptions his classmates or teachers may have.

Documentation checklist

During the hospital stay, document:
- ❐ child's status and assessment findings upon admission
- ❐ changes in the child's status
- ❐ pertinent laboratory and diagnostic findings
- ❐ fluid intake and output
- ❐ nutritional intake
- ❐ child's response to treatment
- ❐ child's and parents' reactions to the illness and hospital stay
- ❐ patient and family teaching guidelines
- ❐ discharge planning guidelines.

Hemophilia A

INTRODUCTION

A congenital bleeding disorder usually transmitted as an X-linked recessive trait (some cases result from spontaneous gene mutation), hemophilia A (classic hemophilia) is caused by a deficiency of factor VIII. This type of hemophilia accounts for 80% of all affected children and may be classified as mild, moderate, or severe.

Mild hemophilia results in prolonged bleeding, easy bruising, and a tendency toward epistaxis (nosebleeds) and bleeding gums. Moderate hemophilia causes more frequent and prolonged bleeding episodes and possible hemarthrosis (bleeding into the joints). The severe form causes excessive bleeding (sometimes spontaneous), subcutaneous and intramuscular hemorrhage, and bleeding into the joint cavities.

Treatment includes the administration of cryoprecipitate and steroids as well as physical therapy. Potential complications include joint deformity, hemorrhage, and death. The prognosis depends on the severity of the disease.

ASSESSMENT

Hematologic
- Hemorrhage and prolonged bleeding
- Superficial bruises
- Splenomegaly

Genitourinary
- Spontaneous hematuria

Musculoskeletal
- Signs and symptoms of deep muscle bleeding (pain, guarding of the affected area, limited range of motion [ROM], and increased temperature and edema at the bleeding site)
- Signs and symptoms of hemarthrosis (pain, limited ROM, and increased temperature and edema at the bleeding site)

Eye, ear, nose, and throat
- Epistaxis
- Bleeding gums

NURSING DIAGNOSIS

Risk for injury (hemorrhage) related to disease

Expected outcome

The child's bleeding stops as evidenced by no observable bleeding, no increase in the circumference of the bleeding site, no increase in pain, age-appropriate vital signs, rising factor VIII level, and a decreasing partial thromboplastin time (PTT).

Interventions

1. Apply direct pressure to the bleeding site (such as an abrasion or a laceration) for at least 15 minutes.

2. Immobilize the bleeding site.

3. Elevate the bleeding site above the level of the heart for 12 to 24 hours.

4. Apply ice to the affected area.

5. Administer cryoprecipitate or factor VIII concentrate (antihemophilic factor), as ordered. Allow the parents or child to administer the agent if they wish to and know how to do so. If they require instruction, teach them how to insert an I.V. line, prepare the skin site, secure the I.V. setup, prepare the mixture, and start the infusion.

Rationales

1. Pressure applied directly to the bleeding site promotes clot formation.

2. Immobilization decreases blood flow to the bleeding site and prevents clot dislodgment.

3. Elevating the bleeding site decreases blood flow to the area and promotes clot formation.

4. Ice promotes vasoconstriction.

5. Administration of cryoprecipitate or factor VIII concentrate completes clot formation. Having the parents or child administer the agent allows them to practice the technique for home use.

6. Monitor the child's vital signs, noting any signs of bradycardia, tachycardia, decreased blood pressure, increased respiratory rate, or elevated temperature. Report any of these signs immediately to the doctor.

6. These signs indicate potential complications, including hypovolemia secondary to bleeding and circulatory overload or transfusion reaction secondary to administration of cryoprecipitate or factor VIII concentrate.

7. Measure the circumference of the bleeding site, marking the skin to ensure consistent measurements. Measure the site again every 8 hours using the same measuring device.

7. Any increase in the circumference indicates continued bleeding, which requires immobilization of the site and the application of ice packs. Marking the skin and using the same measuring device each time ensures consistency.

8. Monitor the child's factor VIII and PTT levels at least once daily. Report any abnormalities to the doctor.

8. Monitoring these laboratory values helps determine the child's clotting status and the need for further intervention.

9. Administer aminocaproic acid (Amicar), as ordered, if the child is scheduled for surgery.

9. This agent (not used routinely) inhibits clot destruction.

10. Follow the Centers for Disease Control and Prevention guidelines for handling blood or body fluids.

10. Hemophiliacs are at high risk for developing acquired immunodeficiency syndrome because of their use of I.V. drugs and blood products.

11. Administer other medications, such as corticosteroids and desmopressin acetate (DDAVP), as ordered.

11. Corticosteroids reduce inflammation; desmopressin acetate stimulates factor VIII activity in mild hemophilia A.

Nursing diagnosis

Pain related to bleeding and swelling

Expected outcome

The child has no signs of pain as evidenced by a relaxed facial expression, expression of comfort, ability to sleep, and no need for analgesics.

Interventions

1. Assess the child's level of pain using pediatric pain assessment tools.

2. Administer analgesics (not salicylates or aspirin-containing products), as ordered

Rationales

1. Such assessment provides essential data for determining the effectiveness of interventions to control pain and for monitoring the child's bleeding status because consistent or increasing pain can indicate continued bleeding.

2. Analgesics relieve pain (the mode of action depending on the specific agent used). Aspirin and other salicylates prolong prothrombin time and inhibit platelet aggregation.

Nursing diagnosis

Impaired physical mobility related to decreased ROM secondary to bleeding and swelling

Expected outcome

The child achieves maximum ROM in the affected joint as evidenced by the ability to perform prescribed exercises.

Interventions

1. Encourage the child to perform isometric exercises, as ordered.

2. Consult the physical therapist on the need for supportive devices, such as braces, and on developing a passive and active ROM exercise program.

3. Assess the child's need for pain medication before beginning each exercise session.

Rationales

1. Isometric exercises help maintain muscle strength by tensing the muscles without moving the joints.

2. Supportive devices help maintain the functional position of muscles and joints and prevent or decrease the degree of physical deformity. Passive and active ROM exercises increase muscle tone and strength around the joint and help prevent muscle atrophy and disability.

3. Administering pain medication before exercise promotes comfort and cooperation.

NURSING DIAGNOSIS

Risk for injury related to hospital stay or procedures (or both)

Expected outcome

The child suffers no injuries resulting from the hospital stay or procedures as evidenced by the absence of hematomas, bruising, and hemorrhaging and by the ability to maintain full ROM.

Interventions

1. Pad the bed's side rails, if appropriate.

2. Make sure the child uses any protective equipment (such as a plastic helmet and elbow and knee pads) that he brought from home. Also ensure that he uses a soft-bristled toothbrush for cleaning his teeth.

3. When collecting blood specimens, perform a fingerstick rather than a venipuncture, when possible. When giving injections, use the subcutaneous (S.C.) (not intramuscular) route, when possible. Afterward, apply pressure to the site for at least 5 minutes.

4. After any bleeding episode, immobilize the bleeding site; then elevate the site above the level of the heart for 12 to 24 hours and apply ice to the area.

5. Inspect the child's toys for sharp edges.

Rationales

1. Padding the side rails decreases the risk of injury, such as bruises, that may result from accidental bumps.

2. Using protective equipment helps decrease the risk of injury from falls caused by accidents or routine play. A soft-bristled toothbrush is less likely to injure the gums.

3. Performing a fingerstick rather than a venipuncture decreases the risk of excessive blood loss because capillaries are smaller than veins and contain less blood. The S.C. route requires a smaller-gauge needle, reducing the risk of blood loss from a larger puncture site. Also, subcutaneous tissue is less vascular than muscle.

4. Immobilization and elevation above the heart decrease blood flow to the bleeding site and prevent clot dislodgment. Ice promotes vasoconstriction and decreases pain.

5. Sharp-edged toys could lacerate or puncture the child's skin.

NURSING DIAGNOSIS

Self-esteem disturbance related to chronic illness and hospital stay

Expected outcome

The child maintains a positive self-image as evidenced by expressing his capabilities as well as his limitations, by participating in self-care, and by continuing his involvement in age-appropriate activities (such as play, schoolwork, and contact with peers).

Interventions

1. Encourage the child to participate in his care, as appropriate. Allow him to perform activities of daily living, administer cryoprecipitate or factor VIII concentrate, and participate in decisions affecting his care, when possible.

2. Encourage the child to express his feelings about the hospital stay and his disease.

3. Provide the child with age-appropriate play activities for use in the playroom or when confined to bed.

4. Encourage the parents to bring in school assignments and to arrange for the child's siblings and peers to visit, if appropriate.

5. Provide information on support groups and regional hemophilia centers. Offer referrals, as needed.

Rationales

1. Encouraging the child to participate in his care promotes independence and fosters a sense of control over the situation.

2. Such encouragement allows the child to vent such feelings as frustration and anxiety that may interfere with positive self-esteem.

3. An essential part of normal growth and development, play can help divert the child's attention from his condition, helping to improve his self-esteem.

4. Contact with others promotes normal interactions and decreases feelings of isolation, improving the child's self-esteem.

5. A support group and hemophilia center can help the child deal with living with a chronic illness, improving his self-esteem.

Nursing diagnosis

Ineffective family coping: compromised related to repeated hospital stays and the child's chronic illness

Expected outcome

The parents and other family members demonstrate effective coping skills as evidenced by interacting with the child and staff members and helping with some of the child's routine care.

Interventions

1. Explore with the parents and other family members their feelings about the child's chronic condition and its impact on their lifestyle.

2. Refer the family to a social worker and other appropriate support groups (such as the National Hemophilia Foundation, 110 Greene Street, Suite 303, New York, NY 10012), as needed.

Rationales

1. Such discussions allow you to assess the family members' needs and their usual coping methods.

2. Families of children with chronic diseases often need extensive emotional and financial support. If still of child-bearing age, the parents also may need genetic counseling to help them understand the hereditary aspects of the disease.

Nursing diagnosis

Knowledge deficit related to home care

Expected outcome

The parents and, as appropriate, the child express an understanding of home care instructions and demonstrate any home care procedures.

Interventions

1. Explain to the parents the importance of providing a safe home environment for the child. Suggest the following safety precautions:
• Pad bed's side rails and sharp corners on furniture.
• Inspect all toys for sharp edges.
• Make the child wear a plastic helmet and elbow and knee pads during play.
• Carpet all floors.

2. Teach the parents to implement the following precautions:
• Have the child wear a medical alert identification bracelet or necklace identifying him as a hemophiliac.

• Ensure that the child undergoes routine dental checkups.
• Consult a dietitian about the child's iron needs.

• Prohibit the use of salicylates and aspirin-containing compounds.
• Confer with the child's teachers, school nurse, and coaches on the child's condition and need for certain restrictions.

• As the child grows older, encourage him to avoid such high-risk behaviors as riding motorcycles, playing football, skateboarding, and rollerblading, and explain why he should avoid such behaviors.
• Promote the child's participation in more appropriate physical activities, such as swimming instead of football.

3. Teach the parents how to control the child's bleeding:
• Apply direct pressure to the bleeding site for at least 15 minutes.
• Immobilize the bleeding site and elevate the area above the level of the heart.

• Apply ice to the bleeding site.

• Administer factor VIII concentrate.

4. Teach the parents the purpose and use of factor VIII concentrate: Include details on administration, dosage, and potential adverse reactions. Also explain how to store and mix the agent, set up an I.V. line, perform a venipuncture, adjust the infusion rate, and document any transfusion reactions.

5. As appropriate, teach the child how to manage his disease.

Rationales

1. These safety measures help decrease the risk of injury and bleeding from bumps, falls, lacerations, and punctures.

2. The family must follow certain precautions to prevent bleeding episodes.
• Wearing a medical alert bracelet or necklace identifies the child as a hemophiliac and alerts rescuers to the child's need for emergency care.
• Routine dental checkups and care help prevent tooth and gum disease that can lead to bleeding.
• The child may need a diet high in iron because hemophilia can cause iron deficiency.
• Salicylates and aspirin-containing products can increase bleeding time and inhibit platelet aggregation.
• The child's teachers, school nurse, and coaches need to understand the seriousness of the child's condition so that they can enforce health and safety precautions and still help the child reach his highest potential.
• As the child reaches adolescence, he may be tempted to take part in high-risk behaviors. Encouraging the child to avoid such behaviors and explaining their dangers helps reduce the risk of injury.
• Encouraging the child to participate in less hazardous sports and activities ensures his developmental growth, yet protects him from injury.

3. Controlling bleeding helps prevent life-threatening hemorrhage.
• Direct pressure stops blood flow to the bleeding site and allows for clot formation.
• Immobilizing the site and elevating the area above the heart reduces the flow of blood to the bleeding site and prevents clot dislodgment.
• Applying ice to the bleeding site promotes vasoconstriction.
• Administering factor VIII concentrate ensures completion of the clotting process.

4. Knowing this information helps ensure correct use and administration for emergency home care.

5. Self-management gives the child some control over interventions and promotes independence.

Documentation checklist

During the hospital stay, document:

- ❏ child's status and assessment findings upon admission
- ❏ changes in the child's status
- ❏ pertinent laboratory and diagnostic findings
- ❏ nutritional intake
- ❏ growth and development status
- ❏ child's response to treatment
- ❏ child's and parents' reactions to the illness and hospital stay
- ❏ patient and family teaching guidelines
- ❏ discharge planning guidelines.

Sickle cell anemia

INTRODUCTION

An incurable autosomal recessive disease that predominantly affects blacks, sickle cell anemia is characterized by the abnormal formation of red blood cells (RBCs) that, under certain circumstances, become sickle-shaped. Because of the cells' fragility and inflexibility, the disease results in occlusion of the small blood vessels and increased RBC destruction.

Treatment for this potentially life-threatening disease usually is supportive unless the child is in sickle cell crisis (usually caused by decreased oxygen levels, stress, infection, or extreme exercise), in which case medical intervention is necessary. Supportive measures include pain control, physical therapy, blood replacement, and rehydration. The prognosis for this disease depends on the extent of the crises and bleeding episodes. Potential complications include splenic infarction, infection, stroke, and death.

ASSESSMENT

Hematologic
- Anemia
- Enlarged spleen

Cardiovascular
- Murmurs

Neurologic
- Headache
- Numbness in the fingers and toes
- Anxiety
- Cerebrovascular accident

Gastrointestinal
- Abdominal pain (in school-age children)
- Thirst
- Vomiting

Hepatic
- Enlarged liver
- Cirrhosis

Genitourinary
- Frequent urination
- Decreased urine concentration
- Enuresis
- Hematuria

Musculoskeletal
- Muscle weakness
- Edematous joints
- Joint and back pain
- Hand-foot syndrome
- Skeletal deformities

Psychosocial
- Delayed growth and development

Integumentary
- Jaundice
- Elevated temperature

NURSING DIAGNOSIS

Altered peripheral tissue perfusion related to blood vessel obstruction secondary to sickling of RBCs

Expected outcome

The child has adequate tissue perfusion as evidenced by decreased cyanosis, warm extremities, and a stable blood pressure.

Interventions

1. Encourage complete bed rest during the acute phase of the illness (pain crisis).

2. Perform passive range-of-motion (ROM) exercises every 4 to 6 hours, or provide other age-appropriate activities that the child can perform in bed, such as isometric exercises.

Rationales

1. Bed rest is necessary because exercise increases cellular metabolism, resulting in tissue hypoxia and increased sickling.

2. Passive ROM and isometric exercises promote mobility without stressing the joints and causing pain.

3. Avoid or limit activities and situations that may cause the child emotional stress.

4. Coordinate caregiving activities to allow the child uninterrupted sleep and rest periods.

3. Emotional stress increases cellular metabolism, resulting in tissue hypoxia and increased sickling. Adrenaline released during stress further constricts vessels.

4. The child needs adequate rest and sleep during the acute phase of the illness.

NURSING DIAGNOSIS

Fluid volume deficit related to decreased fluid intake and the kidneys' inability to concentrate urine

Expected outcome

The child maintains adequate hydration as evidenced by urine output of 1 to 2 ml/kg/hour, moist mucous membranes, decreased thirst, stable weight, age-appropriate serum electrolyte levels, and flat fontanels (in infants).

Interventions

1. Encourage the child to drink fluids every 2 hours for a daily total of 5 oz (150 ml)/kg of body weight.

2. Carefully monitor the child's fluid intake and output, including the administration of any I.V. fluids.

3. Weigh the child daily.

4. Observe the child every 2 to 4 hours for signs of dehydration, including dry skin, poor skin turgor, and decreased urine output. Administer fluids as necessary. Keep the child hydrated 50% over baseline requirements.

5. Monitor laboratory results for pH, hematocrit, hemoglobin, partial pressure of carbon dioxide, and partial pressure of oxygen values.

6. Make sure that the child is not dressed too warmly.

Rationales

1. Adequate hydration prevents increased sickling of RBCs.

2. Careful monitoring allows assessment of the child's fluid balance, which is critical for evaluating kidney function and detecting hemodilution and circulatory overload.

3. Daily weighing is the most accurate measure of the child's hydration status.

4. Dehydration, a common cause of sickling, requires fluid replacement; keeping the child well hydrated can help prevent sickling.

5. Acid-base imbalances may indicate that the child is dehydrated.

6. Dressing too warmly may overheat the child, resulting in fluid loss.

NURSING DIAGNOSIS

Pain related to vascular occlusion and tissue hypoxia

Expected outcome

The child has no signs of pain as evidenced by decreased expression of pain, restful sleep periods, and relaxed facial expressions.

Interventions

1. Assess the child's need for pain medication every 3 to 4 hours. Check for restlessness, tense facial expressions, decreased appetite, crying when touched, and grunting.

Rationales

1. Frequent assessment allows you to determine the degree and type of pain and the child's need for medication.

2. Administer analgesics and narcotics as ordered, and teach the child nonpharmacologic pain-control measures. Evaluate the child's response to pain-control measures.

3. Apply warmth to the affected site every 3 to 4 hours.

4. Maintain the child in a comfortable position, with his joints supported in alignment with the rest of the body. Handle his extremities gently, and avoid bumping or jarring the bed.

2. Pain from sickle cell anemia can be difficult to manage. The doctor may have to try several types of analgesics and narcotics to achieve the desired response; nonpharmacologic pain-control measures can augment analgesic control.

3. Heat causes vasodilation, which allows sickled cells to move through occluded areas, promoting comfort.

4. Proper positioning promotes comfort in painful joints.

NURSING DIAGNOSIS

Risk for infection related to sickling of cells and splenic infarction

Expected outcome

The child has no signs of infection as evidenced by a body temperature less than 100° F (37.8° C), no cough, and an age-appropriate white blood cell count.

Interventions

1. Isolate the child from all known sources of infection.

2. Monitor the child's temperature every 4 hours.

3. Check the child's immunization record and administer vaccines, as ordered.

4. Administer antibiotics, as ordered.

5. Provide a high-calorie, high-protein diet. Serve small, frequent meals.

Rationales

1. The child is especially susceptible to infection because of the spleen's inability to filter bacteria as a result of infarction.

2. An elevated temperature may indicate infection.

3. Children with sickle cell anemia have a markedly increased susceptibility to *Pneumococcus* and *Haemophilus influenzae* infections and should receive scheduled immunizations. (*Note:* Pneumococcal vaccines are recommended at age 2; *Haemophilus* b polysaccharide vaccine, at age 18 months.)

4. Antibiotics help fight and prevent infections; the doctor may prescribe a daily dose of penicillin until the child is 5 years old to prevent infection.

5. A high-calorie, high-protein diet helps the child fight infection and promotes proper growth and development. Serving small, frequent meals helps prevent the child from tiring and ensures that he will eat more of each meal.

NURSING DIAGNOSIS

Knowledge deficit related to home care

Expected outcome

The parents express an understanding of home care instructions.

Hematologic and immunologic systems

Interventions

1. Teach the parents about the anatomy and physiology of normal RBCs, the pathophysiology of sickle cell disease, and the genetic basis of the disease.

2. Teach the parents the signs and symptoms of a developing crisis, including anorexia, joint pain, epigastric pain, fever, and vomiting. Also teach them the signs and symptoms of infection, which increases the risk of a sickle cell crisis, and stroke, which may occur during a crisis.

3. Teach the parents the importance of taking the following measures during a sickle cell crisis:
• Maintain adequate hydration.
• Prevent infection by isolating the child from known sources of infection.
• Administer antibiotics, as ordered.
• Avoid exposing the child to low-oxygen environments (such as flying in an unpressurized airplane) and to cold.
• Watch for and immediately report signs and symptoms of stroke or infection.

Rationales

1. Understanding the normal functioning of RBCs and the nature and course of the disease should help the parents to comply with the overall treatment plan; understanding the genetic basis of the disease helps them recognize the risk of passing on the disease to subsequent children.

2. Knowing this information should prompt the parents to seek medical help when necessary.

3. Taking such measures helps prevent further complications associated with sickle cell crisis.

Documentation checklist
During the hospital stay, document:
❐ child's status and assessment findings upon admission
❐ changes in the child's status
❐ pertinent laboratory and diagnostic findings
❐ fluid intake and output
❐ nutritional intake
❐ child's response to treatment
❐ child's and parents' reaction to the illness and hospital stay
❐ patient and family teaching guidelines
❐ discharge planning guidelines.

Part 9

Endocrine system

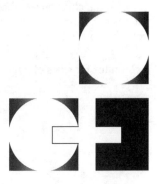

Cushing's syndrome

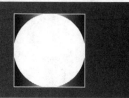

INTRODUCTION

Cushing's syndrome results from the prolonged over-production of glucocorticoid (in particular, cortisol) and is characterized by truncal obesity, short stature, and hypertension. Although rare in children (more common in girls), this disorder usually results from prolonged or excessive administration of adrenocorticotropic hormone (ACTH), but also may result from long-term steroid use, oversecretion of the adrenal glands, or an adrenal neoplasm. Depending on the specific cause, excessive mineralocorticoids and androgens also may be excreted.

Usual treatment includes the gradual decrease of steroid use and surgery (when necessary). Potential complications include osteoporosis, hypertension, arteriosclerosis, amenorrhea, and psychoses.

ASSESSMENT

Endocrine
• Obesity
• Hyperglycemia
• Amenorrhea

Cardiovascular
• Hypertension

Musculoskeletal
• Fatigue
• Loss of muscle mass

Hematologic
• Hyperglycemia
• Hyperkalemia
• Elevated serum ACTH level on dexamethasone suppression test

Integumentary
• Characteristic fat distribution (moon face, buffalo hump)
• Fragile skin
• Edema
• Hirsutism
• Bruising
• Poor wound healing

NURSING DIAGNOSIS

Risk for injury (hyperglycemia) related to the anti-insulin properties of glucocorticoids

Expected outcome

The child suffers no injury, such as nerve injury, poor wound healing, or poor circulation, from hyperglycemia as evidenced by maintaining serum glucose levels between 60 and 100 mg/dl.

Interventions

1. Monitor the child's serum glucose levels at least twice daily.

2. Begin the child on a diabetic diet, and instruct the parents to continue the diet after the child is discharged from the hospital.

3. Monitor for signs of hypertonic dehydration.

Rationales

1. The child may develop hyperglycemia as a result of the anti-insulin properties of glucocorticoids.

2. The child may need a diabetic diet, which uses a balance of complex carbohydrates, protein, and fat to help control hyperglycemia while meeting the child's daily metabolic needs, until the syndrome resolves.

3. Hyperglycemia can cause fluids to be pulled away from the circulatory system into interstitial tissue, resulting in dehydration.

NURSING DIAGNOSIS

Risk for infection related to the immunosuppressive action of glucocorticoids

Expected outcome

The child remains free from infection as evidenced by maintaining a body temperature less than 100° F (37.8°. C) and age-appropriate vital signs.

Interventions	Rationales
1. Take necessary measures to protect the child from potential sources of infection. Screen all visitors for respiratory or other infections.	**1.** Because glucocorticoids suppress the body's normal response to infection, the child should be protected from all possible sources of infection.
2. Assess the child daily for signs of infection, including slight temperature elevation, rhinitis, cough, and ear or wound drainage.	**2.** Signs of infection in a child with excessive glucocorticoid levels may be subtle because steroids can suppress the normal inflammatory response. As a result, the child may not have such normal signs of infection as elevated temperature and swelling.

NURSING DIAGNOSIS

Fluid volume excess related to high serum corticosteroid levels

Expected outcome

The child maintains fluid homeostasis as evidenced by good skin turgor and a capillary refill time of 3 to 5 seconds.

Interventions	Rationales
1. Measure and record the child's blood pressure every shift.	**1.** Hypertension may result from an exaggerated response to catecholamines, the constriction of peripheral vessels, and sodium retention.
2. Weigh the child daily, and assess for pitting edema in dependent areas every shift.	**2.** Weighing the child and assessing for edema help to determine whether the child is retaining fluid.
3. Monitor the child's daily fluid intake and output.	**3.** Excessive mineralocorticoid activity can result in sodium and fluid retention, causing decreased urine output.
4. Monitor the child's serum electrolyte levels.	**4.** Excessive mineralocorticoid activity causes sodium retention and potassium depletion.
5. Restrict the child's sodium intake, as ordered.	**5.** The child may require sodium restriction to prevent fluid retention.

NURSING DIAGNOSIS

Risk for injury related to excessive corticosteroid production

Expected outcome

The child suffers no injuries as evidenced by the absence of soft tissue damage or trauma.

Interventions

1. Protect the child from injury by padding the sharp corners of all furniture in the child's room. Also, inspect all toys for sharp edges or other potentially dangerous features.

2. After giving an injection, apply pressure to the venipuncture site for 3 to 5 minutes.

3. Monitor the healing process of any wounds or incisions.

Rationales

1. Such precautions help protect the child, whose skin is extremely fragile from the protein catabolism associated with excessive corticosteroid levels. The child is especially susceptible to hemorrhage because of the fragility of blood vessel walls.

2. This prevents hemorrhage and hematoma formation.

3. Steroids suppress the healing response and slow the formation of scar tissue.

NURSING DIAGNOSIS

Body image disturbance related to excessive corticosteroid levels

Expected outcome

The child exhibits an improved self-concept as evidenced by expressing an acceptance of his current body image.

Interventions

1. Explain to the child, in age-appropriate terms, the reason for the changes in his physical appearance, stressing that such changes are usually temporary.

2. Encourage the child to express his feelings about his altered appearance.

3. Teach the child's siblings about the effects Cushing's syndrome can have on appearance, including weight gain, moon face, buffalo hump, and hirsutism; give the family information they can use to help educate the child's peers.

Rationales

1. Knowing that changes in his physical appearance are temporary and result from controllable factors should help to improve the child's self-esteem.

2. Expressing his feelings and discussing his condition can help the child better accept his altered body image.

3. Understanding the effects Cushing's syndrome can have on the child's appearance can help his siblings and peers accept such changes, which can in turn help the child to better accept such changes.

NURSING DIAGNOSIS

Knowledge deficit related to home care

Expected outcome

The parents express an understanding of home care instructions.

Interventions

1. Teach the parents the importance of maintaining the child on a diabetic diet and limiting the number of snacks.

2. Teach the parents the importance of preventing infection by having the child avoid crowds and infected individuals, carefully managing wounds, and observing for signs and symptoms of infection (ear or wound drainage, fever, rhinorrhea, swelling, and pain).

Rationales

1. The prescribed diet helps control glucose levels, reducing the risk of hyperglycemia.

2. The child is at increased risk for infection because of his immunosuppressive state.

Documentation checklist

During the hospital stay, document:

❏ child's status and assessment findings upon admission
❏ changes in the child's status
❏ pertinent laboratory and diagnostic findings
❏ fluid intake and output
❏ growth and development status
❏ child's response to treatment
❏ child's and parents' reactions to the illness and hospital stay
❏ patient and family teaching guidelines
❏ discharge planning guidelines.

Diabetes mellitus

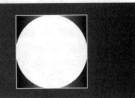

INTRODUCTION

Diabetes encompasses a group of disorders characterized by glucose intolerance resulting from insulin deficiency. Type 1 (insulin-dependent) diabetes mellitus can occur at any age but usually manifests during adolescence, between ages 11 and 12, and affects about 10% to 20% of the entire diabetic population. Type 2 (non-insulin-dependent) diabetes mellitus usually manifests after age 40.

Although the exact cause of type 1 diabetes has not been confirmed, it may result from an autoimmune disorder activated by a virus. Treatment for this type includes a diabetic diet, use of insulin, glucose monitoring, and exercise. Potential complications include blindness, renal disease, and peripheral vascular disease. Life expectancy may be reduced by 10 to 20 years.

ASSESSMENT

Endocrine
- Lack of endogenous insulin production
- Unstable serum glucose levels

Neurologic
- Irritability

Gastrointestinal
- Increased appetite
- Increased thirst
- Weight loss
- Abdominal pain

Genitourinary
- Frequent urination
- Urinary tract infections
- Glucose and acetones in urine
- Enuresis

Musculoskeletal
- Malaise
- Lethargy

Neurologic
- Irritability

Integumentary
- Dry skin
- Poor wound healing
- Dehydration

NURSING DIAGNOSIS

Risk for injury related to noncompliance with the prescribed diet

Expected outcome

The child follows the prescribed diet as evidenced by maintaining a serum glucose level within acceptable limits.

Interventions

1. Teach the child and parents the importance of the prescribed diet. Explain that the child must follow the diet consistently and must eat food at regular intervals. Arrange a referral to the hospital dietitian, as appropriate.

2. Consult the hospital dietitian about the child's food preferences and current eating patterns.

3. Provide the child and parents with a list of appropriate food exchanges and a sample menu that includes acceptable food choices. Stress the importance of reading labels on all food items.

Rationales

1. The child and parents need to understand the link between following the diet and maintaining serum glucose and insulin levels within acceptable ranges. The hospital dietitian can provide detailed instruction as needed.

2. The hospital dietitian can include some of the child's favorite foods in each meal, promoting compliance with the prescribed diet.

3. The child and parents need to know what foods the diet plan includes to help them make appropriate choices. They also need to understand the importance of reading labels to identify foods that might alter the glucose-insulin balance.

NURSING DIAGNOSIS

Risk for injury related to disease and insulin use

Expected outcome

The child suffers minimal injury from the disease and insulin use as evidenced by the absence of severe hypoglycemia and ketoacidotic responses.

Interventions

1. Monitor the child's blood glucose levels three or four times a day.

2. Assess the child for signs and symptoms of hypoglycemia (weakness, ataxia, anxiety, irritability, short attention span, rapid heart rate, tremors, and pale, moist skin) or hyperglycemia (fruity breath, glycosuria, lethargy, decreased level of consciousness, polydipsia, dehydration, and polyuria). Take the following measures, as necessary:
• If the child is hypoglycemic, give him glucose tablets or paste, milk, or crackers. Repeat every 10 to 15 minutes.
• If the child is hyperglycemic, check his glucose level and give the ordered amount of insulin.

3. If hyperglycemia progresses to diabetic ketoacidosis (marked by increased thirst, increased urine output, hypertonic dehydration, electrolyte imbalance, and a sweet or fruity breath odor), administer a continuous infusion of insulin and provide fluid and electrolyte replacement, as ordered.

4. Instruct the child to wear a medical alert bracelet or necklace identifying him as a diabetic.

Rationales

1. Frequent monitoring helps determine the effectiveness of insulin therapy and diet.

2. Hypoglycemia (which may result from excessive insulin levels, lack of food, extreme exercise, or illness) requires prompt action to raise the child's glucose level quickly. Hyperglycemia (which may result from improper eating, a missed insulin dose, or illness) requires the prompt administration of insulin to raise the child's insulin level.

3. Ketoacidosis, which results from low insulin levels, may be life-threatening if not treated promptly.

4. Wearing a medical alert necklace or bracelet allows medical personnel to provide appropriate treatment in an emergency.

NURSING DIAGNOSIS

Risk for injury related to exercise

Expected outcome

The child does not experience hypoglycemia during exercise as evidenced by maintaining a serum glucose level between 90 and 120 mg/dl.

Interventions

1. Encourage the child to participate in a regular exercise program.

2. Instruct the child to eat a snack (something high in protein and carbohydrates, such as cheese or peanut butter and crackers) before exercising.

Rationales

1. Regular exercise promotes normal growth and development and can reduce the child's need for insulin.

2. A snack before exercise helps prevent a sudden drop in blood glucose.

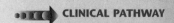

CLINICAL PATHWAY

Diabetes

Categories of care	Day 1	Day 2
Medical treatment	• Begin to stabilize fluid, pH, and blood glucose levels: hydration, laboratory studies, vital signs (VS), insulin, intake and output (I&O), daily weight	• Improved fluid, electrolyte, pH levels; blood glucose level less than 200 mg/dl: hydration, laboratory studies, VS, insulin, I&O, daily weight
Activity	• Bed rest with bathroom privileges	• Ambulatory as tolerated • Exercise in physical therapy if blood glucose level less than 250 mg/dl
Patient/Parent involvement in skills	• Observes routine: insulin injection, blood glucose monitoring, urine ketone testing	• Particpates in routines with nurse assistance: insulin injection, blood glucose monitoring, urine ketone testing
Teaching/learning topics By dietitian:	• Follows American Diabetes Association (ADA) diet as tolerated	• Follows ADA diet as tolerated • Patient/parent continues filling out menus and learning meal plan.
By nurse (or Diabetes Nurse Educator):	•Patient/family verbalizes understanding of plan of care and teaching plan: videotapes and written material made available; explanation of map and teaching protocol.	• Patient/family verbalizes understanding of hypoglycemia and hyperglycemia (prevention, symptoms, and treatment), use of glucagon, record keeping in diary, acceptable blood glucose levels, times to test blood glucose level.
Social	Patient/family will verbalize awareness of resources for effective coping: parent resource, social worker, care conference scheduled for morning of discharge.	• Patient/family will verbalize awareness of resources for effective coping: parent resource, social worker, questions and concerns addressed.

NURSING DIAGNOSIS

Ineffective family coping: compromised related to new diagnosis of chronic illness

Expected outcome

The child and family demonstrate effective coping skills as evidenced by complying with treatment.

Interventions

1. Encourage the child and parents to express their feelings about the child's illness and its effect on their lifestyle.

Rationales

1. The child and parents may have fears and anxieties that hinder their ability to cope with their new situation. Younger children may fear blood tests and insulin injections. Parents may fear not only the immediate threats of the disease but the long-term effects on the child's health as well.

Day 3	Day 4
• Improved fluid, electrolyte, and pH levels; blood glucose level less than 200 mg/dl: hydration, laboratory studies, VS, insulin, I&O, daily weight	• Blood glucose level stable; less than 200 mg/dl: VS, insulin, I&O, daily weight
• Ambulatory as tolerated • Exercise in physical therapy if blood glucose level less than 250 mg/dl	• Ambulatory as tolerated • Exercise in physical therapy if blood glucose level less than 250 mg/dl
• Participates in routines under supervision: insulin injection, blood glucose monitoring, urine ketone testing	• Independently demonstrates insulin injection, blood glucose monitoring, urine ketone testing
• Follows ADA diet as tolerated • Patient/parent continues filling out menus and learning meal plan.	• Follows ADA diet as tolerated • Patient/parent continues filling out menus and learning meal plan.
• Patient/parent verbalizes understanding of sick day rules; skin and foot care; medic alert information; importance of alerting all doctors, dentists, ophthalmologist in future; need to call school and day-care personnel; disposal of insulin syringes.	• Patient/family verbalize understanding of effects of exercise, effects of alcohol, need for continuing education, community resources. •Patient/parent fills out questionnaire to evaluate learning. • Care team conference to summarize information and address alteration in family.
•Patient/family verbalize awareness of resources for effective coping: diabetes support group, diabetes summer camp.	• Patient/family has discharge information: care conference, phone support from diabetes services.

Adapted with permission from Northwest Community Hospital, Arlington Heights, Illinois.

2. Teach the child and parents what steps they can take to control the disease, including diet, insulin use, and regular exercise. Explain that adhering to a strict regimen may help to prevent the onset or reduce the severity of complications.

3. Refer the parents to a local support group or chapter of the American Diabetes Association (ADA) or Juvenile Diabetes Foundation, and provide information on ADA summer camps. If possible, arrange for the parents and child to meet a family with a diabetic child of the same age.

2. The child and parents may associate diabetes with the onset of complications or even death. Emphasizing that they have control over some aspects of the disease should help them cope with the illness.

3. Such groups provide support and information, which should help the family to cope with the child's illness; going to an ADA summer camp can provide further support and can help the child establish relationships with other diabetic children. Meeting another family that is coping well with the disease shows the child and parents that the disease can be managed.

NURSING DIAGNOSIS

Knowledge deficit related to home care

Expected outcome

The child and parents express an understanding of home care instructions and demonstrate home care procedures.

Interventions

1. Assess the child's and parents' knowledge of the disease and their readiness to learn.

2. Arrange specific teaching sessions for the child and parents. Encourage all family members to participate.

3. Provide information on ways to manage the child's disease, including:
• diet (eating a well-balanced diet, using the proper number of exchanges from each food group)
• insulin use (administered by subcutaneous injection and rotated among sites on the arm, thigh, or abdomen or by a metered pump)
• glucose testing (checking the glucose level in blood, usually by fingerstick)
• preventive care (snacking before exercise, managing sores or wounds, preventing infection).

4. Explain to the child and parents the action of insulin within the body. Explain to the younger child that insulin is the key that opens cell doors to glucose.

5. Teach the child and parents the signs and symptoms of hypoglycemia (weakness, ataxia, anxiety, irritability, short attention span, rapid heart rate, tremors, and pale, moist skin) and hyperglycemia (fruity breath, glycosuria, lethargy, decreased level of consciousness, polydipsia, dehydration, and polyuria). Explain what measures to take if the child suddenly exhibits signs of either of these conditions.

6. Teach the child and parents how to mix insulin and give injections. For a younger child, demonstrate the injection procedure on a cloth doll and ask the child to repeat your actions. Have the parents practice by administering saline solution injections to each other. If the child will use a continuous infusion pump, demonstrate the proper administration technique.

7. Show the child and parents the proper injection sites (common sites include the arm, thigh, or abdomen). Explain that they should use the same anatomic area, rotating the site so that each subsequent injection is 1" (2.5 cm) away from the previous one until all sites have been used, and then move to the next anatomic area. Instruct the child to keep a chart of the sites used.

Rationales

1. Families displaying high levels of fear, denial, and stress may need to discuss their feelings before they can learn new information.

2. Unlike many diseases, diabetes requires the development of specific management skills. Encouraging all family members to attend the teaching sessions helps stress the importance of learning these skills and ensures compliance with the home care regimen.

3. Providing such information helps ensure compliance with the treatment regimen.

4. Age-appropriate analogies can help the child and parents understand the need for insulin and the importance of complying with treatment.

5. The child and parents need to know the signs and symptoms of hypoglycemia and hyperglycemia to ensure prompt treatment.

6. Administering injections is an important part of home care. Encouraging the child and parents to practice giving injections reinforces what they learned during the teaching session and ensures compliance with insulin therapy.

7. Rotating the sites helps to prevent hypertrophy of the muscles.

8. Teach the child and parents the purpose and procedure for home glucose monitoring. Have the parents demonstrate the procedure to the child by testing their own blood.

8. Home glucose monitoring allows the child and parents to check the child's blood glucose levels regularly, helping to ensure that levels remain within the acceptable range (usually between 80 and 120 mg/dl). Watching the parents rather than a nurse demonstrate the procedure may frighten the child less, helping ensure compliance with the technique.

9. Teach the child and parents sick-day management and urine ketone testing.

9. During illness, the child may need his insulin dosages adjusted to compensate for his decreased appetite and unstable glucose levels. Urine ketone testing, together with blood glucose monitoring, determine the child's insulin needs during this time.

10. Help the parents to plan for the child's return to school by creating a daily schedule for glucose testing, insulin administration, and meals and snacks. Encourage them to meet with the child's teacher or school nurse to explain the child's condition.

10. A schedule helps prioritize the child's daily needs and helps ensure compliance with the home care regimen. Meeting with the child's teacher or school nurse alerts the proper authorities to the child's condition in case he needs emergency care.

11. Explain to the child and parents the importance of maintaining proper hygiene. Advise the child to avoid walking in bare feet and to keep his toenails cut straight across, being careful not to nick the skin. Also advise him to keep his perineal area clean and dry.

11. Diabetics heal slowly and are more susceptible than the general population to infection, making proper hygiene more important.

12. Emphasize to the parents the importance of having the child's eyes checked at least yearly.

12. Yearly eye examinations can detect the early signs of vision problems, such as diabetic retinopathy.

13. Advise the child to wear a medical alert necklace or bracelet that identifies him as a diabetic.

13. Such identification ensures that medical personnel know the child's diabetic status if he needs emergency treatment.

Documentation checklist
During the hospital stay, document:
❏ child's status and assessment findings upon admission
❏ changes in the child's status
❏ fluid intake and output
❏ nutritional intake
❏ blood and urine glucose levels
❏ insulin dosages and injection sites
❏ child's response to treatment
❏ child's and parents' reactions to the illness and hospital stay
❏ patient and family teaching guidelines
❏ discharge planning guidelines.

Part 10

Psychosocial and other problems

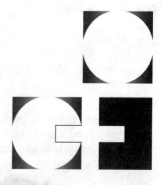

Anorexia nervosa

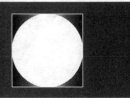

INTRODUCTION

Anorexia nervosa is a complex emotional disorder characterized by severe weight loss and body image disturbances, preoccupation with food, and a morbid fear of obesity. Although the exact etiology is unknown, the disorder, which usually affects adolescent girls, can usually be linked to some underlying psychological or behavioral problem.

Treatment may include nasogastric feedings, total parenteral nutrition, and long-term psychotherapy. Potential complications include cardiovascular damage, hypothermia, dehydration, and death. The expected outcome varies because anorexics are difficult to treat and frequently have relapses.

ASSESSMENT

Psychosocial
• Intense fear of becoming obese
• Refusal to maintain weight
• Distorted body image (overestimation of weight)
• Moodiness
• Social isolation
• Feelings of insecurity and helplessness
• Poor self-esteem

Cardiovascular
• Bradycardia
• Hypotension
• Arrhythmias

Musculoskeletal
• Loss of more than 25% of body weight

Endocrine
• Amenorrhea

Integumentary
• Lanugo
• Dry skin
• Hypothermia

NURSING DIAGNOSIS

Altered nutrition: less than body requirements related to fear of obesity

Expected outcome

The adolescent has an improved nutritional intake as evidenced by a weekly weight gain of ½ to 2 lb (0.25 to 1 kg).

Interventions

1. Provide a well-balanced, high-calorie diet.

2. Weigh the adolescent daily without revealing weight gain to the adolescent.

3. Stay with the adolescent during and after meals.

4. Enforce bed rest until the life-threatening period (marked by fluid and electrolyte imbalance, bradycardia, and extreme weakness) has passed.

Rationales

1. The adolescent needs a high-calorie diet to reverse the physical effects of the disorder and to ensure that she gains weight. However, taking in more than 3,000 calories/day can lead to cardiac arrest.

2. Daily weighing allows assessment of the adolescent's nutritional status. Keeping the actual weight gain from the adolescent helps prevent any manipulative behavior (such as eating meals, then purging) that could lead to a setback.

3. Your presence during and after meals ensures that the adolescent does not dispose of food or resort to self-induced vomiting.

4. Bed rest conserves energy required to maintain vital organs and promotes steady weight gain.

5. Establish a written contract that clearly defines the adolescent's responsibilities as well as those of the hospital staff regarding diet and activities. Avoid any discussion of food.

6. Use a nasogastric tube to feed the adolescent, as ordered, if weight loss continues.

5. A written contract provides limits and structure. Discussions of food may increase the adolescent's anxiety or lead to power struggles with nursing and other staff members.

6. The adolescent may need to be tube fed to ensure that she receives enough calories and nutrients to sustain life.

NURSING DIAGNOSIS

Body image disturbance related to the psychological effects of the disorder

Expected outcome

The adolescent demonstrates a positive self-image as evidenced by making positive comments about herself and performing activities of daily living.

Interventions

1. Encourage the adolescent to engage in activities that will help her become aware of body sensations, such as discussions on appetite before and after meals.

2. Use analogies and storytelling that demonstrate appropriate communication and coping skills.

3. Encourage the adolescent in a warm, caring manner to recognize her strengths, talents, and skills in a warm, caring manner.

4. Make sure the adolescent receives consistent care from a health care team throughout the hospital stay, and reinforce the care plan developed by the psychiatrist or psychologist.

Rationales

1. The anorexic may not be aware of such body sensations as hunger and satiety and may need to be reminded that they exist.

2. The adolescent's distorted self-image may prevent her from responding to direct discussions about her appearance and the disorder.

3. Such encouragement helps the adolescent build self-confidence and self-acceptance, and overcome the intense feelings of rejection typically associated with this disorder. It also allows her to focus on her inner strengths instead of on her physical appearance.

4. Anorexics require consistent care and a highly structured environment to achieve behavioral change.

NURSING DIAGNOSIS

Social isolation related to role conflict

Expected outcome

The adolescent exhibits decreased social isolation as evidenced by the ability to perform age-appropriate role behaviors.

Interventions

1. Discuss with the adolescent her perceived family and social roles, and assess the appropriateness of her role behaviors.

2. Use role playing to help the adolescent learn appropriate family and social role behaviors. Provide positive reinforcement.

Rationales

1. Such discussions and assessments allows you to determine the adolescent's cognitive state and to evaluate her feelings of isolation in relation to role conflicts.

2. Role playing can effectively teach the adolescent new age-appropriate behaviors, helping to decrease feelings of isolation.

Psychosocial and other problems

3. Help the adolescent select role behaviors that meet her personal needs instead of the perceived needs of others.

4. Teach the adolescent to use problem-solving skills to help her accomplish age-appropriate developmental tasks.

3. Selecting behaviors that concentrate on fulfilling personal needs should help the adolescent feel less threatened and isolated.

4. Mastering such skills promotes a feeling of competence in dealing with life's demands and problems.

NURSING DIAGNOSIS

Impaired social interaction related to low self-esteem

Expected outcome

The adolescent demonstrates improved social interaction as evidenced by communicating effectively with parents and significant others.

Interventions

1. Encourage the adolescent to express her feelings and needs.

2. Help the adolescent to distinguish between dependent and independent behaviors and to strive for a balance between the two.

3. Teach the adolescent effective communication and socialization skills.

4. Provide consistent verbal and nonverbal feedback when interacting with the adolescent.

5. Coordinate the support of the adolescent's family and friends.

Rationales

1. Getting the adolescent to talk about herself opens the lines of communication and forces her to acknowledge her feelings and needs.

2. Striking a balance between dependent and independent drives improves the adolescent's ability to love and be loved.

3. Learning these skills helps the adolescent to develop a mastery over herself and her environment and allows her to interact in a socially acceptable manner.

4. Consistent feedback helps the adolescent to build a trusting therapeutic relationship.

5. A strong support system provides nurturing, which the adolescent must have to develop a sense of identity and self-esteem.

Documentation checklist

During the hospital stay, document:
❏ adolescent's status and assessment findings upon admission
❏ changes in the adolescent's status
❏ pertinent laboratory and diagnostic findings
❏ fluid intake and output
❏ nutritional intake
❏ behavioral contract
❏ weight gain
❏ family involvement and therapy
❏ patient and family teaching guidelines
❏ discharge planning guidelines
❏ long-term follow-up plans.

Autism

INTRODUCTION

Autism is a developmental disability usually manifested before age 2½ and characterized by disturbances in speech and language, mobility, perception, and interpersonal relationships. The autistic child typically lacks awareness of others and fails to form interpersonal relationships, even with his parents. The disorder occurs in 5 out of every 10,000 children, affecting more boys than girls.

Treatment includes behavioral modification therapy and a structured environment, usually provided in a specialized care unit. Potential complications include abuse, neglect, and the breakdown of family relationships.

ASSESSMENT

Psychosocial
- Withdrawal from and unresponsiveness to parents
- Extreme resistance to change
- Inappropriate attachment to objects
- Self-stimulating behavior
- Irregular sleep patterns
- Stereotypic play
- Destructive behavior toward self and others
- Frequent tantrums
- Attention to soft sounds rather than speech
- Decreased verbalization
- Refusal to eat lumpy foods

Neurologic
- Inappropriate responses to stimuli
- Poor sucking reflex
- Failure to cry when hungry

Gastrointestinal
- Decreased appetite
- Weight loss

NURSING DIAGNOSIS

Impaired communication related to stimulus confusion

Expected outcome

The child communicates his needs using simple, concrete words or gestures; the infant effectively communicates his needs (for food, sleep, comfort, and so on).

Interventions

1. When communicating with the child, speak in one-to three-word sentences and repeat commands, as necessary. Tell the child to look at you when you speak, and closely observe his body language.

2. Use rhythms, music, and body movements to foster communication until the child can understand language.

Rationales

1. Simple, repetitive sentences may be the only way to communicate because the autistic child may not progress beyond the stage of concrete operational thought. Direct eye contact forces the child to focus his attention on the speaker and helps him to correlate speech with language and communication. Because of the child's inarticulateness, body language may be his only means of communicating his acknowledgment or comprehension of speech.

2. Physical movements and sound help the child recognize body integrity and boundaries, helping to reinforce his separateness from objects and other people.

3. Help the child recognize the relationship between cause and effect by naming specific feelings and identifying the cause of or stimulus for them.

3. Understanding the concept of cause and effect helps the child to establish a sense of separateness from objects and other people and encourages him to express his needs and feelings in words.

4. When communicating with the child, differentiate reality from fantasy in clear, simple terms.

4. Typically, autistic children do not differentiate between reality and fantasy and fail to acknowledge pain or other sensations and life events in a meaningful way. Emphasizing the difference between reality and fantasy helps the child express his needs and feelings.

5. Touch and hold the infant, but only as tolerated.

5. Touching and holding may not comfort the autistic infant.

NURSING DIAGNOSIS

Risk for violence: self-directed or directed at others related to hospital stay

Expected outcome

The child exhibits decreased tendencies toward violent or self-destructive behavior as evidenced by fewer tantrums and episodes of aggression or destruction and increased ability to cope with frustration.

Interventions

1. Provide a structured environment and as much routine as possible throughout the hospital stay.

2. Perform nursing interventions in short, frequent sessions. Approach the child in a gentle, friendly manner, and explain what you are about to do in clear, simple terms. If necessary, demonstrate the procedure on the parents.

3. Use physical restraint during procedures, when necessary, to ensure the child's safety and to redirect his anger and frustration. For example, to prevent the child from banging his head repeatedly against a wall, restrain his upper body but allow him to slap a pillow.

4. Use appropriate behavior modification techniques to reward positive behavior and punish negative behavior. For example, reward positive behavior by giving the child a favorite food or toy; punish negative behavior by revoking a privilege.

5. When the child behaves destructively, ask him if he is trying to tell you something, such as that he would like something to eat or drink or that he needs to go to the bathroom.

Rationales

1. Autistic children thrive on structure and routine and usually cannot cope with changes in their lives. Maintaining order helps prevent feelings of frustration that could lead to violent outbursts.

2. Short, frequent sessions allow the child to become familiar with the nurse and the hospital environment. Maintaining a calm, friendly manner and demonstrating procedures on parents can help the child accept interventions as nonthreatening measures, helping to prevent destructive behavior.

3. Physical restraint help prevent the child from engaging in self-destructive behavior. Allowing the child to engage in less harmful behavior, such as pillow slapping, allows him to redirect his anger and safely express his frustration.

4. Reward and punishment can help alter the child's behavior and prevent violent episodes.

5. Any increase in aggressive behavior may indicate feelings of increased stress, possibly from the need to communicate something.

NURSING DIAGNOSIS

Risk for altered parenting related to the disorder

Expected outcome

The parents demonstrate appropriate parenting skills as evidenced by expressing their concerns about the child's condition and seeking advice and help.

Interventions

1. Encourage the parents to express their feeling and concerns.

2. Refer the parents to a local autism support group and to a specialized school, as necessary.

3. Encourage the parents to contact the Autism Society of America, 7910 Woodmont Ave, Suite 650, Bethesda, MD, 20814-3015.

Rationales

1. Allowing the parents to express their feelings and concerns about the child's chronic condition may help them cope better with the frustrations involved in raising an autistic child.

2. A support group allows the parents to meet with parents of other autistic children to share information and provide emotional support. A specialized school provides a structured environment for implementing behavioral modification therapy.

3. Contact with a national organization helps keep the parents informed about current issues and developments related to autism.

Documentation checklist

During the hospital stay, document:
- ❐ child's status and assessment findings upon admission
- ❐ change in the child's status
- ❐ fluid intake and output
- ❐ nutritional intake
- ❐ environmental structure
- ❐ behavior modification therapy
- ❐ family involvement and therapy
- ❐ discharge planning guidelines
- ❐ guidelines for long-term therapy and parenting.

Psychosocial and other problems

Bulimia

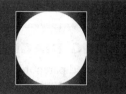

INTRODUCTION

Bulimia refers to a syndrome characterized by a powerful urge to overeat (binging) followed by self-induced vomiting or laxative use (purging). The patient, typically an older adolescent girl, usually has an obsessive fear of obesity and may even resort to intermittent periods of starvation to avoid weight gain.

Treatment usually involves I.V. fluid replacement, total parenteral nutrition, psychotherapy, and behavior modification. Potential complications include fluid and electrolyte imbalances, cardiovascular disorders, muscle weakness, and anemia. The outcome varies because bulimics are usually difficult to treat.

ASSESSMENT

Psychosocial
- Recurrent binging involving high-calorie foods
- Self-induced vomiting
- Laxative and diuretic abuse
- Hiding of food
- Morbid fear of the inability to control food intake
- Depression after binges

Cardiovascular
- Arrhythmias

Gastrointestinal
- Gastric dilation
- Esophagitis
- Cramping
- Decreased bowel function

Musculoskeletal
- Weight fluctuations

Eye, ear, nose, and throat
- Erosion of enamel on inner surface of teeth
- Dental caries
- Sore throat

Endocrine
- Painless swelling of salivary glands
- Menstrual irregularities

NURSING DIAGNOSIS

Altered nutrition: less than body requirements related to binge-purge behavior

Expected outcome

The adolescent maintains an adequate nutritional intake as evidenced by eating the prescribed diet, maintaining weight within standard limits, and refraining from self-induced vomiting.

Interventions

1. Establish a written contract with the adolescent that spells out diet and activity guidelines.

2. Stay with the adolescent during and after meals.

3. Encourage the adolescent to discuss her feelings and how they relate to her binging and purging.

Rationales

1. A written contract provides the structure and limits the bulimic adolescent needs while decreasing manipulative behaviors (such as eating, then vomiting or taking laxatives).

2. Staying with the adolescent provides needed support and ensures that she does not resort to self-inducing vomiting.

3. An important part of the overall therapy, discussing her feelings allows the adolescent to begin to recognize how she uses eating as a means of coping with problems.

NURSING DIAGNOSIS

Personal identity disturbance related to body weight

Expected outcome

The adolescent demonstrates an improved self-concept as evidenced by expressing an acceptance of her body and weight.

Interventions

1. Encourage the adolescent to discuss her feelings about her family, friends, and self.

2. Look for signs and symptoms of sexual abuse (such as overt sexual behavior and language, increased masturbation, isolation, and withdrawal from adults).

3. Assess the adolescent's usual coping mechanisms.

4. Help the adolescent establish and achieve realistic short- and long-term goals.

5. Reinforce the adolescent's strengths and skills.

6. Teach the adolescent necessary role behaviors that can enhance her sense of competency.

7. Coordinate the support of family and friends to provide realistic, positive feedback.

Rationales

1. Such discussions help you assess the adolescent's cognitive and emotional state and begin building a therapeutic relationship with her.

2. The bulimic adolescent may have a history of sexual abuse that may account for her negative self-concept and low self-esteem.

3. Such assessment helps you detect maladaptive coping mechanisms that may contribute to the adolescent's condition and negative self-concept.

4. Achieving clearly defined, realistic, and measurable goals promotes normal growth and development, especially in an adolescent suffering from chronic low self-esteem.

5. Reinforcement helps the adolescent focus on the positive aspects of her personality instead of on the negative aspects that might be contributing to her bulimia.

6. Role adequacy promotes self-esteem.

7. A strong support system helps nurture the adolescent, promoting self-esteem.

Documentation checklist

During the hospital stay, document:
- ❏ adolescent's status and assessment findings upon admission
- ❏ change in the adolescent's status
- ❏ fluid intake and output
- ❏ nutritional intake
- ❏ behavioral contract
- ❏ weight gain
- ❏ family involvement and therapy
- ❏ discharge planning guidelines.

Psychosocial and other problems

Burn injuries

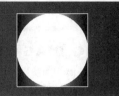

INTRODUCTION

Thermal injuries caused by intense heat, electrical shock, chemicals, or radiation are the third leading cause of accidental death in children. About 80% of all burn injuries occur within the home, most from exposure to flames or scalding with extremely hot water.

Major burns affect not only the integumentary system but also the respiratory, cardiovascular, musculoskeletal, and other body systems and present a special challenge to the health care team.

Treatment usually involves fluid replacement, burn care (using sterile dressings, debridement, and topical ointments), and physical therapy. Potential complications include contractures, kidney damage, respiratory disease, and death. The expected outcome depends on the severity of the burn.

ASSESSMENT

Integumentary
• Reddened, blistered, or blackened skin
• Edema
• Exudate
• Hypothermia

Cardiovascular
• Decreased cardiac output (initially)
• Shock

Respiratory
• Respiratory distress
• Hoarseness

Genitourinary
• Decreased urine output initially, followed by increased urine output
• Hematuria

Eye, ear, nose, and throat
• Singed nasal hairs
• Soot-coated tongue

Hematologic
• Anemia

Psychosocial
• Impaired body image

NURSING DIAGNOSIS

Impaired gas exchange related to edema of the upper airway and smoke injury

Expected outcome

The child's respiratory status remains stable as evidenced by normal rate, depth, and ease of breathing.

Interventions

1. Assess the child for singed nasal hair, soot-coated tongue, wheezing, soot-laden sputum, or hoarseness. Determine where and how the injury occurred. Note whether the child has a history of respiratory problems.

2. Monitor the child's respiratory status hourly, noting the rate and depth of respirations, hoarseness, nasal flaring, retractions, and changes in arterial blood gas (ABG) levels (such as increased partial pressure of arterial oxygen and decreased partial pressure of arterial carbon dioxide levels).

3. Gently suction the child, as needed.

4. Assist with endotracheal intubation, as necessary.

Rationales

1. These signs indicate injury from smoke inhalation, direct thermal injury to the respiratory tract, or shock. Knowing the exact cause of the injury is essential to providing immediate and appropriate treatment.

2. Increased respiratory rate and effort and developing hoarseness indicate increasing airway obstruction. ABG studies indicate the child's current oxygen, carbon dioxide, and pH levels.

3. The child may need suctioning because respiratory injury increases secretions and decreases ciliary action.

4. A child with known smoke inhalation or facial burns may require prophylactic intubation.

NURSING DIAGNOSIS

Fluid volume deficit related to fluid loss through thermal burns

Expected outcome

The child maintains adequate fluid balance as evidenced by good skin turgor, a brisk capillary refill time, no mental confusion, moist mucous membranes, and a urine output of 1 ml/kg/hour.

Interventions

1. Maintain I.V. patency and administer I.V. fluids, as ordered.

2. Monitor the child's urine output and urine specific gravity hourly, watching for trends.

3. Monitor the child's mental state, vital signs, peripheral perfusion, and urine volume.

4. Monitor the child's weight.

Rationales

1. The child must have a patent I.V. line for fluid replacement during the first 24 to 48 hours after a burn injury. During this time, profuse amounts of plasma begin leaking from the vasculature to the interstitial spaces, resulting in decreased circulatory volume.

2. Changes in urine output may indicate renal failure, fluid shifts, or diuresis related to various stages of burn injury. Specific gravity (normal is 1.005 to 1.030) increases with significant protein breakdown. Trends that last over 2 hours are more significant than a single reading.

3. Such monitoring helps determine the child's fluid status and the need to adjust fluid replacement.

4. Daily weight is a major indicator of the child's fluid status.

NURSING DIAGNOSIS

Impaired skin integrity related to the burn wound (pregrafting)

Expected outcome

The child has no indication of impaired skin integrity as evidenced by new skin growth and reduction in the size of the burn and no signs of infection.

Interventions

1. Bathe the child with an antiseptic solution, such as povidone-iodine or bleach solution, one or two times daily.

2. Remove the eschar using a soft sponge, forceps, and scissors.

3. Observe the wound for changes in the amount, color, or odor of drainage. Monitor for other signs of bacterial infection such as fever.

4. Apply a topical antimicrobial ointment or solution, such as silver sulfadiazine or silver nitrate, as ordered.

5. After debridement, inspect the homograft, xenograft, or synthetic wound dressing for purulence or further necrosis.

Rationales

1. Bathing promotes gentle separation of the eschar and dilutes and removes surface bacteria.

2. Removing eschar decreases the risk of bacterial infection.

3. Changes in the wound's appearance may indicate developing sepsis and may signal problems with the potential graft site.

4. Topical antimicrobials can decrease the risk of bacterial infection.

5. Purulent dressings should be removed to prevent bacterial invasion and sepsis.

Psychosocial and other problems

NURSING DIAGNOSIS

Ineffective thermoregulation related to skin damage and heat loss

Expected outcome

The child maintains normal thermoregulation as evidenced by a body temperature less than 100° F (37.8° C).

Interventions

1. Monitor the child's temperature hourly until stable.

2. Maintain a warm environment. Make sure that the water temperature for hydrotherapy remains at 98° F (36.7° C) and that the room temperature remains at 88° F (31.1° C).

3. Use an overhead radiant heat lamp and cover the child with blankets; make sure to tent the blankets around the child's body instead of lying them directly on the skin.

Rationales

1. Frequent monitoring ensures the early detection and prompt treatment of hypothermia to prevent the risk of life-threatening conditions, such as sepsis and renal failure.

2. A warm environment and constant water temperature minimize the reduction of core body temperature by reducing radiant heat loss.

3. Use of an overhead heat lamp and blankets further reduces radiant heat loss and increases body temperature; blankets that touch the wound can cause pain, irritate the wound area, and increase the risk of infection.

NURSING DIAGNOSIS

Risk for infection related to changes in skin integrity

Expected outcome

The child has no signs of systemic infection as evidenced by age-appropriate vital signs and normal wound cultures.

Interventions

1. Monitor the child's vital signs every 1 to 2 hours, noting any changes in the heart and respiratory rate or body temperature.

2. Monitor the child for nausea, vomiting, and abdominal distention.

3. Test the child's stools for occult bleeding using a guaiac preparation (such as Hemoccult).

4. Assess the child for changes in neurologic status or behavior.

5. Assess the burn wound for changes in color, drainage, and odor.

6. Assist with obtaining skin biopsies for culturing, as ordered.

Rationales

1. Increased heart and respiratory rates and increased or decreased body temperature may be early signs of sepsis.

2. Impaired intestinal motility commonly occurs soon after a burn injury. Ileus that occurs later may indicate sepsis.

3. Occult bleeding may indicate a stress ulcer, which is commonly associated with septicemia.

4. A change from alertness to lethargy, confusion, or delirium may indicate sepsis.

5. Changes such as foul odor and purulent drainage may indicate bacterial infection.

6. The child may need surgery to remove the source of infection if biopsy reports indicate 7 to 10 microorganisms per gram of vital tissue.

7. Administer antibiotics and fluid, electrolyte, and plasma replacements, as ordered.

7. Such supportive measures usually are instituted as soon as sepsis is suspected. Antibiotics help fight infection. Fluid, plasma, and electrolytes help stabilize the circulatory system so it can supply the tissues with needed nutrients.

8. Screen all visitors for signs and symptoms of infection before they enter the child's room, and institute isolation precautions, as necessary.

8. Such precautions reduce the risk of infection.

NURSING DIAGNOSIS

Impaired skin integrity related to the burn wound (postgrafting)

Expected outcome

The child has no signs of impaired skin integrity as evidenced by an intact graft and pink skin color.

Interventions

1. Determine what type of graft (autograft, homograft, xenograft, or isograft) was applied to the burn wound.

2. Roll sheet grafts every 1 to 2 hours with a cotton-tipped applicator.

3. Assess the color, amount, and type of drainage from the graft, and note whether the graft appears to be adhering to the wound.

4. Blot any excess blood or plasma from the graft.

5. Use a bed cradle or position the child so that the graft does not touch sheets or bed linens.

Rationales

1. The type of graft determines the specific nursing care required.

2. Rolling sheet grafts removes excess plasma and helps the graft adhere to the wound.

3. Within 48 to 72 hours after graft placement, the graft should become vascularized. Purulent or bloody drainage and swelling indicate that the wound is not fully vascularized.

4. Removing excess blood minimizes crust formation and promotes adherence.

5. Rubbing interferes with the new graft's adherence to the wound.

NURSING DIAGNOSIS

Pain related to skin damage and destruction

Expected outcome

The child has minimal pain as evidenced by age-appropriate vital signs, decreased expression of pain, and decreased restlessness and irritability.

Interventions

1. Assess the child for tachycardia, tachypnea, crying, withdrawal, decreased appetite, and inability to sleep.

2. Administer pain medication such as morphine, as ordered.

Rationales

1. Because children are sometimes too embarrassed to complain about pain, they may try to hide their discomfort. Changes in vital signs, emotional state, appetite, and ability to sleep may signal increased discomfort.

2. Pain medication effectively controls the degree of pain.

Psychosocial and other problems

3. Prepare the child for all treatments by explaining the procedures beforehand.

4. Allow the child to practice self-care, such as allowing him to bathe himself and remove dressings, whenever possible.

5. Institute additional pain-relief measures, such as relaxation and hypnosis, as needed.

6. Administer pain medication such as morphine before such procedures as bathing and debridement.

7. Provide age-appropriate diversional activities.

8. Use a bed cradle to keep bed linens away from the wound site.

3. Knowing what to expect gives the child a greater sense of control over the situation and increases his tolerance of pain.

4. The child's participation in routine care helps promote a sense of control over the situation and increases his tolerance of pain.

5. Nonpharmacologic pain-control measures have proven effective in relieving pain from burn injuries.

6. The child needs pain medication before these painful procedures.

7. Diversional activities help distract the child from his pain.

8. Keeping the wound site free from contact with other surfaces helps prevent pain.

NURSING DIAGNOSIS

Altered nutrition: less than body requirements related to increased caloric requirements

Expected outcome

The child maintains adequate nutritional status as evidenced by maintaining or increasing weight and by eating at least 80% of all meals.

Interventions

1. Obtain a dietary history, including the child's usual food intake, food allergies, food preferences, and chewing and swallowing difficulties.

2. Administer oral fluids or nasogastric feedings, as necessary.

3. Administer enteral fluids through a soft plastic (Silastic) feeding tube.

4. Check gastric residual volumes before each feeding or every 4 hours if the child is being fed continuously by a nasogastric tube. Also assess bowel sounds.

5. Administer total parenteral nutrition, as necessary.

6. Offer the child a diet high in calories, protein, and carbohydrates.

7. Weigh the child daily.

8. Monitor the child's fluid intake and output hourly.

Rationales

1. Such information, usually obtained from the parents (or the child, if appropriate), helps in the development of a nutritional plan.

2. High-calorie fluids (such as PediaSure) can help meet the child's caloric requirements.

3. A soft plastic feeding tube is less irritating to the child's esophagus and helps to ensure that he receives adequate nutrition.

4. Checking for residual volume prevents unnecessary gastric dilation and vomiting. The child should not receive the feeding if the residual volume is greater than half the amount of the proposed feeding or if bowel sounds are absent. Bowel sounds indicate that the bowel is functioning.

5. If the child cannot tolerate enteral feedings, he may need high-protein, high-calorie parenteral feedings.

6. Extra calories and protein promote optimal tissue growth. Extra carbohydrates help combat malnutrition.

7. Daily weighing directly measures the child's nutritional status.

8. Such monitoring determines whether the child requires fluid replacement.

NURSING DIAGNOSIS

Impaired physical mobility related to scar formation

Expected outcome 1

The child maintains physical mobility before grafting as evidenced by having full range of motion (ROM) and minimal contractures.

Interventions	Rationales
1. Position the child as follows to prevent or minimize contractures: • Slightly extend the neck with no pillow. • Place the ankles on a footboard at a 90-degree angle. • Place the elbows and knees in a three-point splint to keep the joint extended. • Place the hands in a thermoplastic splint to maintain a functional position. • Elevate the burned extremity 20 to 30 degrees. Also, encourage ambulation several times daily (if not contraindicated by the extent or severity of burns).	**1.** Proper positioning prevents contractures by applying force to overcome the intrinsic pull of myofibroblasts.
2. Depending on the degree of pain or edema, perform ROM exercises every 4 hours for 15 minutes; then reapply splints.	**2.** ROM exercises prevent joints from becoming stiff.

Expected outcome 2

The child maintains physical mobility after healing as evidenced by having full ROM and minimal contractures.

Interventions	Rationales
1. Apply splints and pressure bandages to all areas of deep second- and third-degree burns.	**1.** Constant pressure help minimize scar formation.
2. Perform ROM exercises, as ordered.	**2.** ROM exercises help increase muscle tone and prevent contractures.

NURSING DIAGNOSIS

Knowledge deficit related to home care

Expected outcome

The parents express an understanding of home care instructions and demonstrate home care procedures.

Interventions	Rationales
1. Teach the parents proper wound care, including details on medication administration, cleaning techniques, debridement, dressing changes, and sterile technique. Have them demonstrate such care before the child is discharged.	**1.** Learning this information and demonstrating techniques before discharge allows the parents to provide adequate home care.

2. Teach the parents to perform ROM exercises, such as moving all joints (knees, elbows, wrists, shoulders, and ankles) through their normal range of motion, every 4 hours for 15 minutes.

3. Explain to the parents the need for a diet high in calories, protein, and carbohydrates.

4. Encourage the parents to provide emotional support by allowing the child to perform self-care (when appropriate), encouraging him to express his feelings, and providing nonpharmacologic pain-control measures (such as hypnosis and guided imagery).

2. An important part of home care, ROM exercises promote the return of mobility to injured muscles and limbs.

3. A high-calorie, high-protein diet provides essential nutrients to repair damaged tissue. A high-carbohydrate diet supplies the additional calories the child needs to combat malnutrition.

4. Burn injuries can be physiologically and psychologically devastating to the child, who requires much patience and support to work through his feelings of fear, anger, frustration, and body-image difficulties.

Documentation checklist

During the hospital stay, document:
- ❐ child's status and assessment findings upon admission
- ❐ changes in the child's status
- ❐ pertinent laboratory and diagnostic findings
- ❐ fluid intake and output
- ❐ nutritional intake
- ❐ child's response to treatment
- ❐ graft response
- ❐ child's emotional status and the child's and family's support systems
- ❐ patient and family teaching guidelines
- ❐ discharge planning guidelines.

Child abuse and neglect

INTRODUCTION

Child abuse and neglect involves long-term physical, mental, or emotional maltreatment of an infant or a child, usually resulting in physical trauma, sexual molestation, or nutritional or medical neglect. One type of abuse on the rise is shaken-baby syndrome, in which a child suffers head injuries from being shaken.

In recent years, the number of reported child abuse cases has risen sharply—as many as 25% of all children are considered abused or neglected in some way. Such abusive behavior may be triggered by stress, socioeconomic pressures, or other psychosocial problems. In many cases, the abusive parent or caregiver was abused as a child.

Treatment involves immediate medical attention to correct the child's physical problems (such as fractures, burns, or head or spinal cord injuries) and psychotherapy or family therapy. Part of the nurse's duty involves reporting all cases of known or suspected abuse to the proper authorities. Potential complications include brain damage, muscle and bone damage, coma, and death.

This plan focuses on the psychosocial aspects of child abuse and neglect. For more information on the physical aspects, see the individual plans on fractures, head injury, spinal cord injury, and burn injuries in this book.

ASSESSMENT

Psychosocial
• Evidence of neglect (dirty clothes and hair, diaper rash, foul smell)
• Failure to thrive
• Delayed cognitive, psychomotor, and psychosocial development
• Withdrawal from adults

Musculoskeletal
• Fractures
• Sprains
• Dislocated joints

Genitourinary
• Urinary tract infection
• Vaginal tears
• Vaginal bleeding

Integumentary
• Circular lesions (usually caused by cigarette burns)
• Scalded skin or burns
• Bruises or abrasions
• Unexplained human bite marks
• Unexplained injuries
• Soft-tissue swelling

NURSING DIAGNOSIS

Ineffective family coping: compromised related to factors that contribute to child abuse

Expected outcome

The family demonstrates improved coping mechanisms within 6 months of diagnosis.

Interventions

1. Identify factors leading to the breakdown of the family's coping mechanisms, such as the parents' age, the number of children in the family, the parents' socioeconomic status, the developmental level of all family members, the use or lack of support systems, and any other triggering events.

Rationales

1. Identifying such factors allows the determination of the need for interventions and referral to appropriate health care and social services organizations.

2. Consult appropriate health care personnel and social service workers about the family's problems. Offer referrals for individual or family therapy, as needed.

3. Encourage the child and family members to express their feelings about what might be causing the abusive behavior.

4. Teach the parents the normal development and management of children at various ages; teach specific parenting skills and appropriate discipline techniques.

2. Families affected by child abuse or neglect usually require care by a multidisciplinary team. Support groups, such as Parents Anonymous and Alcoholics Anonymous, can help with specific problems.

3. Such encouragement allows family members to discuss their problems and explore ways of modifying their behavior.

4. The parents may have unrealistic expectations about the normal growth and development of children, possibly affecting their ability to cope with the stresses of parenting.

NURSING DIAGNOSIS

Altered growth and development related to inadequate caregiving

Expected outcome

The child demonstrates age-appropriate cognitive, psychomotor, and psychosocial development within 6 months of diagnosis.

Interventions

1. Administer age-appropriate developmental tests to determine the child's current developmental level.

2. Discuss test findings with the parents and child.

3. Initiate activities (such as reading, bicycling, and discussions on feelings) with the parents and child to enhance the development of deficient cognitive abilities, psychomotor skills, and psychosocial functioning.

4. Reassess the child's developmental level at appropriate intervals, such as 1 month, 2 months, 6 months, and 1 year.

5. Involve the developmentally delayed in a stimulation program to promote development.

Rationales

1. Test results serve as a baseline to gauge the child's progress over the projected course of teaching and therapy.

2. The parents and child should be aware of test findings so that they can plan for short- and long-term goals.

3. Abused children typically experience developmental delays because of impaired family functioning. Such activities help to correct developmental problems that result from dysfunctional relationships.

4. Periodically assessing the child's developmental level helps determine whether the child is progressing as expected.

5. A stimulation program helps promote normal growth and development.

NURSING DIAGNOSIS

Risk for violence (abusive family member): directed at others related to maladaptive behavior

Expected outcome

The abusive family member demonstrates a decreased level of violence within 2 to 4 weeks of diagnosis.

Interventions

1. Identify the abuser's violent behavior patterns, such as demonstrating abusive behavior while using alcohol or drugs or while unemployed.

Rationales

1. Identifying such abusive behavior patterns helps to determine appropriate interventions and to assess improvement.

2. Explore with the abuser the factors that may have triggered the violent episodes, such as alcohol or drug use.

3. Provide multidisciplinary counseling, including referral to a psychologist and appropriate community organizations (such as Alcoholics Anonymous and Parents Anonymous).

4. Refer the family to an appropriate family therapist.

5. Report all incidents of actual or suspected abuse to the proper authorities.

2. Identifying such factors makes the abuser more aware of what types of situations trigger violent behavior, helping him to prevent recurrences.

3. Counseling helps the abuser develop effective coping skills to deal with the triggering factors that lead to abusive behavior.

4. Family therapy stresses the involvement and support of the entire family to prevent violent behavior patterns.

5. Nurses have a legal responsibility to report all such cases and to keep accurate records of physical evidence for further investigation.

NURSING DIAGNOSIS

Altered parenting related to the abusive parent's inability to attach to or bond with the child

Expected outcome

The abusive parent demonstrates effective parenting behaviors as evidenced by appropriate touching and the ability to communicate without yelling or screaming.

Interventions

1. Discuss normal attachment and bonding with the abusive parent.

2. Provide role models for the parent.

3. Encourage the parent to enroll in classes that teach appropriate parenting skills.

4. Refer the parent to appropriate support services (such as Parents Anonymous, Alcoholics Anonymous, or Al-Anon) for intervention and counseling, as needed.

Rationales

1. Making the parent aware of the normal attachment and bonding process may help him to become interested in developing appropriate parenting skills.

2. Role models allow the parent to emulate appropriate parenting behavior.

3. Such classes provide examples and practice forums for developing effective parenting skills.

4. The parent may need to rely on support services during crises to help him cope with stressful situations that might trigger abuse.

Documentation checklist

During the hospital stay, document:
❑ child's status and assessment findings upon admission
❑ parental involvement in the child's care
❑ child's response to the family
❑ social services involvement
❑ reports of abuse to the appropriate authorities
❑ discharge planning guidelines.

Psychosocial and other problems

Depression

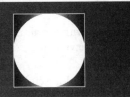

INTRODUCTION

A mood disturbance disorder characterized by feelings of sadness, despair, and discouragement, depression usually results from some loss or disappointment. The disorder is more common among adolescents than younger children and tends to run in families.

Acute depression that lasts from days to weeks may be normal and usually requires no medical or therapeutic intervention. Chronic depression, however, requires therapeutic measures, including psychotherapy and use of antidepressants. Potential complications include anorexia, bulimia, and suicide.

ASSESSMENT

Psychosocial
- Impulsiveness
- Self-destructive or self-demeaning behaviors
- Attention-getting behaviors
- Feelings of hopelessness, helplessness, and worthlessness
- Withdrawal
- Loss of interest in usual activities

Neurologic
- Excessive sleep or insomnia

Gastrointestinal
- Weight gain or loss

NURSING DIAGNOSIS

Self-esteem disturbance related to stress or loss

Expected outcome

The adolescent demonstrates improved self-esteem as evidenced by increased interest in interpersonal interactions, school, and social activities and an increased ability to cope with the future.

Interventions

1. Establish a trusting therapeutic relationship with the adolescent.

2. Encourage the adolescent to recognize and express his feelings, especially those of shame and loss, and to forgive himself and others.

3. Teach the adolescent acceptable social skills (such as communication skills, proper hygiene, and appropriate dress) and role behaviors (family and social) and provide positive feedback.

4. Carefully examine the child's belief systems and expectations about the future.

5. Identify the child's maladaptive coping mechanisms and encourage him to use alternative methods in times of crisis.

6. Coordinate peer and family support.

Rationales

1. A trusting relationship must be in place before treatment can begin; the adolescent must feel comfortable enough to discuss his problems.

2. A depressed adolescent tends to internalize feelings. Getting him to express feelings of shame and loss and to forgive allows the adolescent to progress through the normal stages grieving.

3. Learning to interact successfully with others and receiving positive feedback should increase the child's self-esteem and encourage him to feel hopeful about the future.

4. Unrealistic expectations may cause anxiety and stress and contribute to the child's depression.

5. Using appropriate coping mechanisms increases the child's self-control, which should help improve his self-esteem.

6. A strong support system provides the security, love, and sense of belonging necessary to building self-esteem.

NURSING DIAGNOSIS

Risk for violence: self-directed or directed at others related to the inability to cope with negative feelings

Expected outcome

The adolescent demonstrates decreased aggressiveness and violence as evidenced by not harming himself or others.

Interventions

1. Assess the child's potential for destructive behavior, and take necessary precautions to ensure his safety and the safety of others (including observing the adolescent on an hourly basis and removing potentially harmful objects from his room).

2. Encourage the adolescent to use alternative methods for coping with his negative feelings.

3. Help the adolescent to recognize the cause-and-effect relationship of his violent behavior.

4. Teach the adolescent appropriate problem-solving skills.

Rationales

1. External controls and safety measures may be needed until the adolescent learns self-control.

2. Using alternative coping skills helps prevent violent episodes, improving social relationships and increasing self-esteem.

3. Getting the adolescent to recognize the causes and consequences of his violent behavior should encourage him to accept responsibility for his actions and acknowledge the need for change.

4. Learning to solve problems fosters self-control and feelings of adequacy and reduces frustration.

Documentation checklist

During the hospital stay, document:
❑ child's status and assessment findings upon admission
❑ behavioral contracts
❑ therapy and group involvement
❑ family involvement
❑ discharge planning guidelines.

Psychosocial and other problems

Failure to thrive

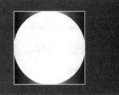

INTRODUCTION

Failure to thrive is a chronic, potentially life-threatening condition characterized by failure to maintain weight and sometimes height above the fifth percentile on age-appropriate growth charts (see appendix C, Physical growth charts). Most children with this condition are diagnosed before age 2.

The condition, which can result from physical causes or emotional or psychological problems, may be classified as follows:
- organic — caused by a serious illness, such as gastroesophageal reflux, malabsorption syndrome, congenital heart defects, or cystic fibrosis
- inorganic — the most common type, caused by psychosocial problems between the child and primary caregiver (usually the mother), such as failure to bond
- mixed — results from a combination of organic and inorganic causes

Treatment may include nutritional therapy, total parenteral nutrition, family therapy, and a structured environment. Potential complications include impairment of the child-parent relationship, impaired or delayed physical and psychosocial growth, and mental retardation.

ASSESSMENT

Psychosocial
- Maternal deprivation resulting from child's low birth weight, sex, or appearance
- Factors affecting the parents' ability to bond with child, including:
  - Marital discord (spouse may be unsupportive, frequently absent, or a substance abuser)
  - Inadequate income
  - Maternal age (under age 16)
  - Neglect or lack of attention as a child
  - Poor self-esteem
  - Limited ability to perceive the needs of others
  - Limited capacity for concern
  - Depression or other psychological problems

Cardiovascular
- Tetralogy of Fallot
- Transposition of the great vessels

Neurologic
- Cerebral palsy

Gastrointestinal
- Malabsorption syndrome
- Chronic diarrhea
- Pernicious vomiting

Musculoskeletal
- Muscular dystrophy

NURSING DIAGNOSIS

Altered growth and development related to inadequate weight gain

Expected outcome

The child demonstrates improved growth and development as evidenced by maintaining body weight during the hospital stay.

Interventions

1. Weigh the child upon admission.

2. Assess the child's growth and development using age-appropriate growth charts and developmental screening tests (such as the Denver Developmental Screening Test).

Rationales

1. An initial weight serves as a baseline to assess the infant's progress throughout the hospital stay.

2. Such assessments determine the child's developmental level compared with other children of the same age.

3. Observe the interaction between the parents (particularly the mother) and child, including the establishment of eye contact and the parents' handling of and communication with the child.

4. Assess the child's neurologic and cardiovascular status, checking especially for alertness and signs of arrhythmias, murmurs, or developmental delays.

5. Provide ongoing assessments of the child's feeding and elimination patterns by:
• assigning one nurse for feeding
• establishing a routine feeding time
• providing a calm environment
• holding the child during feedings.

6. Weigh the child daily, and carefully monitor his intake and output.

7. Provide the infant with visual and auditory stimulation by exposing him to bright colors, different shapes, and music. Provide the older child with age-appropriate stimulation, including books, games, and toys.

8. Place the infant on the floor to encourage crawling and head raising.

3. Failure to interact appropriately with the child may signal the parents' inability to form an emotional attachment to the child, which may be the cause of the child's failure to thrive.

4. Such assessment helps determine whether the child's failure to thrive has a physiologic cause.

5. Ongoing assessments help determine if the child has any feeding difficulties, vomiting, pain, constipation, cramping, diarrhea, or other problems that might cause his failure to thrive. Consistent feeding patterns and a nurturing environment can help the child form normal attachments and trusting relationships.

6. Daily weighing and intake and output monitoring allows for direct evaluation of the child's nutritional status and developmental progress.

7. Visual and auditory stimulation promote normal sensory development but may lead to hyperactivity in some children.

8. This helps to stimulate development of the large muscles.

Nursing diagnosis

Altered parenting related to inability to form normal maternal attachment to child

Expected outcome

The parents demonstrates improved parenting skills as evidenced by asking appropriate questions about the child's condition and participating in the child's care.

Interventions

1. Teach the parents (especially the mother) normal parenting skills by demonstrating proper holding, stroking, and feeding techniques and by communicating with the child using age-appropriate words and gestures.

2. Help the parents to develop organizational skills.

3. Provide counseling, as necessary, to help the parents overcome feelings of mistrust or neglect resulting from personal childhood experiences.

4. Monitor the parents' progress and provide reinforcement, when necessary.

Rationales

1. Parenting is a learned response, usually based on skills demonstrated by other parents or role models.

2. Parenting requires increased energy and effective planning to meet the child's needs adequately.

3. The parents may be responding to the child based on the way they were treated as children. Counseling can make them aware of the cause of the child's failure to thrive, which can improve their parenting skills.

4. Continued monitoring and reinforcement gives the parents a chance to practice parenting skills and allows the detection of deficiencies that require further intervention.

NURSING DIAGNOSIS

Knowledge deficit related to home care

Expected outcome

The parents demonstrate an understanding of home care instructions.

Interventions

1. Teach the parents age-appropriate growth and development milestones (see appendix A, N2ormal growth and development).

2. Demonstrate appropriate feeding techniques, including details on how to hold the child, how long to feed him, and which foods to provide.

3. Encourage the parents to spend as much time as possible at the hospital during the child's stay.

Rationales

1. Such instruction gives the parents realistic expectations of what the child may or may not be able to do.

2. The parents may need such instruction, particularly if the child's failure to thrive stemmed from inorganic causes, such as the parents' inability to form normal attachments to the child. Also, stressing the importance of proper nutrition and feeding techniques encourages the parents to comply with therapeutic measures begun during the child's hospital stay.

3. This allows the nursing staff to observe the parents' behavior and to provide further teaching and reinforcement as necessary.

Documentation checklist

During the hospital stay, document:
- ❐ child's status and assessment findings upon admission
- ❐ fluid intake and output
- ❐ nutritional intake
- ❐ child's or infant's response to treatment
- ❐ family therapy
- ❐ discharge planning guidelines.

Suicidal behavior

INTRODUCTION

Suicidal behavior refers to the conscious decision or deliberate attempt to cause self-inflicted harm that will result in death. Suicidal tendencies occur most frequently among adolescents (suicide is the third leading cause of death in children ages 15 to 18), usually stemming from overwhelming feelings of hopelessness, powerlessness, and the inability to meet increased demands and expectations. Often, the adolescent blames himself for problems that are out of his control but cannot bring himself to ask for help. Such problems as depression, illness, family conflicts, and substance abuse commonly are involved. Usual treatment includes psychotherapy and the use of antidepressant medications.

ASSESSMENT

Psychosocial
• Dispersal of personal items
• Triggering crisis
• Previous suicidal threats
• Depression
• Withdrawal

NURSING DIAGNOSIS

Risk for violence: self-directed related to loss of self-esteem

Expected outcome

The adolescent makes no further suicide attempts and expresses feelings of increased self-esteem and hope for the future.

Interventions

1. Ensure the adolescent's safety by removing all potentially harmful objects from the room. Also, remove his clothing so that he cannot leave the hospital. Frequently observe his behavior—at least once every 15 minutes—if he is not under constant supervision.

2. Explain to the adolescent that all procedures and restrictions are necessary to protect him, and to help him sort out his feelings and thoughts.

3. Provide a warm, accepting, supportive environment, and identify and reinforce the adolescent's strengths.

4. Teach the adolescent appropriate social skills (such as communication skills, hygiene, and appropriate dress) and role behaviors.

5. Discuss with the adolescent his feelings of depression, shame, guilt, and loss.

6. Identify maladaptive coping mechanisms and suggest alternative ways to deal with negative feelings.

7. Assess the adolescent's response to therapy.

Rationales

1. Such measures help ensure the adolescent's safety and provide a sense of security until the adolescent can maintain self-control.

2. Offering such explanations promotes a sense of trust that is basic to a therapeutic relationship.

3. This affirms the adolescent's sense of self-worth and encourages him to concentrate on positive thoughts.

4. Learning appropriate social skills and role behaviors should help the adolescent to establish successful interpersonal relationships, increasing his self-esteem.

5. Discussing these feelings may reveal the reason for the attempted suicide. Accepting these feelings and forgiving himself is crucial to building the adolescent's self-esteem.

6. An adolescent who has demonstrated an inability to cope with problems needs to learn alternative ways to manage negative feelings and build self-esteem.

7. This helps to determine the effectiveness of therapy and the need for further intervention.

Documentation checklist

During the hospital stay, document:

❏ adolescent's status and assessment findings upon admission
❏ adolescent's feelings about suicide
❏ observations of the adolescent's activities
❏ family involvement
❏ group and individual therapy
❏ discharge planning guidelines.

Part 11

Perioperative care

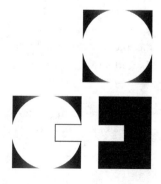

Anesthesia (induction phase)

INTRODUCTION

The perioperative period, especially anesthesia induction and surgery itself, can be particularly frightening to a child. I.V. anesthetic agents can sometimes cause pain, and inhalational agents commonly have an unpleasant odor and can alarm the child.

Depending on the child's age, anesthesia-related anxieties may range from mild agitation to a fear of death. Infants may become irritable and fretful in response to parental anxieties about anesthesia induction. Toddlers usually fear separation from their parents at this time. Children under age 5 usually worry about what will happen when they awake after surgery. School-age children often associate anesthesia with being "put to sleep" and fear that they will never awaken. Adolescents usually fear loss of control and worry about what they might say or do while under anesthesia.

Potential complications of anesthesia include respiratory distress, coma, and death.

ASSESSMENT

Psychosocial
- Crying
- Withdrawal
- Fear (stated verbally or implied through facial expressions)

NURSING DIAGNOSIS

Anxiety related to anesthesia induction

Expected outcome

The child will experience minimal anxiety as evidenced by minimal crying, screaming, and irritability.

Interventions

1. Use age-appropriate relaxation techniques, such as distraction, guided imagery, medical play, storytelling, and music, to calm the child. As appropriate, teach the child what will happen during anesthesia induction and surgery.

2. When administering an anesthetic by mask, use a clear mask and introduce the mask slowly; you might try to make the child think of it as a game. Avoid negative description, such as "smelly gas" when talking about the anesthetic.

3. Do not undress the child until after he is anesthetized.

4. When addressing the child, speak in a soft, calm, monotonous voice and move slowly.

5. Start all I.V. lines after the child is anesthetized, unless otherwise instructed.

6. Place a pleasant strong-smelling extract, such as chocolate, lemon, or vanilla, on the mask before administering the anesthetic.

Rationales

1. Relaxation techniques help the child focus on something other than his fears, reducing his anxiety. Understanding what will happen also helps reduce fear and anxiety.

2. A clear mask is less frightening to a child than an opaque or black mask. Introducing the mask slowly and helping the child think of the process as a game decreases his anxiety and promotes relaxation. Avoiding negative descriptions helps prevent the child's anxiety from escalating.

3. Removing the child's clothes may frighten him more than the surgery itself.

4. A soft voice and slow movements promote a more relaxed atmosphere.

5. Anesthesia prevents the child from being aware of this painful and potentially frightening invasive procedure.

6. Strong-smelling extracts can mask the noxious smell of most anesthetic agents, making anesthesia induction more pleasant.

7. Encourage the adolescent to participate in the anesthesia-induction process by allowing him to select the administration route (gas versus I.V.) and to hold the mask or select the I.V. site.

7. Making such decisions fosters a feeling of self-control in the adolescent, who typically fears losing control while under anesthesia.

NURSING DIAGNOSIS

Ineffective breathing pattern related to anesthesia induction

Expected outcome

The child will have no signs of respiratory compromise as evidenced by maintaining a respiratory rate of 16 to 30 breaths/minute and by exhibiting no signs of respiratory distress.

Interventions

1. Closely monitor the child's respirations and skin color during the induction phase.

2. Closely observe the child for vomiting until an endotracheal tube is inserted.

3. Be prepared to apply cricoid pressure if instructed to do so by the anesthesiologist.

Rationales

1. The induction phase is the most dangerous period of anesthesia. Close monitoring promotes early detection and prompt treatment of such complications as respiratory distress, cardiac arrest, and anaphylactic shock.

2. The child is at risk for aspiration until intubated.

3. Cricoid pressure occludes the esophagus and prevents passive regurgitation.

NURSING DIAGNOSIS

Risk for injury related to anesthesia induction

Expected outcome

The child will suffer no injury or trauma during the induction phase.

Interventions

1. Be prepared to apply soft arm or leg restraints during the induction phase.

2. Position the child appropriately, and secure him to the operating table, as necessary, by placing a strap across his abdomen or chest until the induction phase is complete.

Rationales

1. A child typically experiences an excitement phase before losing consciousness. He may need restraints to prevent him from injuring himself.

2. Securing the child ensures that he does not fall off the table.

Documentation checklist

During the perioperative period, document:
- ❏ child's status upon admission to the operating room
- ❏ vital signs
- ❏ nothing-by-mouth status
- ❏ preoperative medications
- ❏ preoperative teaching.

Perioperative care

Anxiety (preoperative)

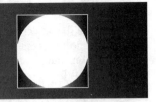

INTRODUCTION

Because of the strangeness of the hospital environment and the upcoming surgery, most children experience some degree of anxiety during the preoperative period. Orienting the pediatric patient to the operating room, postanesthesia care unit, and intensive care unit (if applicable), and explaining surgical and postoperative care procedures should help alleviate this anxiety.

Developmentally appropriate teaching should include explanations and demonstrations using illustrations, videotapes, and sample equipment, when available. It also should include a tour of the operating room and adjunct facilities. The younger child may benefit from play demonstrations of the actual surgical procedure using dolls or puppets.

ASSESSMENT

Psychosocial
- Hyperactivity
- Crying
- Withdrawal
- Acting out
- Regression
- Expressions of fear of death

NURSING DIAGNOSIS

Anxiety (child) related to surgery

Expected outcome

The child will demonstrate minimal anxiety as evidenced by continuing to interact with parents and significant others.

Interventions

1. Explain to the child the events surrounding surgery, using simple, age-appropriate terms and illustrations, dolls, puppets, and sample equipment (when available).

2. Provide age-appropriate emotional support when the child enters the surgical suite. Such support may include cuddling the infant, providing familiar toys for the small child, or talking casually with the older child.

3. Allow the parents to accompany the child to the entrance of the operating room, and involve them in the recovery process as early as possible.

4. Help the parents cope with their own anxieties by providing preoperative teaching, counseling, and a supportive environment.

5. Use such relaxation techniques as deep breathing, distraction and redirection, or focusing and guided imagery (alone or in combination) to help reduce the child's and parents' anxiety.

6. Give the child age-appropriate information about the recovery room.

Rationales

1. Such explanations allow the child to anticipate the preoperative and postoperative events, reducing his anxiety.

2. Providing emotional support during the preoperative period helps ensure a positive surgical experience.

3. Parents are a familiar, stabilizing force for the child. Their presence immediately before and after surgery promotes the child's emotional well-being.

4. The parents' anxiety directly affects the child. Reducing the parents' anxiety should, in turn, reduce the child's anxiety.

5. Relaxation techniques help the child and parents concentrate on matters other than the upcoming surgery, which reduces their anxiety.

6. Understanding what the recovery room will be like should help decrease the child's fear of the unknown, reducing his anxiety.

Documentation checklist

During the perioperative period, document:

❏ child's status upon admission to the operating room
❏ questions the child may ask
❏ child's expressions of fear or anxiety
❏ child's understanding of the surgical procedure.

Hypothermia

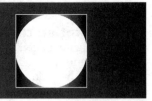

INTRODUCTION

Hypothermia refers to a low body temperature that usually results from exposure of the skin to cool air or solutions. During the perioperative period, infants are generally at greater risk than older children for hypothermia because they have a proportionally greater body surface area.

Hypothermia usually results in increased heart and respiratory rates and decreased glucose levels. Usual treatment involves covering as much of the child's body as possible with blankets, warming pads, and a head cap.

ASSESSMENT

Integumentary
• Decreased temperature
• Cyanosis
Cardiovascular
• Tachycardia
Respiratory
• Increased respiratory rate

NURSING DIAGNOSIS

Ineffective thermoregulation related to surgery

Expected outcome

The child will maintain normal thermoregulation as evidenced by maintaining an axillary temperature of 97.6° to 99° F (36.4° to 37.2° C).

Interventions

1. Ensure that the operating room temperature is set at 96.8° to 98.6° F (36° to 37° C) 30 minutes before the child's arrival.

2. Place an aquathermia pad set at 101.3° F (38.5° C) on the operating table. Remove the pad before placing the child on the table.

3. Provide the child with warm blankets upon his arrival in the operating room.

4. Avoid any unnecessary or prolonged exposure of the child's skin during the preoperative period and the induction and emergence phases of anesthesia.

5. Monitor and document the child's temperature throughout the procedure.

6. Use thermal lamps, as necessary, during the induction and emergence phases of anesthesia. Monitor closely to prevent overheating.

7. Warm all solutions to be used on the surgical field in a normal saline solution or sterile water bath.

8. Cover the child's extremities with plastic bags.

Rationales

1. Maintaining the room at this temperature decreases the risk of hypothermia from environmental causes.

2. An aquathermia pad warms the operating table, reducing the risk of heat loss through conduction during the surgical procedure.

3. Warm blankets reduce the risk of heat loss through conduction.

4. Prolonged skin exposure leads to decreased body temperature and increased metabolic activity.

5. Frequent monitoring allows for early detection and prompt treatment of significant fluctuations in the child's body temperature.

6. Thermal lamps provide radiant heat and help to maintain body temperature.

7. Cold solutions can decrease body temperature; a cold solution used as a flush can lower core body temperature.

8. Plastic bags provide extra insulation.

9. After the surgical procedure is completed, dry the child thoroughly.

9. Drying prevents chilling by evaporation.

10. If the child will be transported in a self-contained incubation unit, warm the unit 45 minutes before transfer.

10. Warming the unit prevents heat loss by convection and conduction.

Documentation checklist
During the perioperative period, document:
❐ child's vital signs
❐ preoperative teaching
❐ child's and parents' responses to teaching.

Hypovolemia

INTRODUCTION

A decrease in the extracellular fluid (plasma) volume, hypovolemia can cause lowered blood pressure and poor perfusion of vital organs. During the perioperative period, it may result from the child's nothing-by-mouth (NPO) status (withholding of fluids), the surgical procedure itself, or third-space fluid shifting. Other possible causes include fluid loss from diarrhea, fever, vomiting, systemic infection, and impaired ability to concentrate urine.

ASSESSMENT

Cardiovascular
• Decreased blood pressure
• Increased pulse rate
• Decreased central venous pressure
• Decreased capillary refill time
• Little or no neck vein distention (when placed in supine position)
Genitourinary
• Decreased urine output
Integumentary
• Skin tenting
• Flushing
• Dry skin
• Cool extremities

NURSING DIAGNOSIS

Fluid volume deficit related to surgery

Expected outcome

The child will maintain adequate hydration as evidenced by good skin turgor and a capillary refill time of 3 to 5 seconds.

Interventions

1. Monitor the child's vital signs throughout the perioperative period, noting any changes in pulse rate and blood pressure. Also assess the child's skin for dryness and coolness.

2. Monitor the amount of blood lost during surgery.

3. Monitor the child's hemoglobin and hematocrit values and capillary refill time before surgery.

4. Administer I.V. fluids and electrolytes, as ordered, and document the amount administered.

Rationales

1. Increased pulse rate, decreased blood pressure, and dry, cool skin indicate a fluid deficit, which requires the administration of replacement fluids.

2. Such monitoring is essential to detect hypovolemia during surgery. (A child undergoing surgery can lose 10% to 20% of his total blood volume.)

3. Preoperative blood values help determine the need for blood or fluid replacement. Capillary refill time is prolonged in hypovolemia.

4. Careful documentation of all I.V. fluids and electrolytes administered during the perioperative period helps determine the child's overall fluid status.

5. Evaluate for additional fluid loss from:

• NPO status

• vomiting or diarrhea

• nasogastric suctioning

• diuretic use

• third-space fluid shifts

• elevated temperature

• mechanical ventilation.

5. Any of these conditions or procedures can cause hypovolemia during the perioperative period.
• NPO status prevents replacement of normal fluid losses through the skin, lungs, and bowel.
• Vomiting and diarrhea increase the amount of fluid lost through the alimentary tract and bowel.
• Nasogastric suctioning removes the stomach contents, including fluids.
• Diuretics increase total urine output, contributing to total fluid loss.
• Third-space fluid shifts result from internal mechanisms in which fluid moves to inflammatory sites, causing a general reduction in the total circulating volume.
• Elevated temperature increases the amount of fluid lost through the skin and lungs.
• Unless warm, humidified air is used, mechanical ventilation can dry mucous membranes and increase the amount of fluid lost through the lungs. Careful monitoring ensures that the ventilator is functioning properly and that the child has ventilatory readings within normal limits.

Documentation checklist

During the perioperative period, document:
❏ child's status and assessment findings upon admission to the operating room
❏ vital signs
❏ NPO status
❏ medications administered
❏ skin turgor and capillary refill time
❏ amount of I.V. fluids and electrolytes administered.

Perioperative care

Pain (postoperative)

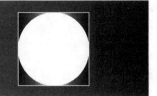

INTRODUCTION

Postoperative pain is caused by the disruption of tissue and nerve endings, usually from an incision. A child's response to pain depends on his age and individual pain threshold.

Infants generally respond to pain by crying and flailing their arms and legs, but how they perceive pain and how much they can remember of the experience remains controversial. Toddlers and preschoolers usually are influenced by their previous experiences and may react violently or attempt to escape painful situations, making them difficult to control. However, as children grow older, they develop increasingly individual ways of dealing with pain. School-age children use various methods, including deep breathing, counting out loud to 10, and yelling "ouch." Adolescents tend to be more reserved and usually do not verbally express feelings of anxiety or pain, fearing loss of self-control.

ASSESSMENT

Neurologic
- Crying
- Guarding
- Verbal expressions of pain
- Withdrawal

Cardiovascular
- Increased blood pressure
- Increased heart rate

Respiratory
- Increased respiratory rate

NURSING DIAGNOSIS

Pain related to surgery

Expected outcome

The child will have minimal postoperative pain as evidenced by decreased restlessness and irritability and by age-appropriate blood pressure and pulse and respiratory rates.

Interventions

1. Objectively assess the child's pain:

• Ask the child if he is comfortable. If he indicates that he is uncomfortable, ask him to describe his pain by using a face interval, numeric rating, or pain color scale (depending on the child's developmental level).

• Watch for guarding, rigidity, restlessness, and crying.

• Monitor the child for increased heart rate and blood pressure.

2. Administer narcotics along with other pain medication, as ordered; carefully observe and document the child's response.

Rationales

1. Depending on the child's age and usual response to pain, objective indicators may provide the most reliable assessment of the child's pain.

• A negatively phrased question, such as asking the child if he is in pain, may influence his answer; asking the child if he is comfortable allows him to respond more objectively. He may need a pain-rating scale to indicate his level of pain, especially if he is too young to describe the pain's severity in words.

• The child may be too young or feel too embarrassed to say that he is in pain. In that case, nonverbal cues, such as guarding, rigidity, restlessness, or crying, may signal the child's increased discomfort.

• These autonomic responses may indicate that the child is feeling pain.

2. During the immediate postoperative phase, narcotics must be administered carefully because of the potential residual effects of anesthetic agents, such as respiratory depression and hypotension.

e the parents in managing the child's pain as
ossible after surgery.

ition the child, as needed, to maximize his

5. Speak to the child in a soothing voice, and provide a quiet, nonstimulating environment.

6. Use other techniques, such as distraction, biofeedback, and imagery, to help control the child's pain.

3. Parents are most familiar with the child's normal response to pain and know which pain-control techniques have worked in the past.

4. Repositioning relieves pressure on skin and reduces muscle cramping.

5. A calm, soothing voice and quiet surroundings can effectively calm the child, reducing his tension and thus reducing his pain.

6. The use of biofeedback and of toys, stories, imagery, and other distractions may draw the child's attention away from his pain, decreasing his perception of it.

Documentation checklist
During the perioperative period, document:
❑ child's status and ongoing assessment
❑ vital signs
❑ medications administered
❑ responses to pain.

Respiratory compromise (postoperative)

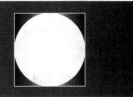

INTRODUCTION

During the postanesthesia recovery period, the residual effects of anesthetics and irritation from the endotracheal tube put the child at risk for respiratory compromise. Infants are at particular risk because they are obligatory nose and diaphragmatic breathers. Treatment of this condition includes oxygen administration and reintubation, when necessary.

ASSESSMENT

Respiratory
• Increased respiratory rate
• Sternal retractions
• Decreased tidal volume
Integumentary
• Cyanosis

NURSING DIAGNOSIS

Ineffective breathing pattern related to anesthetic administration

Expected outcome

The child will maintain an effective breathing pattern and an adequate level of oxygenation as evidenced by maintaining pink mucous membranes, unlabored respirations (16 to 30 breaths/minute), and an oxygen saturation level above 95%.

Interventions

1. Administer up to 40% humidified oxygen at a rate of 2 to 3 L/hour by face mask until the child is awake and responsive.

2. Monitor the child's oxygen saturation level with a pulse oximeter until he is awake and stable.

3. Place the child in a semiprone or lateral position unless contraindicated by the surgical procedure.

4. Carefully assess the child's respirations (noting rate, depth, and effort) and skin color every 15 minutes. Take into account the anesthetic agent used during surgery when making evaluations.

5. Assess the child every 15 minutes for signs of airway obstruction, including a crouplike cough, hoarseness, inspiratory stridor, and cyanosis.

Rationales

1. Administering oxygen during the postanesthesia recovery period increases the total oxygen concentration in circulation until the child's respiratory rate is fully established. Humidified air helps keep the mucous membranes moist. Administering humidified oxygen at levels higher than 40% places the child at risk for retrolental fibroplasia.

2. Because the child's respiratory control center is easily fatigued after surgery, his oxygen saturation level may drop; levels should be above 90%, preferably above 95%. Such monitoring is especially important for an infant, who may breathe irregularly.

3. These positions help maintain airway patency, provide easy access for suctioning, and reduce the risk of the child's tongue obstructing the airway — a risk that increases with the supine position.

4. If the child received a muscle relaxant—a common practice in pediatric surgery—he is at increased risk for respiratory depression (marked by decreased respiratory rate, cyanosis, and decreased oxygen saturation levels).

5. Postintubation croup may result from edema caused by the tube's irritating effects on the child's small airway.

minister 100% oxygen by manual resuscitation r face mask if the child has signs and symptoms of y obstruction.

refully suction the child's mouth when airway ob- tion becomes evident, avoiding contact with the cal site.

ke necessary measures to open the child's airway, such as inserting an oral or nasal airway, using the jaw-thrust maneuver, or inserting an endotracheal tube.

6. High levels of oxygen reduce the risk of hypoxia in the child with a compromised airway.

7. The pooling of secretions near the obstructed airway can cause laryngospasm.

8. If airway blockage occurs, such measures can ensure a patent airway.

Documentation checklist

During the perioperative period, document:
❑ child's ongoing status
❑ vital signs
❑ signs and symptoms of respiratory distress
❑ oxygen saturation level
❑ amount and rate of oxygen administered.

Part 12

Diagnostic studies

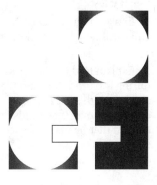

Computed tomography

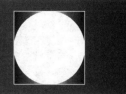

INTRODUCTION

In computed tomography (CT), multiple X-rays pass through a specified body area and are measured while detectors record differences in tissue attenuation. A computer reconstructs this data as a three-dimensional image on an oscilloscope screen. Attenuation varies with tissue density and appears as shades of gray on the screen. A contrast medium may be used to accentuate differences in density.

Indications for testing
- Abscesses
- Cysts
- Cerebral hematomas
- Intracranial hemorrhages
- Cerebral edema
- Tumors
- Hydrocephalus
- Liver disease
- Renal calculi

NURSING DIAGNOSIS

Knowledge deficit related to procedure

Expected outcome

The child and parents will express an understanding of the procedure.

Interventions

1. Explain to the child and parents the purpose of the test. Also explain that the test will take place in the radiology department and that the radiologist will determine if the parents can remain in the room during the test. Explain that, depending on the area scanned, the test should take from 30 to 60 minutes.

2. Describe the equipment to the child in age-appropriate terms. Tell him that he will be placed on a table that slides in and out of a scanner (tell the young child that the scanner looks like a big donut and that the table slides in and out of the hole). Show him a picture of the scanner, if possible. Tell him the room may feel cool, but that he will be given a blanket.

3. Explain that the child will need to remove all metallic objects, such as barrettes, jewelry, or eyeglasses, before the test.

4. Explain that while the X-rays are being taken the child will hear loud clicking noises.

5. Explain to the child that he will need to lie very still during the procedure and that he may need to be restrained with straps or body wraps to ensure that he does not move. If he needs chest or abdominal scans, explain that he may be asked to hold his breath for a short while.

Rationales

1. Such explanations help alleviate any fears or anxieties and help ensure the child's cooperation during the test.

2. The CT scanner can appear ominous and frightening, especially to a young child. Describing the equipment to the child or showing him a picture of the scanner should prepare him for what the machine looks like, helping to ensure his cooperation during the test.

3. The high density of metallic objects can cause images to appear darker on the screen, interfering with test results.

4. Such noises, caused by the X-ray tube rotating within the cylinder, may alarm the child if he does not expect them.

5. Any movement, including respirations, during the filming of X-rays can cause blurred images on the screen. Understanding the need for lying still ensures the child's cooperation.

6. If the test involves a contrast medium, offer the following information, using age-appropriate terms:
• To prevent vomiting and aspiration from use of the contrast medium, the child must not eat or drink for 4 to 6 hours before the test.
• Contrast medium enhances the image of body parts so that they are more visible on the screen.
• If the child does not already have an I.V. line in place, the contrast medium will be injected through a small needle placed under his skin. The needle will be removed after the injection.
• The contrast medium may cause a burning or stinging sensation at the injection site, warmth, nausea, or a salty or metallic taste. These effects last only a few minutes.

6. Preparing the child for injection of the contrast medium and its effects helps make the procedure less stressful and frightening. (*Note:* Do not use the word *dye* to refer to contrast medium; the child may misinterpret the word as *die*.)

NURSING DIAGNOSIS

Risk for injury related to sedative use

Expected outcome

The child will suffer no adverse reactions to the sedatives.

Interventions

1. If you think the child will not lie still during the procedure, consult the doctor about administering a sedative-hypnotic, such as chloral hydrate (Noctec) or pentobarbital (Nembutal). Withhold food and fluids for 6 hours before administering the medication.

2. Observe the child closely during the procedure to ensure adequate breathing.

3. Monitor the child's vital signs until he is fully awake.

Rationales

1. A child under age 5 may have a hard time lying still during the procedure. Administering a sedative-hypnotic 20 to 30 minutes before the study usually keeps the child sedated for the time required. Withholding food and fluids for 6 hours empties the stomach, which helps prevent vomiting and aspiration of gastric contents.

2. Sedatives can depress the respiratory drive and cause apnea.

3. Such assessment can identify adverse reactions to the sedative, such as respiratory depression.

NURSING DIAGNOSIS

Risk for injury (allergic reaction) related to the use of contrast medium

Expected outcome

The child will exhibit no signs of allergic reaction to the contrast medium.

Interventions

1. Check the child's record for a history of hypersensitivity to iodine-containing contrast media or for a history of asthma or other severe allergies. Ask the parents if the child has ever had a reaction to iodine or iodine-containing foods (such as seafood). Alert the doctor to any positive findings.

Rationales

1. The iodine contained in the contrast medium may trigger an allergic reaction, especially if the child has a history of such allergy or a history of asthma. If the contrast medium is essential to the test, the doctor may order antihistamines or steroids to prevent an allergic reaction.

Diagnostic studies

2. Alert the radiology department if the child is at risk for allergic reaction, and ensure that emergency drugs (precalculated to the child's weight) and equipment are on hand.

3. Observe the child for signs and symptoms of allergic reaction (including skin rash, hives, urticaria, headache, vomiting, sneezing, flushing, respiratory distress, hoarseness, tachycardia, and palpitations). Administer diphenhydramine for a mild reaction or epinephrine for a severe reaction, as ordered.

4. Teach the parents the signs and symptoms of a delayed allergic reaction, including headache, itching, skin rash, nausea, and vomiting. Tell them to immediately call the doctor if such a reaction occurs.

2. Emergency drugs, such as epinephrine (Adrenalin) and diphenhydramine hydrochloride (Bendadryl), and emergency equipment should be readily available in case of an allergic reaction.

3. The release of histamine causes capillary dilation, increased permeability of the blood vessels, contraction of smooth muscle, and stimulation of mucus-secreting glands.

4. The child may experience an allergic reaction after leaving the radiology department and going home. If the reaction is severe, he needs immediate medical attention. If the reaction is mild, the doctor may order an oral antihistamine.

Documentation checklist

After the procedure, document:
- ❏ child's status
- ❏ vital signs
- ❏ allergic reaction
- ❏ level of consciousness.

Excretory urography

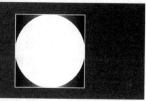

INTRODUCTION

Excretory urography, also called intravenous pyelography, is the radiographic examination of the kidneys, ureters, and bladder after injection of a contrast medium. The contrast medium is excreted through the kidneys, allowing visualization of the urinary tract. X-rays are taken to identify suspected renal or urinary tract disease, space-occupying lesions, congenital anomalies, or trauma to the urinary system.

Indications for testing
- Polycystic kidney
- Renal calculi
- Tumors

NURSING DIAGNOSIS

Knowledge deficit related to procedure

Expected outcome

The child and parents will express an understanding of the procedure.

Interventions

1. Explain to the child and parents that food and fluids may be restricted at midnight the day of the procedure. Tell them the child will receive a suppository the evening before and morning of the procedure and, if necessary, an enema. If the patient is a young child, briefly describe suppository and enema administration in age-appropriate terms.

2. Tell the parents they will be asked to sign a consent form.

3. Explain to the child that he will go to the radiology department for the procedure, and let the parents know if they can accompany the child.

4. Tell the child he will wear a hospital gown, and remove all metal objects from the child.

5. Describe the X-ray equipment and, if possible, show the equipment to the child and parents before the test. Use age-appropriate terms in your descriptions. For example, if the patient is a young child, describe the equipment as a special camera that will take his picture. Explain that the machine will be placed close to his body but will not touch him.

6. Tell the child he will be asked to urinate just before the test and then lie flat on the X-ray table while the machine takes one picture of his stomach before he receives the contrast medium.

Rationales

1. Fluid restrictions promote concentration of the contrast medium. Food restrictions, suppositories, and enemas help clean the bowel of feces, allowing visualization of the kidney. A young child may feel less threatened by unfamiliar experiences if he receives a clear explanation beforehand. (*Note:* Diet restrictions, suppositories, and enemas may be contraindicated in a child under age 2.)

2. Because the contrast medium is injected, excretory urography is considered an invasive procedure.

3. Such factors as limited space, physical constraints, or the mother's pregnancy may prevent one or both parents from accompanying the child.

4. Because X-rays cannot penetrate metal, objects such as jewelry or diaper pins can obscure the view of urinary structures.

5. A clear explanation helps ease the family's fears, particularly those of a young child, who may imagine that the X-ray machine is a monster.

6. Retained urine dilutes the contrast medium and impairs visualization of the bladder. A "scout" film is taken to detect gross abnormalities of the urinary system before the contrast medium is injected.

7. Explain that a small needle will be placed under the child's skin to inject the contrast medium and will be removed as soon as the injection is complete. Tell him that the contrast medium may cause a burning, stinging, or warm sensation; nausea; and a salty or metallic taste for a few minutes. Reassure him that the sensation should pass quickly.

7. Preparing the child for the test by providing clear explanations can enhance his cooperation and may alleviate some of his anxiety.

8. Tell the child he may be asked to drink a carbonated beverage during the test.

8. Carbonation produces gas in the stomach, which enhances visualization of the kidneys.

9. Caution the child that the X-ray technician may press on his abdomen with a compression board (a board with half of a ball attached to it). Assure the child it will not hurt.

9. The round part of the ball is pressed into the abdomen to promote better visualization of the kidneys or renal pelvis.

10. Tell the child that he must lie still while the technician takes the X-rays and that the test lasts about 30 minutes. Assure a young child that he will not be left alone.

10. Movement distorts the X-ray image. Knowing how long the test will last and having someone with him during the procedure should make the procedure easier for the child to bear.

Nursing diagnosis

Risk for injury related to the contrast medium

Expected outcome

The child will exhibit no signs of allergic reaction to the contrast medium.

Interventions

1. Check the child's history for hypersensitivity to iodine or to food (such as shellfish) or contrast media that contain iodine. Also check for a history of asthma or other severe allergies.

2. Notify the doctor if the child's history is positive for any of the above conditions.

3. Alert the radiology department to the potential for an allergic reaction.

Rationales

1. These conditions may cause an allergic reaction to the contrast medium.

2. If the child must have the test, he may receive antihistamines or steroids before the test.

3. Emergency equipment and drugs, such as epinephrine (Adrenalin) and diphenhydramine (Benadryl) should be available in case of a reaction.

Documentation checklist
After the procedure, document:
❑ child's status
❑ site used for administering contrast medium
❑ allergic reaction
❑ vital signs.

Magnetic resonance imaging

INTRODUCTION

Magnetic resonance imaging (MRI, also called nuclear magnetic resonance) is a noninvasive procedure used to diagnose such conditions as cerebral infarction, tumors, abscesses, edema, and hemorrhage. Like computed tomography (CT), MRI produces cross-sectional images of the brain and spinal cord in multiple layers without bone interference. Unlike CT, however, MRI does not rely on ionizing radiation or injected contrast media to produce the images. The child lies on his back on a narrow table in the MRI scanner, which uses a strong magnetic field and short bursts of energy in the form of radio waves. Radio receivers detect the energy released from hydrogen ions in the body as they are exposed to the radio waves. The MRI computer processes the signals and displays the high-resolution images on a video monitor. The test is painless, and no harmful effects have been documented.

Indications for testing
- Hemorrhage
- Neoplasm
- Cystic lesion
- Hydrocephalus
- Head trauma
- Cerebrovascular accident
- Atrophy
- Birth defects
- Tethered cord
- Hydromyelia
- Vascular and structural abnormalities

NURSING DIAGNOSIS

Knowledge deficit related to procedure

Expected outcome

The child and parents will express an understanding of the procedure.

Interventions

1. Explain MRI and its purpose to the parents and child. Tell them that the procedure can detect and examine abnormalities in the body. Use age-appropriate terms in your descriptions. For example, if the patient is a young child, describe the scanner as a long tunnel open at both ends and the radio frequency coil as a hard shell or helmet. If possible, show the family a picture of the scanner. Tell them the procedure will take 30 to 60 minutes, depending on the body area being examined.

2. Remove any jewelry, electrocardiography pads, or diaper pins from the child, and have him wear pajamas without metal snaps. If the parents want to accompany the child, tell them to remove credit cards, watches, beepers, loose jewelry, belts with metal buckles, keys, and other metal objects.

3. Tell the child he must lie still during the procedure. Explain that he will hear repetitive knocking sounds at different pitches; consider giving him earplugs if necessary.

Rationales

1. Clearly explaining the procedure and equipment can enhance the family's cooperation and may alleviate some of their anxiety.

2. Metal objects should not be brought into the magnetic field. The magnet would pull any loose objects (such as jewelry or keys) toward it, creating a hazard. The powerful magnetic field can damage credit cards, watches, and beepers.

3. The slightest movement can distort the video images. The sounds heard during the procedure (caused by the radio frequencies) may disturb the child and make him restless (although the monotony sometimes lulls young children to sleep).

NURSING DIAGNOSIS

Risk for injury related to procedure

Expected outcome

The child will show no signs of discomfort or injury.

Interventions

1. Assess the child to determine his suitability for MRI. Contact the radiology department if the child has:
• a winged needle device for I.V. access
• an infusion pump
• spring-action cassettes in I.V. tubing
• a stainless steel implantable infusion port

• implanted metal objects, such as intracranial surgical clips, aneurysm clips, artificial heart valves, or rods

• a history of foreign bodies in the eyes
• claustrophobia

• a history of nausea or headaches

• a need for mechanical ventilation

• a critical illness.

2. If you think the child will not lie still during the procedure, consult the doctor about administering a sedative-hypnotic, such as chloral hydrate (Noctec) or pentobarbital (Nembutal). Give the child nothing by mouth for 6 hours before administering the medication.

3. Observe the child closely during the procedure to ensure adequate breathing. Use a cardiac output monitor or a pulse oximeter designed for use with MRI, if available.

4. Monitor the child's vital signs until he is fully awake.

Rationales

1. Various factors may prevent a child from undergoing MRI.
• The magnetic field can cause the needle to dislodge.
• The magnetic field can cause equipment to fail.
• Stainless steel springs may inhibit fluid flow.
• The magnetic field may pull on a stainless steel infusion port within the chest wall. (*Note:* Plastic infusion ports have been developed for use in MRI. Infusion ports in place for longer than 3 months pose little safety hazard but may degrade image quality.)
• Magnetic pull on implanted objects can cause tissue damage. Certain rods and clips may not be contraindicated if they have been in place longer than 3 months and adhesions have developed.
• Movement of objects can cause tissue damage.
• A child with claustrophobia may not tolerate the scanner's narrow diameter.
• The sounds generated during MRI may exacerbate nausea or headaches.
• Mechanical ventilators cannot be taken into the magnetic field. The child would need manual ventilation.
• Restricted access to the child and the metal components in most resuscitation equipment make resuscitation during MRI difficult — and potentially dangerous for the child and staff.

2. A child under age 5 may have a hard time lying still for the procedure. Administering a sedative-hypnotic 20 to 30 minutes before the study usually keeps the child sedated for the time required. Withholding food and fluids for 6 hours helps prevent vomiting and aspiration of gastric contents.

3. Sedatives can depress the respiratory drive and cause apnea. However, monitoring a child inside the scanner is difficult. Visibility is not ideal, and metallic components and interference from radio waves prevent the use of cardiac or apnea monitors.

4. Such monitoring can identify adverse reactions to the sedative.

Documentation checklist

After the procedure, document:
❏ child's status
❏ results of the test.

Nuclear medicine

INTRODUCTION

Nuclear medicine studies use radioactive isotopes to image tumors, abscesses, or other abnormalities in the bones, thyroid, kidney, liver, heart, brain, or lung. The radioisotope is usually administered I.V. and concentrates in certain body organs based on the radiopharmaceutical used. Gamma camera detectors record the radiation emitted from the organ. Nuclear medicine scans involve very low radiation doses and pose minimal risk to the patient and staff.

Indications for testing
Cardiovascular disorders
- Structural defects
- Cardiomegaly

Neurologic disorders
- Brain tumors

Respiratory disorders
- Lung tumors

Musculoskeletal disorders
- Osteomyelitis
- Metastatic neoplasms
- Degenerative processes
- Fractures

Thyroid disorders
- Goiters
- Nodules
- Substernal masses
- Hyperthyroidism
- Hypothyroidism
- Thyroid cancer
- Metastases

Genitourinary disorders
- Trauma
- Acute or chronic renal failure
- Cysts
- Transplant rejection
- Impaired renal function

NURSING DIAGNOSIS

Knowledge deficit related to procedure

Expected outcome

The child and parents will express an understanding of the procedure.

Interventions

1. Briefly explain the procedure and its purpose to the child and parents. Use age-appropriate terms. Tell them a needle will be placed under the child's skin to inject the contrast medium. Assure them that the injection will hurt for just a minute and that the needle will be removed once the contrast medium has been injected.

2. Avoid using the word *dye* to describe the contrast medium.

3. Tell the child he will be asked to void before the study. (*Note:* If the patient is an infant, his diapers may need changing during the procedure.)

4. Explain that the camera will be brought close to the child's body but will not touch it. Assure the child that the camera will not fall on him.

5. Tell the child he may need to change positions during the test but should lie still while the camera takes pictures. Explain that he can move between pictures.

Rationales

1. Clearly explaining the procedure helps the family prepare for what will happen to the child, can improve their cooperation, and may alleviate some of their anxiety.

2. The child may misinterpret the word *dye* for *die*.

3. The kidneys usually excrete the isotope. Bladder activity and wet diapers may distort the image.

4. The gamma camera detector is a large, round cylinder placed over the organ being imaged. Preparing the child for the experience can alleviate his fear.

5. Movement distorts the image. The duration for each image may vary. The child may need to change positions if an organ must be imaged from different angles.

6. Explain to the parents that the amount of radiation received is less than that from X-rays.

6. This information can allay the concerns of parents worried by the terms *nuclear* and *radiation*.

7. Tell the child to remove metal objects, such as jewelry, before the procedure.

7. Metal objects obstruct the view of organs.

NURSING DIAGNOSIS

Risk for injury related to sedative use

Expected outcome

The child will suffer no adverse reactions to the sedatives.

Interventions

1. If you think the child will not lie still during the procedure, consult the doctor about administering a sedative-hypnotic, such as chloral hydrate (Noctec) or pentobarbital (Nembutal). Withhold food and fluids for 6 hours before administering the medication.

2. Observe the child closely during the procedure to ensure adequate breathing.

3. Monitor the child's vital signs until he is fully awake.

Rationales

1. A child under age 5 may have a hard time lying still for the procedure. Administering a sedative-hypnotic 20 to 30 minutes before the study usually keeps the child sedated for the time required. Withholding food and fluids for 6 hours helps prevent vomiting and aspiration of gastric contents.

2. Sedatives can depress the respiratory drive and cause apnea.

3. Such monitoring can identify adverse reactions to the sedative.

NURSING DIAGNOSIS

Risk for injury related to radiation exposure

Expected outcome

The child, parents, staff members, and other patients will receive minimal radiation exposure.

Interventions

1. Wear gloves when coming in contact with the child's body fluids, and dispose of urine and other excretions in the toilet. Wash hands thoroughly.

2. If the child has an indwelling urinary catheter, empty the collection bag every hour for 24 hours.

3. Double-bag linens before putting them in the hospital laundry. Double-bag disposable waste, especially soiled diapers, before discarding in the trash.

4. If you are pregnant or must hold the child for longer than 1 hour, wear a lead apron. Caution the parents to do likewise.

Rationales

1. Most radioisotopes are excreted in the urine, which can be disposed of safely in the toilet.

2. Radioactive substances in the urine concentrate in the collection bag if the bag is not emptied hourly.

3. Double bagging helps prevent contamination of laundry bins and trash receptacles.

4. Although radiation emission is minimal, prolonged exposure may be harmful.

Documentation checklist

After the procedure, document:
- ❏ child's status
- ❏ vital signs.

Radiologic and ultrasound studies

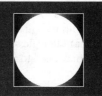

INTRODUCTION

Radiologic studies involve radiographic examination of one or more body areas, depending on the specific study ordered. The four densities of the body—air, water, fat, and bone—absorb varying degrees of radiation. For instance, air is the least dense and results in dark images on the film. Bone causes light images or white structures on film (the calcium in bone absorbs much of the radiation, preventing radiation from striking the X-ray film). The resulting light and dark images allow the detection of abnormalities; for example, white areas in a normally dark lung field might indicate pneumonia.

Ultrasonography produces pictures of structures in the body with sound waves, which reflect off tissues to produce an image on the screen. The test is noninvasive.

Indications for testing
Chest
- Atelectasis
- Pneumonia
- Lung abscess
- Tumor
- Pneumothorax
- Scoliosis
- Kyphosis
- Cardiomegaly
- Vessel anomalies

Abdomen
- Masses
- Small-bowel obstruction
- Ascites
- Tissue trauma

Kidney, ureter, bladder
- Abnormal size and structure
- Renal calculi
- Kidney or bladder masses

Skull
- Trauma
- Fracture
- Congenital anomalies
- Bone defects

NURSING DIAGNOSIS

Knowledge deficit related to procedure

Expected outcome

The child and parents will express an understanding of the specific study ordered.

Interventions

1. Explain food or fluid restrictions, if applicable.

2. Tell the child and parents that the study will take place in the radiology or ultrasound department, unless a portable X-ray or ultrasound has been ordered. Let the parents know if they can accompany the child.

Rationales

1. Most studies do not require food or fluid restrictions, although the child may be placed on a restricted diet for tests administered after general X-rays. A low-fat diet is usually required before a gallbladder ultrasound. Fluids are usually encouraged before a pelvic or abdominal ultrasound so the bladder remains full and visible during the test.

2. Portable equipment usually produces a less-detailed image but may be necessary for an acutely ill or immobilized child. Such factors as limited space and physical constraints may prevent one or both parents from accompanying the child.

3. Tell the child he will wear a hospital gown; if he is undergoing a radiologic study, he must remove all metal objects and may need to wear a lead shield over his lower pelvic area.

4. Explain the equipment to be used, and show it to the child and parents before the study, if possible. Use age-appropriate terms in your descriptions. For example, for a young child undergoing a radiologic study, describe the equipment as a special camera that will take his picture. Explain that the machine will be placed close to his body but will not touch him. Tell him the study usually takes 10 to 15 minutes. For a young child undergoing ultrasonography, explain that the technician will apply some gel to part of his body and gently rub a wand over the area; reassure him that it will not hurt. Tell him the procedure should take about 30 to 45 minutes.

5. Explain that the child may be asked to change positions during the study. Remind the child that he must remain still while the technician takes the picture or passes the transducer over his body. Assure him that he can move between pictures and when the transducer is not on his body. A young child may need sedation for an ultrasound study.

6. For a chest X-ray, tell the child he may be asked to take a deep breath and hold it while the X-ray is taken. If the patient is a young child, demonstrate the task, have him practice it, and provide feedback.

3. Metal objects (such as jewelry, snaps, and belt buckles) block X-rays and can obscure anatomic structures. Reproductive organs are generally shielded to prevent unnecessary exposure to X-rays.

4. A clear explanation helps ease fears, particularly those of a young child, who may imagine that the X-ray machine is a monster or that the ultrasound transducer may hurt him.

5. The child may need to assume various positions to provide the best images, depending on the study, the body area involved, or the angle desired. For example, the child usually stands for posteroanterior chest films and may sit or lie down for anteroposterior views. Movement can distort the X-ray or ultrasound image. Sedation allows the young child to remain still for the longer time needed for an ultrasound study.

6. Holding a deep breath enhances visualization of lung expansion. Practice and feedback can help a young child master an unfamiliar task and lessen his fear of the procedure.

Documentation checklist
After the procedure, document:
❐ child's status
❐ results of the test.

Upper GI and small-bowel series

INTRODUCTION

An upper GI and small-bowel series involves the fluoroscopic examination of the esophagus, stomach, and small intestine after the ingestion of barium sulfate (barium swallow). This test is indicated for children with upper GI symptoms (swallowing difficulty, regurgitation, and burning or gnawing epigastric pain), signs of small-bowel disease (diarrhea and weight loss), and signs of GI bleeding (hematemesis and melena).

When performing a complete GI series, barium enema should always precede this test because retained barium may cloud anatomic structures on X-rays.

Indications for testing
Upper GI
- Pyloric stenosis
- Ulcers
- Abdominal pain
- Diarrhea

Small-bowel follow-through
- Malabsorption syndrome
- Small-bowel strictures.

NURSING DIAGNOSIS

Knowledge deficit related to the procedure

Expected outcome

The child and parents will express an understanding of the procedure.

Interventions

1. Explain to the child that he will be allowed nothing to eat or drink beginning at midnight on the day of testing (beginning 3 hours before testing for children under age 2).

2. Explain that if the child has undergone other diagnostic testing involving barium sulfate (such as barium enema or barium swallow) within the last few days, he may require laxatives or enemas.

3. Explain to the child that the test will take place in the radiology department and that the technicians will be wearing lead aprons. Tell him that he will need to wear a hospital gown and remove all metal objects, such as necklaces, that might interfere with the X-rays.

Rationales

1. Withholding food and drink promotes the complete digestion of barium. Limiting fasting in very young children to 3 hours before testing helps prevent hypoglycemia.

2. Laxatives and enemas clear the digestive tract of any residual barium. However, they are contraindicated in children with inflammatory bowel disease, ulcerative colitis, or Crohn's disease because of their irritating effects on the GI system.

3. Such explanations help prepare the child for what the radiology room will look like; it may be particularly frightening to a young child. Metal objects would distort the image because X-rays cannot penetrate metal.

4. Explain the following events to the child, using age-appropriate terms:

• Explain that he will be given some barium sulfate to swallow. Tell him that the barium is thick like a milk-shake but that it may not taste as good.

• Reassure a young child that he will not fall off the table.
• Explain that he may need a nasogastric tube inserted to instill the remaining barium directly into his stomach. Tell him that the doctor may press on his stomach.
• Reassure the child that his parents or a nurse will remain with him throughout the procedure.

4. The child should understand the details of the procedure, which can be especially frightening to a young child.
• Infants are given the barium from a bottle; young children may sip the liquid through a straw. Some hospitals flavor the barium with strawberry or chocolate to improve the taste.
• The child may be placed in various positions on a tilted table while the X-rays are taken.
• The radiologist, wearing a lead-lined glove, may compress the child's stomach to ensure that the barium adequately coats the gastric mucosa.
• The child may need to wait between X-rays and can be in the radiology room for 2 to 4 hours before the small-bowel series is completed.

Nursing diagnosis

Constipation related to barium retention

Expected outcome

The child will maintain usual bowel elimination patterns as evidenced by having a normal bowel movement within 24 hours after the procedure.

Interventions

1. Notify the doctor if the child is taking anticholinergics or narcotics. Administer laxatives, as ordered.

2. After confirming with the radiology department that all tests have been completed, begin the child on a regular diet.

3. Assess the quantity and quality of the child's stools for the first few days after the procedure. Warn the child and parents that the stools will be white or light colored (possibly pink if a strawberry flavoring was used) during this time.

4. Administer castor oil or milk of magnesia, as ordered.

5. Inform the doctor if the child has not expelled all of the barium within 3 days.

6. If appropriate, encourage the child to increase his fluid intake.

Rationales

1. Anticholinergics and narcotics may decrease peristalsis and impede the elimination of barium from the GI tract, possibly leading to constipation.

2. A well-balanced diet promotes normal bowel elimination.

3. Such assessments determine if the child is constipated and needs a cathartic.

4. Cathartics, such as castor oil or milk of magnesia, help eliminate any remaining barium from the child's system.

5. Barium may absorb water in the colon and solidify feces, causing constipation and impaction.

6. Liberal fluid intake promotes the elimination of barium from the child's system.

Documentation checklist
After the procedure, document:
❏ child's status
❏ bowel sounds
❏ bowel movements.

Part 13

Home health care

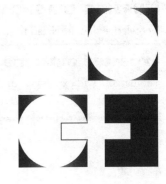

Antibacterial or antifungal therapy

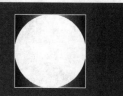

INTRODUCTION

Long-term home antibacterial or antifungal therapy is sometimes necessary to treat infection (such as pulmonary infection, cystic fibrosis, human immunodeficiency virus infection, and osteomyelitis), even after a prolonged hospital stay. This plan focuses on the care required for children on home I.M. or I.V. therapy. The parents or another caregiver, such as a home health nurse, may provide the care.

ASSESSMENT

Respiratory
• Wheezing
• Dyspnea
Integumentary
• Rash
• Hives
• Urticaria
• Elevated temperature.

NURSING DIAGNOSIS

Impaired tissue integrity related to bacterial or fungal infection

Expected outcome

The child will maintain tissue integrity as evidenced by decreases in temperature, white blood cell count, heart rate, and (if the infection is localized) purulent drainage and odor.

Interventions

1. If appropriate, instruct the parents to administer medications I.V. (through an I.V. access by continuous infusion or intermittent infusion with a heparin lock) instead of I.M. during the course of therapy.

2. Make sure the parents know to administer medications around the clock, as indicated.

3. Inform the parents that the home health nurse will routinely monitor the child's blood work (including the complete blood count, erythrocyte sedimentation rate, and any necessary bacterial or fungal cultures) and assess vital signs and affected body systems daily or every 2 days, as indicated.

Rationales

1. Using the I.V. route, when appropriate, alleviates the trauma, anxiety, and pain sometimes associated with I.M. administration.

2. Administering medications around the clock helps maintain appropriate serum levels, helping to ensure optimal bacteriostatic or fungistatic action.

3. Routine monitoring and assessment help determine the need for dosage adjustments or the discontinuation of therapy.

NURSING DIAGNOSIS

Knowledge deficit related to home care

Expected outcome

The parents will express an understanding of home care instructions and will demonstrate any home care procedures.

Interventions

1. Teach the parents how to:
- flush a heparin lock
- prime and administer medications with or without an infusion pump
- care for an I.V. dressing
- care for injection sites (if medications are given I.M.)
- administer I.M. injections.

2. Teach the parents the importance of:
- gathering all supplies ahead of time
- inspecting the I.V. access device for patency
- double-checking all medications for correct dose
- checking for any unusual color or precipitates in solutions
- preparing the administration set
- setting the infusion pump for the desired rate (if applicable)
- swabbing the cap of the heparin lock system with alcohol or iodine, inserting the needle into the cap, and securing the needle with tape (if applicable).

3. Review with the parents the potential adverse effects of each prescribed medication.

Rationales

1. The parents need to know how to perform these tasks to provide proper home care, especially if the child requires daily medication administration and a home health nurse is unavailable.

2. Gathering supplies ahead of time and taking the time to prepare for the administration procedure help prevent mistakes that can cause adverse reactions.

3. Knowing the potential adverse effects should prompt the parents to seek medical help when necessary.

Documentation checklist

During the home care session, document:
- ❏ child's status
- ❏ child's response to antibiotic or antifungal therapy
- ❏ adverse reactions to medications
- ❏ I.V. or I.M. site used.

Colostomy and ileostomy

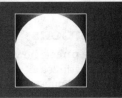

INTRODUCTION

Colostomy is the surgical creation of an opening between the colon and the outside surface of the body. Ileostomy is the surgical creation of an opening into the ileum.

Children require ostomies for various reasons, including congenital anomalies (such as imperforate anus, intestinal atresia, or Hirschsprung's disease) or some other disease or condition (such as necrotizing enterocolitis, ulcerative colitis, or trauma from an automobile accident).

ASSESSMENT

Gastrointestinal
• Brown or brownish green stool
• Normal stool consistency (loose stools with an ileostomy; formed stools with a colostomy)

Integumentary
• Pinkish or pale red skin at the stoma site
• Moist mucous membranes forming the stoma
• Intact skin around the stoma site.

NURSING DIAGNOSIS

Impaired skin integrity related to exposure of skin to stool

Expected outcome

The child will have no signs of impaired skin integrity as evidenced by intact periostomal skin.

Interventions

1. Tell the parents (and child, if appropriate) to use a properly fitting ostomy bag and to secure it to the skin with a skin barrier (such as Hollihesive, Stomahesive, or Comfed) to prevent leakage from the bag. For an infant, instruct the parents to apply the bag before diapering.

2. Instruct the parents to check the ostomy bag for leakage every 2 hours and to change the bag as soon as they suspect or note leakage.

3. Teach the parents the importance of emptying the ostomy bag when it is one-fourth to one-third full.

4. Tell the parents to change the ostomy bag at least every 24 hours until the skin heals (usually within 1 to 3 days).

5. Teach the parents how to clean the skin around the stoma using water or normal saline solution.

6. If skin breakdown (marked by redness or excoriation) occurs, instruct the parents to treat the skin using the method and medications ordered by the doctor, enterostomal therapist, and ostomy nurse.

Rationales

1. Using a properly fitting bag and an effective skin barrier protects the skin from the caustic effects of stool. An enterostomal therapist can advise the parents on which product would best suit the child's needs. Diapering without a bag usually causes skin breakdown.

2. Prolonged contact of skin with stool increases the risk of skin breakdown.

3. Allowing the bag to become too full increases the risk of leakage because the weight of the stool pulls against and breaks the seal.

4. Daily changing allows for frequent observation and treatment, when necessary.

5. Removing stool from the skin surface prevents irritation.

6. The degree of skin breakdown determines the specific treatment required.

NURSING DIAGNOSIS

Risk for infection related to contamination of incision with stool

Expected outcome

The child will remain free from infection as evidenced by maintaining a normal temperature and having no signs of erythema, induration, or drainage from the incision.

Interventions

1. Instruct the parents (and child, if appropriate) to change the ostomy bag daily until the incision heals (if the bag covers the incision). Tell them to change the ostomy bag immediately if they note or suspect leakage (especially important if the skin barrier and bag partially or completely cover the incision).

2. Make sure the parents understand that they should assess the incision for signs of infection — including redness, skin breakdown, purulent drainage — and elevated body temperature, whenever they change the bag.

Rationales

1. Daily changing allows for frequent observation of the incision for signs of contamination and infection. Leakage permits prolonged contact of skin with stool, which can lead to skin breakdown and infection.

2. Regular assessment allows for early detection and prompt treatment of infection.

NURSING DIAGNOSIS

Altered nutrition: less than body requirements related to colostomy or ileostomy

Expected outcome

The child will maintain adequate nutritional intake as evidenced by eating at least 80% of all meals.

Interventions

1. Instruct the parents to serve the child small, frequent meals.

2. Stress the importance of limiting or eliminating foods from the child's diet that cause gas or diarrhea, including cabbage, spicy foods, beans, brussels sprouts, and fruits or fruit juices.

Rationales

1. Serving the child small, frequent meals ensures that he receives adequate nutrition without overfilling his stomach.

2. Limiting or eliminating these foods helps prevent gas, which can cause distention and disinterest in eating.

NURSING DIAGNOSIS

Constipation related to water absorption

Expected outcome

The child will have normal bowel elimination as evidenced by soft bowel movements and lack of pain during elimination.

Colostomy irrigation

When irrigating an ostomy, perform the irrigation at the same time each day, allowing 1 hour for the entire procedure. Proceed as follows:

• Fill the irrigation bag with warm water or another solution as instructed by the doctor or enterostomal therapist. Use warm water — not cold — to decrease the risk of cramping.

• Fasten an irrigation sleeve around the stoma, and place the end of the sleeve in the toilet. This lets the irrigation solution drain directly into the toilet.

• Before inserting the 1⅛" to 1⅝" plastic irrigation tube into the stoma, dilate the stomal opening with a lubricated, gloved finger and apply lubricant to the tube (this helps prevent forcing the tube into the stoma and possibly perforating the bowel). Then insert the tube.

• After the tube is in place, begin instilling the solution. Reduce the rate if cramping occurs. Hold the irrigation cone against the stomal opening to prevent the water from flowing back into the irrigation bag.

• Let most of the fluid drain into the toilet (this usually takes about 10 to 15 minutes). After draining, close the end of the sleeve and instruct the child to wear the bag for another hour. Tell him to move around during this time to help the rest of the solution drain into the bag.

• After the colostomy has completely drained, remove the irrigation bag and apply an ostomy bag and skin barrier to contain any feces produced later in the day.

Interventions

1. Tell the parents (and child, if appropriate) to irrigate the colostomy or ileostomy early in the morning (see *Colostomy irrigation*).

2. Provide a high-fiber diet.

3. Increase the child's fluid intake, as ordered.

Rationales

1. Irrigation early in the morning empties the bowel and helps prevent constipation later in the day.

2. A high-fiber diet increases stool bulk, helping to prevent constipation.

3. Increased fluid intake increases the water content of stools, promoting normal elimination.

NURSING DIAGNOSIS

Body image disturbance related to colostomy or ileostomy

Expected outcome

The child will demonstrate an improved self-concept as evidenced by talking about the colostomy or ileostomy, changing the bag, and showing increased interest in self-care.

Interventions

1. Encourage the child to participate in self-care. Advise him to change or rinse the ostomy bag at least daily to prevent odor.

2. Encourage the child to express his feelings.

3. Encourage the child to join an age-appropriate ostomy support group.

Rationales

1. Such encouragement promotes continued interest in hygiene and personal appearance, helping to improve the child's self-concept. Changing or rinsing the bag daily helps prevent foul odors that can make the child self-conscious.

2. Allowing the child to express his feelings helps him face his altered body image without fear of rejection.

3. Group support promotes acceptance and allows the child to share experiences with others in similar situations.

Documentation checklist

During the home care session, document:
❑ condition of the stoma site
❑ elimination pattern
❑ nutritional intake
❑ fluid intake and output
❑ comments by the child or family.

Mechanical ventilation

INTRODUCTION

Mechanical ventilation is a means of artificially controlling or assisting respiration. In home care, it usually involves a volume-cycled or pressure-cycled ventilator that has been somewhat modified for home use. Conditions that require ventilatory assistance include bronchopulmonary dysplasia, coma, and musculoskeletal disorders.

ASSESSMENT

Respiratory
• Normal respiratory rate and rhythm
• Clear breath sounds
• Absence of crackles or rhonchi

Cardiovascular
• Normal heart rate and rhythm

Neurologic
• Quietness
• Level of consciousness appropriate to diagnosis: opens eyes, moves, or blinks eyes on command

Integumentary
• Pale pink color
• Brisk capillary refill time

NURSING DIAGNOSIS

Ineffective breathing pattern related to possible airway obstruction

Expected outcome

The child will maintain effective breathing as evidenced by the absence of respiratory distress.

Interventions

1. Explain to the parents the importance of using humidified oxygen for ventilation.

2. Instruct the parents to preoxygenate and hyperventilate the child with 100% oxygen for 30 to 60 minutes before suctioning.

3. Instruct the parents to instill 0.5 ml of normal saline solution into the endotracheal tube before suctioning.

4. Explain that the child should be suctioned only if he is dyspneic or gurgling.

5. Teach the parents how to monitor the child's heart rate (using a stethoscope or home cardiac monitor) and assess his color during suctioning.

6. Instruct the parents to change the child's tracheostomy tube, as ordered (usually once weekly) or whenever plugging occurs. Tell them to keep two or three extra tubes on hand at all times.

Rationales

1. Moist, warm air prevents the thickening of mucous secretions.

2. Preoxygenation may prevent hypoxia associated with suctioning. Hyperventilation opens the alveoli and decreases the risk of atelectasis.

3. Instilling saline solution may help liquefy thickened secretions.

4. Suctioning may cause such complications as bleeding, decreased oxygen saturation rate, and increased intracranial pressure and should be performed only when necessary.

5. Such monitoring and assessment may reveal arrhythmias or hypoxemia, potential complications of suctioning.

6. Weekly tube changes decrease the risk of plugging. Dyspnea that does not improve with suctioning indicates the need for emergency tube replacement.

7. Instruct the parents to administer aerosol bronchodilators and perform chest physiotherapy, as ordered.

8. Teach the parents to assess the child's respiratory status every 4 to 8 hours. Most parents receive help from a home health nurse in such assessments.

7. Bronchodilators help relieve bronchospasms. Chest physiotherapy loosens and mobilizes mucous secretions.

8. Frequent assessments allow evaluation of the effectiveness of care. Even if receiving help from a home health nurse, the parents or primary caregiver should be able to assess the child's respiratory status and detect complications.

Nursing diagnosis

Risk for injury (tracheal trauma) related to tracheostomy tube movement and suctioning

Expected outcome

The child will suffer minimal tracheal trauma as evidenced by pink, intact tissue around the tracheostomy and the absence of bleeding during suctioning.

Interventions

1. Tell the parents to secure the ventilator circuit to the tracheostomy tube by tying it in place and to clip the circuit to the child's clothing.

2. Instruct the parents to hold the tracheostomy tube in place when changing tracheostomy ties.

3. Teach the parents to monitor for signs of erosion, such as evidence of bleeding, through surrounding tissue.

Rationales

1. Securing the circuit avoids unnecessary manipulation of the tracheostomy and decreases any tension on the tube that could lead to dislodgment.

2. Holding the tube in place during tie changes minimizes trauma to the trachea.

3. Pressure from the tracheostomy may erode the tissue, causing bleeding and possible hemorrhage.

Nursing diagnosis

Risk for impaired skin integrity related to moisture accumulation and tube manipulation

Expected outcome

The child will maintain normal skin integrity as evidenced by pink skin coloring and the absence of erythema.

Interventions

1. Instruct the parents to change the child's tracheostomy ties whenever they become wet and to observe the skin for rash, redness, and swelling.

2. Tell the parents to place a shoulder roll or a rolled towel under the shoulder.

3. Have the parents clean the tracheostomy site with cotton-tipped applicators saturated in hydrogen peroxide and rinse with saline solution or sterile water. Tell them to avoid getting solution into the stoma.

Rationales

1. Continuous exposure to moisture may cause the skin around the tracheostomy to break down. Redness, rash, or swelling may indicate stomal infection.

2. A shoulder roll or rolled towel extends the neck and decreases the risk of skin irritation from the tracheostomy tube.

3. Proper cleaning rids the tracheostomy site of secretions and prevents skin irritation.

NURSING DIAGNOSIS

Impaired gas exchange related to respiratory disorder

Expected outcome

The child will maintain normal gas exchange as evidenced by a capillary refill time of 3 to 5 seconds, an oxygen saturation level above 90%, and pink mucous membranes.

Interventions

1. Tell the parents to observe the child for symmetric chest wall movement and to auscultate for bilateral breath sounds.

2. Have the parents monitor the child's heart rate, respiratory rate, and oxygen saturation level (if the home ventilator level device is capable of such monitoring). Otherwise, tell them to monitor the child's skin color, capillary refill time, and mucus production.

3. Instruct the parents to ventilate the child using a hand-held resuscitation bag if he has signs and symptoms of hypoxia.

Rationales

1. Symmetric chest movements indicate that the child is receiving adequate ventilation. A decreased pitch over a lung field may indicate atelectasis.

2. Cyanosis, decreased oxygen saturation level, and increased respiratory rate, capillary refill time, and mucus production indicate hypoxia.

3. Manual ventilation provides adequate ventilation until the unit's circuit can be checked.

NURSING DIAGNOSIS

Risk for infection (stoma or lower respiratory tract) related to the artificial airway

Expected outcome

The child will remain free from infection as evidenced by the absence of foul odor and purulent drainage from the stoma and the absence of fever, coughing, and copious sputum.

Interventions

1. Instruct the parents to clean the stoma with hydrogen peroxide once or twice daily.

2. Tell the parents to suction the child using clean technique. Make sure they understand the need to avoid excessive handling of the suction catheter and to keep the catheter from dropping or touching bed linens.

Rationales

1. Routine cleaning removes surface bacteria, helping to prevent infection.

2. Clean, rather than sterile, technique is adequate for home care because pathogens are less common in the home setting.

NURSING DIAGNOSIS

Altered growth and development related to dependence on mechanical ventilation

Expected outcome

The child will grow and develop normally as evidenced by achieving developmental milestones.

Interventions

1. Explain to the parents the need to provide the child with developmentally appropriate toys and activities.

2. Tell the parents to maintain eye contact when talking or reading to the child.

3. Help the parents develop a communication board for the older child who cannot speak because of his tracheostomy or ventilator dependence. A younger child may use pictures to help him communicate.

Rationales

1. Developmentally appropriate toys and activities encourage normal growth and development without frustrating the child.

2. Watching mouth movements while listening to speech enhances the child's language skills.

3. A communication board or pictures allows the child to express his needs and feelings, which is essential to normal development.

NURSING DIAGNOSIS

Altered nutrition: less than body requirements related to aspiration

Expected outcome

The child will maintain adequate nutritional intake as evidenced by an appropriate weight gain and absence of vomiting.

Interventions

1. When feeding the child, tell the parents to position him upright with his head flexed slightly forward.

2. Instruct the parents to add blue food coloring to foods if they suspect aspiration.

3. Instruct the parents to immediately notify the doctor if they note or suspect aspiration.

Rationales

1. This position promotes swallowing, helping to ensure adequate intake and decreasing the risk of aspiration.

2. This allows for easy identification of aspiration (blue tracheal secretions indicate aspiration).

3. The child may require nasogastric tube feedings to prevent aspiration while ensuring that he receives adequate nutrition.

NURSING DIAGNOSIS

Altered family processes related to the child's increased needs and the continual presence of health care personnel in the home

Expected outcome

The family will suffer only minor disruptions in family processes as evidenced by the ability to carry out activities of daily living and to maintain contacts outside the immediate family.

Interventions

1. Encourage the parents to establish house rules (such as a time schedule and smoking policy) by which all health care personnel must abide.

2. Advise the parents to set aside specific times for family interaction and for interaction with the child's siblings.

Rationales

1. House rules help ensure that the family maintains control of their home.

2. Caring for a ventilator-dependent child may cause the parents to lose sight of their own needs and the needs of their other children. Regularly scheduled family time and time with their other children promotes family unity and reinforces normal family processes.

3. Encourage the discussion of caregiving roles and responsibilities among the parents and other family members.

4. Encourage the training of responsible adults outside the immediate family to act as the child's caregivers.

5. Encourage the child's siblings to participate in his care.

3. Clearly defining and discussing the roles and responsibilities of each caregiver helps prevent family conflict.

4. Training others to provide respite care allows the parents and other family members time away from the ventilator-dependent child without feeling guilty or insecure.

5. Such participation increases the siblings' sense of control and involvement and can help improve the relationship between the child and his siblings.

Documentation checklist

During the home care session, document:
- child's ongoing status
- ventilator settings
- signs and symptoms of infection
- vital signs
- respiratory status
- parent's and child's concerns.

Peritoneal dialysis

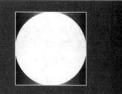

INTRODUCTION

A child receiving treatment for acute or chronic renal failure, acute renal disease (such as glomerulonephritis), or poisoning may need home peritoneal dialysis to remove impurities from the blood and to maintain normal electrolyte levels.

Usually, home peritoneal dialysis involves continuous ambulatory peritoneal dialysis (CAPD) or cycled peritoneal dialysis. CAPD, which can take place any time during waking hours, allows the child to remain ambulatory throughout the dialysis treatment. Cycled peritoneal dialysis, a more convenient method, relies on a dialysis machine to instill and drain dialysate during the night while the child sleeps.

ASSESSMENT

Respiratory
• Increased shallow respirations
Cardiovascular
• Increased heart rate
• Decreased blood pressure
Gastrointestinal
• Abdominal distention, tightness, or pain
• Anorexia
• Nausea, vomiting
• Decreased bowel sounds
Genitourinary
• Decreased urine output
Integumentary
• Elevated temperature
Psychosocial
• Depression
• Anger
• Overprotective parents

NURSING DIAGNOSIS

Knowledge deficit related to home care

Expected outcome

The parents will express an understanding of home care instructions and demonstrate any home care procedures.

Interventions

1. Instruct the parents on the importance of good hand-washing technique.

2. Teach the parents the following guidelines:
• Before administering the dialysate solution, make sure it is the right solution and that the fluid is clear.
• Make sure that all clamps are open to the dialysis catheter and that all drainage clamps are closed.
• Begin infusing the solution at the prescribed rate. If the solution is not running well, try repositioning the child.
• Monitor for signs of cramping. If cramping occurs, slow the infusion rate.
• After the infusion is complete, clamp the infusion lines and leave them in the peritoneal cavity for 15 to 20 minutes.
• Open the drainage catheters and let them drain for 5 to 10 minutes.

Rationales

1. Proper hand washing decreases the risk of infection.

2. Following these guidelines ensures that the child receives the proper amount of dialysate solution to remove impurities from the blood.

3. If appropriate, teach the parents the purpose of and procedure for CAPD. Explain that the procedure is like that performed in the hospital, except for the following:
• The procedure must be performed three or four times in a 24-hour period.
• The solution must remain in the peritoneum for several hours.
• The child must wear a drainage bag at the waist.
• The solution will be drained when the dwelling time is complete.

4. If appropriate, teach the parents the purpose of and procedure for cycled peritoneal dialysis. Explain that the procedure is like that performed in the hospital, except the catheter is hooked to the machine as well as the drainage bag and the machine cycles automatically during the night.

5. Teach the parents to monitor the child daily for signs and symptoms of peritoneal infection, including an enlarging abdomen, fever, and abdominal pain.

6. Explain the importance of using a 1:2 solution of hydrogen peroxide in water to clean any exudate from around the catheter site.

7. Teach the parents to monitor the child's daily fluid intake and output.

8. Teach the parents the purpose and use of all prescribed medications; include details on administration, dosage, and potential adverse reactions.

3. CAPD accomplishes the same function as regular peritoneal dialysis, yet allows the child to remain ambulatory throughout the dialysis procedure.

4. Cycled peritoneal dialysis allows the child greater freedom during the day and eliminates the need to disconnect the catheter periodically during the infiltration time.

5. Peritoneal infection may result from the introduction of bacteria into the abdominal cavity through the catheter.

6. Exudate buildup promotes bacterial infection and skin breakdown.

7. Such monitoring lets them determine the amount of urine produced; urine output directly indicates kidney functioning.

8. Understanding the purpose and use of all medications helps ensure compliance with the medication regimen. Knowing the potential adverse reactions should prompt parents to seek medical help when necessary.

Nursing diagnosis

Altered growth and development related to chronic illness

Expected outcome

The child will grow and develop normally as evidenced by maintaining social contacts and achieving developmental milestones.

Interventions

1. Encourage the parents to allow the child's peers to visit him at home.

2. Advise the parents to encourage the child to continue with his school work.

Rationales

1. Contact with peers helps the child maintain social ties and encourages the development of age-appropriate skills.

2. Keeping up with school assignments lets the child advance with his classmates.

Documentation checklist

During the home care session, document:
❏ child's ongoing status
❏ abdominal girth
❏ fluid intake and output
❏ amount of dialysate instilled and drained
❏ catheterization site
❏ parent's and child's concerns.

Total parenteral nutrition

INTRODUCTION

A child who cannot gain or maintain optimal weight on enteral feedings alone may require total parenteral nutrition (TPN). TPN involves the infusion of a solution of dextrose, proteins, electrolytes, vitamins, and trace elements in amounts that exceed the child's energy expenditure, thus achieving anabolism. Because of the solution's concentration, TPN must be delivered into a high-flow central vein to avoid injury to the peripheral vasculature.

ASSESSMENT

Gastrointestinal
• Weight gain
Genitourinary
• Adequate urine output
Integumentary
• Good skin turgor
• Insertion site that is free from swelling or redness

NURSING DIAGNOSIS

Altered nutrition: less than body requirements related to ongoing disease

Expected outcome

The child will maintain adequate nutritional intake as evidenced by stable or increased weight and good skin turgor.

Interventions

1. Instruct the parents to monitor the child's daily fluid intake (including oral and parenteral feedings) and output.
2. Instruct the parents to maintain a weekly weight record.

Rationales

1. Such monitoring directly indicates the child's fluid status and nutritional intake.

2. A weekly weight record shows if the child is maintaining or gaining weight, an indicator of adequate nutrition.

NURSING DIAGNOSIS

Risk for infection related to use of central venous catheter (CVC)

Expected outcome

The child will have no signs of CVC-related sepsis as evidenced by maintaining a body temperature between 97.6° and 99° F (36.4° and 37.2° C), the absence of chills, and an age-appropriate white blood cell count.

Interventions

1. Teach the parents how to follow aseptic technique when performing dressing changes and when connecting and disconnecting the CVC.

2. Instruct the parents to monitor the child's urine glucose level daily.

Rationales

1. Aseptic technique minimizes the risk of introducing bacteria into the CVC.

2. Glucose in the urine may indicate early systemic infection as well as intolerance to the rate of administration or concentration of the TPN solution.

3. Review with the parents the signs and symptoms of infection, including redness, exudate, edema, tenderness, and elevated temperature.

4. Instruct the parents to cover the I.V. site when bathing the child.

5. Explain to the parents the importance of turning the child's head and wearing a mask when changing the child's dressing.

3. Knowing the signs and symptoms of infection should prompt the parents to seek medical help when necessary.

4. Moisture can increase the risk of bacterial infection.

5. These measures help prevent the spread of infection through airborne contaminants.

NURSING DIAGNOSIS

Anxiety (child and parent) related to procedure

Expected outcome

The parents and child will be less anxious as evidenced by demonstrating a degree of comfort with the TPN procedure and by expressing an acceptance of the child's condition.

Interventions

1. Develop a schedule with the home health nurse that gradually reduces the frequency of home care visits.

2. Make sure a primary care nurse is assigned to the family to act as a liaison for information and follow-up care.

3. Encourage the child (if appropriate) to care for his catheter and to participate in other self-care activities.

4. Encourage the family to use cycled infusion therapy (infusing TPN solutions at designated intervals, such as during the night while the child sleeps) when possible.

5. Introduce the parents to the parents of other children undergoing TPN therapy.

Rationales

1. Gradually reducing the frequency of visits (instead of abruptly stopping all visits) allows the family to perform the procedure independently for increasing intervals, helping to increase their confidence and lessen their anxiety.

2. Assigning one nurse to the family ensures that they receive consistent attention and care, which should ease their anxiety.

3. Performing self-care activities helps the child develop a sense of control over his situation, helping to decrease his anxiety.

4. Cycled therapy allows the family to maintain some aspects of their usual lifestyle, helping to ease their anxiety.

5. Meeting other parents who have children undergoing TPN provides a sense of support and helps the parents find ways of dealing with their altered lifestyle.

NURSING DIAGNOSIS

Knowledge deficit related to home care

Expected outcome

The parents will express an understanding of home care instructions and will demonstrate any home care procedures.

Interventions

1. Explain to the parents the purpose of all equipment (including infusion pumps, I.V. pole, infusion tubing, TPN fluid, I.V. fat emulsion, and ancillary supplies), and demonstrate their use.

2. Review with the parents the proper procedures for:
• hand washing
• infusing the TPN solution at the prescribed rate
• maintaining the infusion cycle time
• monitoring the infusion pump
• recording the child's intake and output
• manipulating the infusion tubing
• caring for and troubleshooting the CVC
• changing dressings.

3. Teach the parents the following emergency procedures:
• If the catheter breaks, clamp the line.
• If air gets in the I.V. line, aspirate the air.
• If the child is bleeding from the catheter site, assess the site and, if the bleeding is excessive, apply pressure.

4. Explain to the parents the importance of flushing the system with saline solution if the TPN solution does not properly flow through the catheter. Emphasize that if the solution still does not flow properly after flushing, they should stop the infusion and notify the doctor.

Rationales

1. Such explanations and demonstrations familiarize the parents with the function and design of all equipment so that they will know how to use it when caring for the child at home.

2. Reviewing these procedures reinforces the parents' understanding of TPN and helps ensure their compliance with the treatment regimen.

3. Knowing how to respond in an emergency helps the parents prevent serious complications.

4. Flushing with saline solution may be necessary to clear an obstructed catheter.

Documentation checklist

During the home care session, document:
❑ child's ongoing status
❑ catheterization site
❑ vital signs
❑ signs and symptoms of infection
❑ parent's and child's concerns.

Tracheostomy

INTRODUCTION

A tracheostomy is a surgically created opening into the trachea that provides a patent airway to bypass upper airway obstruction, ensure long-term ventilatory support, or clear mucous secretions from the airway. Indications for tracheostomy include bronchopulmonary dysplasia, subglottic stenosis, and respiratory distress.

ASSESSMENT

Respiratory
- Crackles
- Rhonchi
- Respiratory distress
- Stridor
- Purulent mucus
- Difficulty passing tracheal suctioning catheter
- Cyanosis

Integumentary
- Redness around the stoma
- Purulent drainage
- Elevated temperature

NURSING DIAGNOSIS

Impaired skin integrity related to humidity, moisture, or mucus accumulations

Expected outcome

The child will have good skin integrity as evidenced by maintaining intact skin with no signs of redness, swelling, or fever.

Interventions

1. Instruct the parents (and child, if appropriate) to clean the tracheostomy site with hydrogen peroxide every 8 hours or as needed.

2. Tell the parents to keep the child's neck dry and to remove secretions, as needed.

3. Tell the parents to change the tracheostomy ties daily or as needed.

4. Have the parents change or clean the suction canister, nebulizer, and other equipment every 48 hours or as needed.

5. Stress the importance of cleaning the inner cannula every 8 hours using sterile technique.

Rationales

1. Frequent cleaning decreases the irritating effects of secretions on the skin.

2. Moisture causes irritation that may lead to skin breakdown.

3. Wet ties irritate the skin and provide a warm, moist environment in which infection may develop.

4. Routine changing and cleaning of equipment decreases the risk of skin breakdown that can lead to infection.

5. Frequent cleaning of the inner cannula using sterile technique decreases the risk of bacterial infiltration that can lead to skin breakdown and infection.

Nursing diagnosis

Ineffective breathing patterns related to tracheal tube dislodgment or plugging

Expected outcome

The child will maintain normal breathing patterns as evidenced by bilaterally equal respirations, pink and moist mucous membranes, and the absence of dyspnea, coughing, and choking.

Interventions

1. To prevent tube dislodgment, instruct the parents to tie the tracheostomy ties snugly in knots, not bows. Have them check the ties at least every 8 hours.

2. Tell the parents to make sure the new ties are in place before removing the old ties. Also explain that two people should change the ties whenever possible.

3. Emphasize the importance of keeping a spare tracheostomy tube and scissors near the child at all times.

4. Instruct the parents to change the tracheostomy tube at least monthly (preferably weekly).

5. Have the parents assess the color, amount, consistency, and odor of secretions every 8 hours. Tell them to notify the doctor of any significant changes in secretions.

6. Instruct the parents to suction the child with a bulb syringe or catheter, as needed, if the child gurgles, has difficulty breathing, or produces large amounts of secretions.

7. Have the parents instill 0.5 ml of normal saline solution directly into the tracheostomy tube, as needed, to loosen thick secretions.

8. Have the parents encourage the older child to cough up secretions.

9. Explain the importance of assessing the child's breath sounds before and after suctioning.

10. Instruct the parents to provide humidified air or oxygen, as needed.

11. Tell the parents to instill one or two drops of normal saline solution into the tracheostomy tube, as needed, when the child is away from the humidification source.

12. Tell the parents to encourage the child to drink two to eight 8-oz (240-ml) glasses of fluid (depending on the child's age) unless otherwise restricted.

Rationales

1. Bows can easily loosen or untie, increasing the risk of tube dislodgment and respiratory distress.

2. Making sure the new ties are in place before removing the old ties decreases the risk of accidental tube dislodgment. Two people can change the ties more efficiently than one, especially if the child tends to cough or move.

3. This allows for immediate replacement in case of plugging or accidental tube dislodgment.

4. A clean tube decreases the risk of plugging and infection.

5. Thick, copious secretions increase the risk of plugging and indicate the need for increased fluids or humidity or both. A change in color or odor may indicate infection.

6. A bulb syringe removes secretions from the upper portion of the trachea without causing tracheal trauma. A catheter allows for deep suctioning.

7. Loose secretions are easier to expectorate or suction.

8. Coughing decreases the need for suctioning and the risk of tracheal trauma.

9. Such assessment lets the parents evaluate whether the suctioning effectively cleared secretions.

10. Humidification liquefies secretions and helps decrease respiratory distress. Most children require some humidification as long as they have a tracheostomy in place; however, they usually do not need continuous humidification after the first few postoperative days.

11. Normal saline solution helps to keep secretions loose and moist for easy removal, decreasing the risk of respiratory distress.

12. Adequate fluid intake keeps secretions moist and loose for easy removal, decreasing the risk of respiratory distress.

NURSING DIAGNOSIS

Risk for injury (poor oxygenation) related to suctioning procedure

Expected outcome

The child will remain free from injury as evidenced by maintaining good skin color, clear bilateral breath sounds, and adequate oxygen saturation level (if monitored) during suctioning.

Interventions

1. Instruct the parents to ventilate the child with oxygen for 30 to 60 seconds before and after suctioning, if needed.

2. Instruct the parents to keep the catheter in place no longer than 15 seconds when suctioning the child.

3. Tell the parents to use the correct size catheter when suctioning the child (usually one-half the diameter of the tracheostomy tube).

Rationales

1. Supplemental oxygen helps prevent decreases in oxygen saturation from suctioning.

2. The parents should minimize the time the catheter is in place because suctioning removes oxygen along with secretions.

3. Using a catheter that is too large increases the risk of trauma to the trachea and may cause the catheter to lodge in the tracheostomy tube.

NURSING DIAGNOSIS

Risk for aspiration related to impaired swallowing and vomiting

Expected outcome

The child will not aspirate feedings as evidenced by retaining feedings without vomiting.

Interventions

1. Instruct the parents to position the child upright during feedings.

2. Have the parents suction the child as needed before giving the child any food or drink. However, tell them not to suction the child right after a feeding.

Rationales

1. Sitting upright decreases the risk of aspiration.

2. Suctioning the child right after he eats or drinks may cause irritation and vomiting.

Documentation checklist

During the home care session, document:
- ❏ child's ongoing status
- ❏ child's vital signs
- ❏ signs and symptoms of infection
- ❏ equipment settings and function
- ❏ parent's and child's concerns.

Appendices, selected references, and index

Appendix A: Normal growth and development

Use the following chart as a general guide to some major developmental milestones. If you suspect that your patient has a developmental problem, refer him for further testing with an appropriate screening tool, such as the Denver Developmental Screening Test.

	Physical development	Motor activity	Sensory ability	Social skills	Communication skills
Birth to 1 month (neonate)	• Usually weighs between 5½ and 9½ lb (2,500 and 4,300 g) at birth, gaining about 1½ lb (680 g) during the first month • Usually measures 19" to 21" (48 to 53 cm) at birth, growing about 1" (2.5 cm) during the first month • Head circumference averages 12½" to 14" (32 to 36 cm) at birth • Fontanels are open; sutures may be overriding	• Can track objects and lift head for a short time • Can grasp objects placed in hands for a short time	• Becomes startled by loud sounds • Is attentive to speech, especially mother's voice • Focuses on faces and objects when in direct line of vision	• Is completely dependent on caregivers • Establishes eye contact • Smiles briefly	• Responds to human voices • Makes small gutteral sounds • Establishes patterns of crying • Coos and expresses comfort when fed
2 to 12 months (infant)	• Experiences rapid weight gain, especially during the first 6 months, when growth averages 1½ lb per month; gains about ½ lb (340 g) per month during remaining months • Length increases an average of 1" (2.5 cm) per month during first 6 months, then ½" (1.3 cm) per month during remaining months • Head circumference increases about ½" per month during first 6 months, then ¼" (0.6 cm) per month during remaining months • Posterior fontanel closes completely at about 6 to 8 weeks	• Holds head erect and steady by 3 months • Sits upright by 7 months • Can maneuver from a prone to sitting position by 10 months • Can creep on hands and knees and maneuver while standing and holding onto furniture by 11 months	• Responds to sounds by turning to source by 4 months; responds to name by 10 months • Focuses on near objects by 5 months	• Develops sense of trust in response to having needs met • Begins developing personality • Requires continual stimulation and play • Enjoys shaking, banging, and pulling objects and demonstrating imitative behavior by 4 to 8 months • Develops stranger anxiety by 6 to 9 months	• Begins vocalizing consonants by 3 to 4 months and vowels by 4 to 6 months • Laughs aloud by 4 months • Begins mouthing words by 6 to 9 months • Associates meaning to sound, says single words, and understands the word *no* by 9 to 12 months

	Physical development	Motor activity	Sensory ability	Social skills	Communication skills
1 year	• Weight since birth triples • Length since birth increases about 50% • Head and chest circumferences are equal • Can breathe through mouth when nose is occluded • Rooting, Moro's, and tonic neck reflexes disappear • May have six to eight teeth	• Occasionally attempts to stand alone • Walks with someone holding one hand • Uses thumb and forefinger to pick up objects; pokes at objects with one finger • Sits up for prolonged time without support • Places one object after another into a container	• Responds to name • Localizes sounds; listens for sounds to recur • Eyes follow rapidly moving objects • Plays simple interactive games such as peekaboo • Explores objects by chewing and biting on them	• Is afraid of strange surroundings; clings to mother • Enjoys playing simple ball games • Shows emotions such as jealousy • Appears affectionate; hugs and kisses when asked to do so • Shakes head to signify "no" • Stops activity when told to do so	• Understands simple commands such as "wave bye-bye" • Says one or two other words besides repetitive *momma* and *dadda* • Recognizes objects by names • Imitates animal sounds
1 to 3 years (toddler)	• Anterior fontanel is closed • Able to control anal and urinary sphincters • Height and weight increase at slower rates • Birth weight quadruples by age 30 months • Arms and legs lengthen from ossification and long-bone growth • Primary dentition complete	• Goes up and down stairs alone, placing both feet on a step before climbing to next step • Jumps down steps without losing balance • Kicks ball forward without losing balance • Turns doorknobs • Rides tricycle • Holds crayon with fingers; copies crosses and circles	• Vision is 20/40; accommodation is complete • Hearing (including ability to localize sounds) fully developed	• At 15 months, feeds self with little difficulty, tolerates some separation from mother, begins imitating parents • At 24 months, feeds self well, helps undress himself, becomes possessive of toys; may achieve daytime elimination control • At 36 months, engages in parallel playing (playing in close proximity to others but without interaction), puts things away, pulls people to show them something, wants and displays increased independence from mother, begins to recognize sex differences, and knows own sex; may achieve nighttime elimination control	• From 15 to 18 months, uses own jargon—sounds that he understands but that aren't real words • By 24 months, uses 2- to 3-word phrases and correctly pronounces vowels. Has a 270- to 300-word vocabulary • By age 3, has a 900-word vocabulary and uses 4- to 5-word sentences

Appendices

	Physical development	Motor activity	Sensory ability	Social skills	Communication skills
4 to 5 years (preschooler)	• Pulse and respiratory rates and blood pressure decrease • Height and weight gains remain constant • Height since birth doubles • First permanent teeth erupt • Right- or left-handedness established	• Walks down stairs, alternating feet • Throws and catches ball well • Ties shoelace in bow by age 5 • Hops on one foot • Uses scissors well	• Visual acuity approaches 20/20 *Note:* Amblyopia most often develops at age 4	• At age 4, is very independent and aggressive; shows off and tattles on others. May have imaginary playmate; may live in fantasy world • At age 5, is less rebellious, ready to accomplish tasks at hand. Cares for himself; is independent but trustworthy. Starts to understand rules and conformity; may notice prejudices; identifies with parent of same sex • Egocentric	• At age 5, can follow three commands given in a row, asks meanings of new words, has vocabulary of 2,100 words, counts and identifies coins, uses 6- to 8-word sentences, describes drawings in detail
6 to 12 years (school-age child)	• By age 6, height and weight gains slow; dexterity increases; child is very active • By age 7, grows at least 2" (5 cm) per year; posture becomes more tense and stiff • By ages 10 to 12, height increase slows, weight gain increases; child may become obese at this age. Pubescent changes begin to appear; a girl's body lines start to become soft and rounded	• At age 6, is aware of using hand as a tool; draws, prints, and colors well • At age 7, repeats activities to become proficient at them; uses table knife • At age 8, fine motor control well developed; able to use tools such as hammers and screwdrivers	• Fully developed	• May become highly self-critical. Subject to depression if unable to live up to others' expectations • Develops a strong sense of industry • May assume independent duties and chores • Has defined ideas and attitude toward sex • Enjoys hobbies, physical activity, and sports	• Has a 2,550- to 2,600-word vocabulary • Capable of producing all the sounds in his native language (any articulation problems present at this age need special evaluation) • Uses complex sentence structure • Uses tone and new vocal patterns to express ideas • Uses words to express feelings, desires, and attitudes
13 to 18 years (adolescent)	• Experiences significant changes in bones, muscle, and adipose tissue. Hormonal changes cause shoulder breadth, arm and leg length increases in boys; hip, pelvis, and breast development in girls. *Note:* Approximately 99% of adult height is reached by age 18	• All gross and fine motor skills are developed. Activities now serve to refine motor skills	• Fully developed	• Explores emotional needs; frequent testing of parents' authority may cause barrier between child and parents • Explores sexuality • Feels strong need to conform with peers • May romanticize about daily life or fantasize about death • Begins making long-range plans	• Has an adult's proficiency with language but may frequently use slang or jargon to communicate with peers

Appendix B:
Normal vital sign measurements

The following vital sign measurements are considered normal for pediatric patients.

	Temperature	Heart rate	Respiratory rate	Blood pressure
Birth to 1 month	97° to 100° F (36.1° to 37.8° C)	70 to 180 beats/minute	30 to 80 breaths/minute	40 to 90 (systolic) 16 to 60 (diastolic)
2 months to 1 year	99.1° to 99.7° F (37.3° to 37.6° C)	80 to 160 beats/minute	30 to 60 breaths/minute	70 to 100 (systolic) 45 to 70 (diastolic)
2 to 5 years	98.5° to 99.1° F (36.9° to 37.3° C)	90 to 150 beats/minute	20 to 40 breaths/minute	75 to 115 (systolic) 45 to 80 (diastolic)
6 to 12 years	98° to 98.5° F (36.7° to 36.9° C)	60 to 100 beats/minute	15 to 30 breaths/minute	90 to 130 (systolic) 55 to 80 (diastolic)
13 to 18 years	97.6° to 97.9° F (36.4° to 36.6° C)	50 to 90 beats/minute	12 to 20 breaths/minute	90 to 140 (systolic) 50 to 90 (diastolic)

Appendices

Appendix C:
Physical growth charts

To use the growth charts on the following pages, correlate the child's age with the appropriate growth measurement (head circumference, length/height, or weight). Consider the child's growth normal if the plotted measurement falls between the 5th and 95th percentiles; consider the child's growth abnormal if it falls below the 5th or above the 95th percentile.

BOYS: BIRTH TO 36 MONTHS

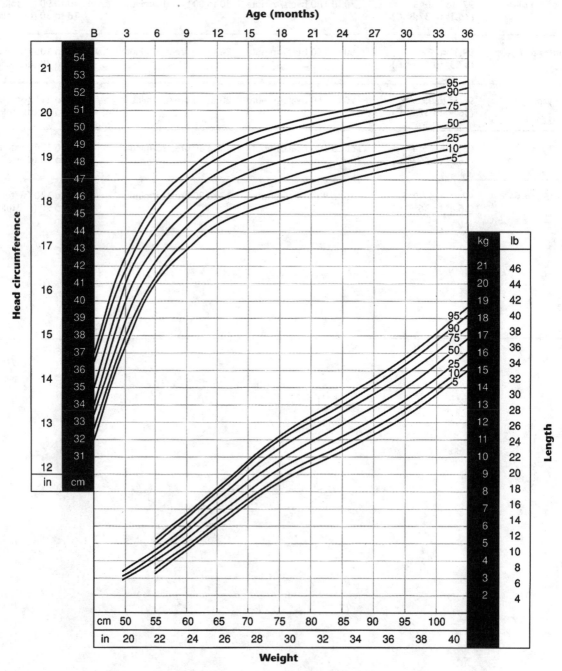

Adapted from National Center for Health Statistics. *NCHS Growth Charts*, Rockville, Md., 1976.

GIRLS: BIRTH TO 36 MONTHS

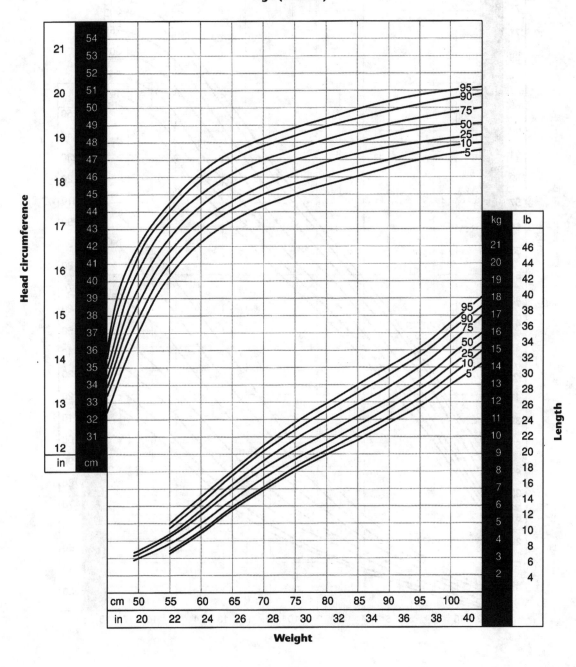

BOYS: 2 TO 18 YEARS

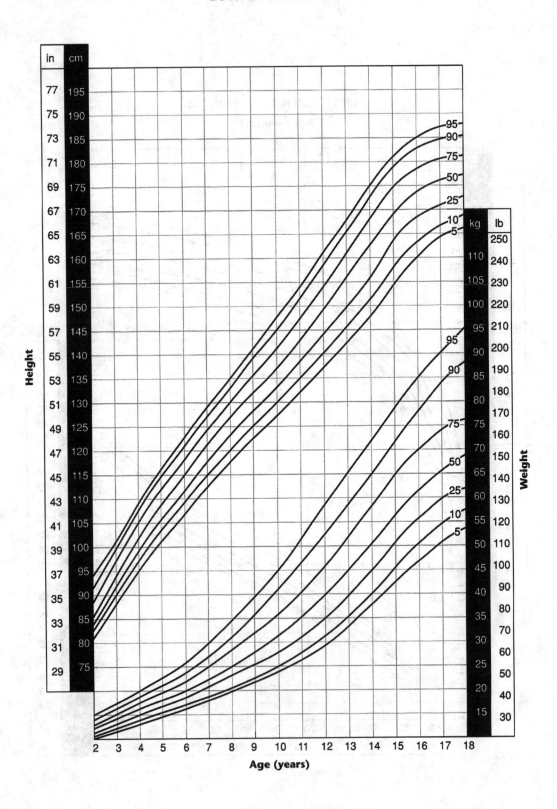

GIRLS: 2 TO 18 YEARS

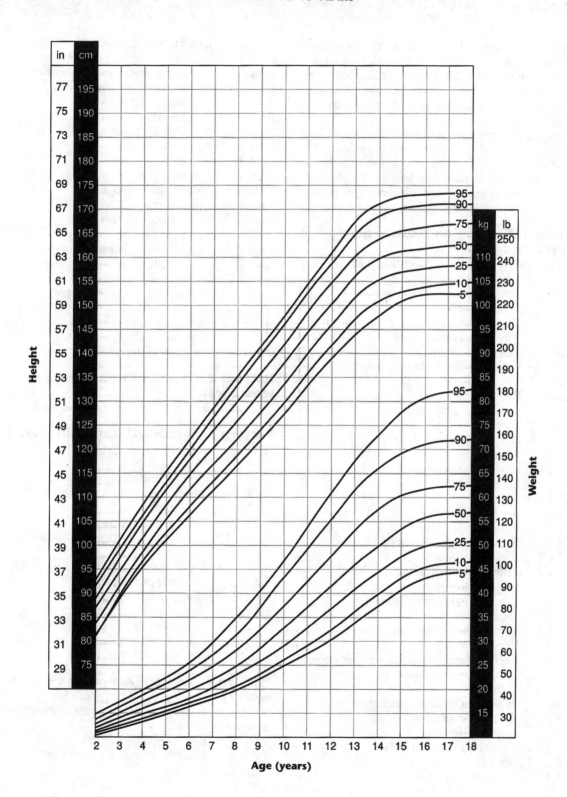

Appendix D:
NANDA taxonomy of nursing diagnoses

The currently accepted classification system for nursing diagnoses is that of the North American Nursing Diagnosis Association (NANDA). It is organized around nine human response patterns: exchanging, communicating, relating, valuing, choosing, moving, perceiving, knowing, and feeling.

The complete taxonomic structure is listed here. The series of numbers before each diagnosis is its classification number, used to determine the placement of the diagnosis within the taxonomy. The number of digits delineates the level of abstraction of the nursing diagnosis (more specific diagnoses are assigned longer numbers).

Pattern 1. Exchanging (Mutual giving and receiving)

1.1.2.1	Altered nutrition: More than body requirements
1.1.2.2	Altered nutrition: Less than body requirements
1.1.2.3	Altered nutrition: Risk for more than body requirements
1.2.1.1	Risk for infection
1.2.2.1	Risk for altered body temperature
1.2.2.2	Hypothermia
1.2.2.3	Hyperthermia
1.2.2.4	Ineffective thermoregulation
1.2.3.1	Dysreflexia
1.2.3.2	Risk for autonomic dysreflexia
1.3.1.1	Constipation
1.3.1.1.1	Perceived constipation
1.3.1.1.2	Colonic constipation
1.3.1.2	Diarrhea
1.3.1.3	Bowel incontinence
1.3.1.4	Risk for constipation
1.3.2	Altered urinary elimination
1.3.2.1.1	Stress incontinence
1.3.2.1.2	Reflex urinary incontinence
1.3.2.1.3	Urge incontinence
1.3.2.1.4	Functional urinary incontinence
1.3.2.1.5	Total incontinence
1.3.2.1.6	Risk of urinary urge incontinence
1.3.2.2	Urinary retention
1.4.1.1	Altered (specify type) tissue perfusion (renal, cerebral, cardiopulmonary, gastrointestinal, peripheral)
1.4.1.2	Risk for fluid volume imbalance
1.4.1.2.1	Fluid volume excess
1.4.1.2.2.1	Fluid volume deficit
1.4.1.2.2.2	Risk for fluid volume deficit
1.4.2.1	Decreased cardiac output
1.5.1.1	Impaired gas exchange
1.5.1.2	Ineffective airway clearance
1.5.1.3	Ineffective breathing pattern
1.5.1.3.1	Inability to sustain spontaneous ventilation
1.5.1.3.2	Dysfunctional ventilatory weaning response (DVWR)
1.6.1	Risk for injury
1.6.1.1	Risk for suffocation
1.6.1.2	Risk for poisoning
1.6.1.3	Risk for trauma
1.6.1.4	Risk for aspiration
1.6.1.5	Risk for disuse syndrome
1.6.1.6	Latex allergy
1.6.1.7	Risk for latex allergy
1.6.2	Altered protection
1.6.2.1	Impaired tissue integrity
1.6.2.1.1	Altered oral mucous membrane
1.6.2.1.2.1	Impaired skin integrity
1.6.2.1.2.2	Risk for impaired skin integrity
1.6.2.1.3	Altered dentition
1.7.1	Decreased adaptive capacity: Intracranial
1.8	Energy field disturbance

Pattern 2. Communicating (Sending messages)

2.1.1.1	Impaired verbal communication

Pattern 3. Relating (Establishing bonds)

3.1.1	Impaired social interaction
3.1.2	Social isolation
3.1.3	Risk for loneliness
3.2.1	Altered role performance
3.2.1.1.1	Altered parenting
3.2.1.1.2	Risk for altered parenting
3.2.1.1.2.1	Risk for altered parent/infant/child attachment
3.2.1.2.1	Sexual dysfunction
3.2.2	Altered family processes
3.2.2.1	Caregiver role strain
3.2.2.2	Risk for caregiver role strain
3.2.2.3.1	Altered family process: Alcoholism
3.2.3.1	Parental role conflict
3.3	Altered sexuality patterns

Pattern 4. Valuing (Assigning relative worth)

4.1.1	Spiritual distress (distress of the human spirit)
4.1.2	Risk for spiritual distress
4.2	Potential for enhanced spiritual well-being

Pattern 5. Choosing (Selecting alternatives)

5.1.1.1	Ineffective individual coping
5.1.1.1.1	Impaired adjustment
5.1.1.1.2	Defensive coping
5.1.1.1.3	Ineffective denial
5.1.2.1.1	Ineffective family coping: Disabling
5.1.2.1.2	Ineffective family coping: Compromised
5.1.2.2	Family coping: Potential for growth
5.1.3.1	Potential for enhanced community coping
5.1.3.2	Ineffective community coping
5.2.1	Ineffective management of therapeutic regimen (individuals)
5.2.1.1	Noncompliance (specify)
5.2.2	Ineffective management of therapeutic regimen: Families
5.2.3	Ineffective management of therapeutic regimen: Community
5.2.4	Effective management of therapeutic regimen: Individual
5.3.1.1	Decisional conflict (specify)
5.4	Health-seeking behaviors (specify)

Pattern 6. Moving (Involving activity)

6.1.1.1	Impaired physical mobility
6.1.1.1.1	Risk for peripheral neurovascular dysfunction
6.1.1.1.2	Risk for perioperative positioning injury
6.1.1.1.3	Impaired walking
6.1.1.1.4	Impaired wheelchair mobility
6.1.1.1.5	Impaired wheelchair transfer ability
6.1.1.1.6	Impaired bed mobility
6.1.1.2	Activity intolerance
6.1.1.2.1	Fatigue
6.1.1.3	Risk for activity intolerance
6.2.1	Sleep pattern disturbance
6.2.1.1	Sleep deprivation
6.3.1.1	Diversional activity deficit
6.4.1.1	Impaired home maintenance management
6.4.2	Altered health maintenance
6.4.2.1	Delayed surgical recovery
6.4.2.2	Adult failure to thrive
6.5.1	Feeding self-care deficit
6.5.1.1	Impaired swallowing
6.5.1.2	Ineffective breast-feeding
6.5.1.2.1	Interrupted breast-feeding
6.5.1.3	Effective breast-feeding
6.5.1.4	Ineffective infant feeding pattern
6.5.2	Bathing or hygiene self-care deficit
6.5.3	Dressing or grooming self-care deficit
6.5.4	Toileting self-care deficit
6.6	Altered growth and development
6.6.1	Risk for altered development
6.6.2	Risk for altered growth
6.7	Relocation stress syndrome

6.8.1	Risk for disorganized infant behavior
6.8.2	Disorganized infant behavior
6.8.3	Potential for enhanced organized infant behavior

Pattern 7. Perceiving (Receiving information)

7.1.1	Body image disturbance
7.1.2	Self-esteem disturbance
7.1.2.1	Chronic low self-esteem
7.1.2.2	Situational low self-esteem
7.1.3	Personal identity disturbance
7.2	Sensory or perceptual alterations (specify visual, auditory, kinesthetic, gustatory, tactile, olfactory)
7.2.1.1	Unilateral neglect
7.3.1	Hopelessness
7.3.2	Powerlessness

Pattern 8. Knowing (Associating meaning with information)

8.1.1	Knowledge deficit (specify)
8.2.1	Impaired environmental interpretation syndrome
8.2.2	Acute confusion
8.2.3	Chronic confusion
8.3	Altered thought processes
8.3.1	Impaired memory

Pattern 9. Feeling (Being subjectively aware of information)

9.1.1	Pain
9.1.1.1	Chronic pain
9.1.2	Nausea
9.2.1.1	Dysfunctional grieving
9.2.1.2	Anticipatory grieving
9.2.1.3	Chronic sorrow
9.2.2	Risk for violence: Self-directed or directed at others
9.2.2.1	Risk for self-mutilation
9.2.3	Post-trauma syndrome
9.2.3.1	Rape-trauma syndrome
9.2.3.1.1	Rape-trauma syndrome: Compound reaction
9.2.3.1.2	Rape-trauma syndrome: Silent reaction
9.2.4	Risk for post-trauma syndrome
9.3.1	Anxiety
9.3.1.1	Death anxiety
9.3.2	Fear

Appendices

Appendix E:
Normal laboratory values

Below is a listing of normal laboratory values for some commonly ordered tests.

Test	Age	Normal values
Bilirubin, serum	Birth to 1 day 1 to 2 days 2 to 5 days 5 days to 18 years	<6 mg/dl (<6 µmol/L) <8 mg/dl (<8 µmol/L) <12 mg/dl (<12 µmol/L) 0.2 to 0.7 mg/dl (0.2 to 1 µmol/L)
Chloride, serum	Birth to 1 month 1 month to 18 years	96 to 110 mEq/L (mmol/L)) 98 to 130 mEq/L (mmol/L)
Cholesterol, serum	Birth to 1 month 1 to 12 months 1 to 12 years 12 to 18 years	45 to 135 mg/dl (1.37 to 3.5 mmol/L) 70 to 175 mg/dl (1.81 to 4.53 mmol/L) 120 to 200 mg/dl (3.11 to 5.18 mmol/L) 120 to 210 mg/dl (3.11 to 5.44 mmol/L)
Glucose, serum	Birth to 1 month 2 months to 12 years 12 to 18 years	30 to 97 mg/dl (1.7 to 5 mmol/L) 60 to 100 mg/dl (3.3 to 5.5 mmol/L) 70 to 120 mg/dl (3.9 to 5.8 mmol/L)
Hematocrit	Birth to 1 month 2 to 12 months 1 to 6 years 6 to 12 years 12 to 18 years	43% to 75% (0.43 to 0.75) 28% to 41% (0.28 to 0.41) 31% to 43.5% (0.31 to 0.435) 36% to 45% (0.36 to 0.45) Males: 37% to 54% (0.37 to 0.54) Females: 36% to 47% (0.36 to 0.47)
Hemoglobin	Birth to 1 month 2 to 3 months 4 to 12 months 1 to 6 years 6 to 12 years 12 to 18 years	14 to 23 g/dl 9 to 14.5 g/dl 10 to 15 g/dl 10 to 16 g/dl 11 to 15.5 g/dl Males: 13 to 18 g/dl (2.02 to 2.48 mmol/L) Females: 11.5 to 16 g/dl (1.86 to 2.48 mmol/L)
Platelet count	Birth to 1 month 2 months to 18 years	85,000 to 450,000/mm³ (85 to 450 ×10⁹/L) 150,000 to 400,000/mm³ (150 to 400×10⁹/L)
Potassium, serum	Birth to 1 month 2 to 12 months 1 to 6 years 6 to 18 years	4 to 5.9 mEq/L (mmol/L) 4 to 5.3 mEq/L (mmol/L) 3.5 to 4.9 mEq/L (mmol/L) 3.5 to 5.2 mEq/L (mmol/L)
Sodium, serum	Birth to 1 month 2 to 12 months 1 to 6 years 12 to 18 years	124 to 146 mEq/L (mmol/L) 138 to 146 mEq/L (mmol/L) 138 to 148 mEq/L (mmol/L) 136 to 146 mEq/L (mmol/L)
Triglycerides, serum	Birth to 5 years 6 to 11 years 12 to 15 years 16 to 18 years	30 to 99 mg/dl (0.3 to 0.98 mmol/L) 31 to 114 mg/dl (0.31 to 1.14 mmol/L) 36 to 138 mg/dl (0.36 to 1.38 mmol/L) 40 to 163 mg/dl (0.4 to 1.63 mmol/L)
White blood cell count	Birth to 1 month 2 to 12 months 1 to 3 years 4 to 12 years 12 to 18 years	9,000 to 30,000/mm³ (9 to 30×10⁹ cells/L) 5,000 to 19,000/mm³ (5 to 19×10⁹ cells/L) 6,000 to 17,000/mm³ (6 to 17×10⁹ cells/L) 4,500 to 13,000/mm³ (4.5 to 13×10⁹ cells/L) 4,500 to 11,000/mm³ (4.5 to 11×10⁹ cells/L)

Appendix F: Guide to food values

Use the information below to help meet your patient's special dietary needs, keeping in mind the following daily calorie requirements: for children weighing up to 22 lb (10 kg), 100 calories/kg; for children weighing 22 to 44 lb (10 to 20 kg), 1,000 calories plus 50 calories/kg; and for children weighing more than 44 lb (20 kg), 1,500 calories plus 20 calories/kg.

HIGH-CALORIE FOODS

Food and amount	Calories	Food and amount	Calories	Food and amount	Calories	Food and amount	Calories
Apple pie (one 4" slice)	375	Cream cheese (1 oz)	105	Macaroni and cheese (1 cup)	505	Shortcake with strawberries (1 cup)	400
Avocado (1½ cups)	245	Custard (1 cup)	205	Malted milkshake (8 oz)	500	Spaghetti (1 cup, cooked)	395
Beef stew (1 cup)	530	Eggnog (8 oz)	235	Peanut butter (2 tbs)	95	Waffle (two 4" squares)	210
Chocolate cake (one 2" slice)	350	Hamburger with bun (3 oz, cooked)	330	Pumpkin pie (one 4" slice)	330		
Chocolate pudding (1 cup)	220	Ice cream shake (8 oz)	420	Raisins (2 cups)	430		

HIGH-PROTEIN FOODS

Food and amount	Protein (g)	Food and amount	Protein (g)	Food and amount	Protein (g)	Food and amount	Protein (g)
Baked beans (1 cup)	7.5	Chicken and gravy (3 oz, cooked)	22	Lima beans (½ cup)	6.5	Spareribs, pork (2½ oz, cooked)	15.5
Bean soup (½ cup)	6	Club sandwich (3 oz)	35.5	Macaroni and cheese (1 cup)	19	Split pea soup (½ cup)	7
Beef brisket (3 oz, cooked)	16	Cottage cheese (1 cup)	22	Malted milkshake (8 oz)	13	Veal cutlet (3 oz, cooked)	24
Beef stew (1 cup)	28	Haddock, fried (3 oz)	23.5	Oyster stew (1 cup)	15	Vegetable beef soup (1 cup)	6
Chicken, fried (3½ oz)	27	Hamburger with bun (3 oz, cooked)	17	Spaghetti (1 cup, cooked)	12.5		

LOW-FAT FOODS

Food and amount	Fat (g)	Food and amount	Fat (g)	Food and amount	Fat (g)	Food and amount	Fat (g)
Angel food cake (one 2" slice)	0.1	Cornflakes (1 oz)	0.1	Orange juice (8 oz)	0.2	Rye crackers (two 2" wafers)	0.1
Apple cider (8 oz)	0	Gelatin, plain (1 cup)	0	Pancake (one 4" cake)	1	Sherbet (1 cup)	0
Apple juice (8 oz)	0	Grapefruit juice (8 oz)	0.1	Peaches, canned (1 cup)	0.1	Soda, carbonated (8 oz)	0
Applesauce (1 cup)	0.2	Honeydew melon (1 cup)	0	Pears (1 cup)	0.1	Squash (1 cup)	0.1
Banana (one medium)	0.2	Jam (1 Tbsp)	0.1	Pineapple (1 cup)	0.1		
Cantaloupe (1 cup)	0.2	Milk, skim (8 oz)	0.2	Potatoes (1 cup)	0.1		
Carrots (1 cup)	0.5	Orange (one medium)	0.2	Rye bread (1 slice)	0.3		

HIGH-CALCIUM FOODS

Food and amount	Calcium (mg)	Food and amount	Calcium (mg)	Food and amount	Calcium (mg)	Food and amount	Calcium (mg)
American cheese (1 oz)	175	Macaroni and cheese (½ cup)	180	Pancakes (two 4" cakes)	120	Waffle (one 4" square)	180
Cheddar cheese (1 oz)	200	Milk, skim (8 oz)	300	Pizza (2 slices)	335	Yogurt, low-fat with fruit (1 cup)	345
Cream-style soup (1 cup)	170	Milk, whole (8 oz)	290	Swiss cheese (1 oz)	275		

LOW-SODIUM FOODS

Food and amount	Sodium (mg)	Food and amount	Sodium (mg)	Food and amount	Sodium (mg)	Food and amount	Sodium (mg)
Apple (one medium)	1	Cauliflower, cooked (1 cup)	12	Orange (one medium)	1	Tuna, canned in water (3½ oz)	40
Apple juice (8 oz)	2	Cranberry juice (8 oz)	3	Popcorn, plain (1 cup)	5		
Applesauce (1 cup)	5	Egg noodles, cooked (1 cup)	3	Potato, boiled (1 cup)	15		
Banana (one medium)	1	Flounder, baked (3½ oz)	75	Strawberries (1 cup)	1		

HIGH-FIBER FOODS

Dried peas and beans
Lentils
Navy, lima, kidney, and pinto beans

Fresh fruits and vegetables
Apples
Oranges
Peaches
Carrots
Broccoli
Peas
String beans

Whole-grain breads and cereals
Bran, oat-flake, or shredded-wheat cereal
Oatmeal
Pasta
Whole-wheat or pumpernickel bread

Selected references

Barnard, K., and Brazelton, T., eds. *Touch: The Foundation of Experience*. Madison, Conn.: International Universities Press, 1990.

Behrman, R.E., and Kliegman, R.M., eds. *Nelson Essentials of Pediatrics*, 3rd ed. Philadelphia: W.B. Saunders Co., 1996.

Burns, C., et al. *Pediatric Primary Care*. Philadelphia: W.B. Saunders Co., 1996.

Carlat, D.J., et al. "Eating Disorders in Males: A Report on 135 Patients," *American Journal of Psychiatry* 154(8):1127-32, August 1997.

Dambro, M. *Griffith's 5 Minute Clinical Consult*. Baltimore: Williams & Wilkins Co., 1997.

Diagnostic and Statistical Manual of Mental Disorders, 4th ed. Washington, D.C.: American Psychiatric Association, 1994.

Doenges, M.E., et al. *Nursing Care Plans: Guidelines for Planning and Documenting Patient Care*, 4th ed. Philadelphia: F.A. Davis Co., 1997.

Ferri, R., et al. "AIDS Update," *Clinician Reviews* 7(3):189-96, March 1997.

Flournay, J. "Incest Prevention: The Role of the Pediatric Nurse Practitioner," *Journal of Pediatric Health Care* 10(6):246-54, November-December 1996.

Fuller, B. "Meanings of Discomfort and Fussy-Irritable in Infant Pain Assessment," *Journal of Pediatric Health Care* 10(6): 255-64, November-December 1996.

Kemper, K. "A Practical Approach to Chronic Asthma Management," *Contemporary Pediatrics* 14(8):86-106, August 1997.

McCarthy, A., et al. "Children with Chronic Conditions: Educators' View," *Journal of Pediatric Health Care* 10(6):272-79, November-December 1996.

1997 Red Book: Report of the Committee on Infectious Disease, 24th ed. Elk Grove Village, Ill.: American Academy of Pediatrics, 1997.

Plaut, T. "Red Light Green Light," *Advances for Nurse Practitioners* 5(2):77-82, February 1997.

Redman, B. *The Process of Patient Education*, 8th ed. St. Louis: Mosby–Year Book, Inc., 1997.

Schwartz, M.W., et al. *Pediatric Primary Care: A Problem-Oriented Approach*, 3rd ed. St. Louis: Mosby–Year Book, Inc., 1997.

Stein, M. "Preparing Families for the Toddler and Preschool Years," *Contemporary Pediatrics* 15:88-108, 1998.

Thomson, S., and Dancey, C. "Symptoms of Irritable Bowel in School Children: Prevalence and Psychosocial Effects," *Journal of Pediatric Health Care* 10(6):380-85, November-December 1996.

"Update on the 1987 Task Force Report on High Blood Pressure in Children and Adolescents: Part 1," *Pediatrics* 98(4):649-58, October 1996.

Wagner, M., and Jacobs, J. "Improving Asthma Management with Peak Flow Meters," *Contemporary Pediatrics* 14(8):111-19, August 1997.

Wong, D. *Whaley and Wong's Essentials of Pediatric Nursing*, 5th ed. St. Louis: Mosby–Year Book, Inc., 1997.

Wong, D.L., and Baker, C.M. "Pain in Children: Comparison of Assessment Scales," *Pediatric Nursing* 14(1):9-17, January-February 1988.

Index

A

Acquired immunodeficiency syndrome, **202-204**
  assessment of, 202
  definition of, 202
  documentation checklist for, 204
  fear and, 203-204
  infection and, 202
  knowledge deficit and, 204
  self-esteem disturbance and, 203
Activity deficit, diversional
  arrhythmias and, 41-42
  congenital hip dysplasia and, 164
Activity intolerance, risk for
  fractures and, 176
  glomerulonephritis and, 144
  hepatitis and, 109
Aganglionic megacolon. *See*
  Hirschsprung's disease.
AIDS. *See* Acquired immunodeficiency syndrome.
Airway clearance, ineffective
  cleft lip and cleft palate and, 190-191
  epiglottitis and, 27
  pneumonia and, 32
Anesthesia, **254-255**
  anxiety and, 254-255
  assessment and, 254
  definition of, 254
  documentation checklist for, 255
  ineffective breathing pattern and, 255
  injury and, 255
Anorexia nervosa, **228-230**
  altered nutrition and, 228-229
  assessment of, 228
  body image disturbance and, 229
  definition of, 228
  documentation checklist for, 230
  impaired social interaction and, 230
  social isolation and, 229-230
Antibacterial or antifungal therapy, **282-283**
  assessment and, 282
  definition of, 282
  documentation checklist for, 283
  impaired tissue integrity and, 282
  knowledge deficit and, 282-283
Anxiety, **256-257**
  anesthesia and, 254-255
  assessment of, 256

Anxiety *(continued)*
  asthma and, 6
  bronchiolitis and, 11
  bronchopulmonary dysplasia and, 16
  cleft lip and cleft palate and, 190
  congenital heart defects and, 49, 54
  craniosynostosis and, 166
  croup and, 19-20
  cystic fibrosis and, 24
  definition of, 256
  documentation checklist for, 257
  epiglottitis and, 28-29
  glomerulonephritis and, 145
  head injury and, 67
  heart failure and, 59
  Hirschsprung's disease and, 114
  hydrocephalus and, 74
  hypospadias and epispadias and, 147, 149
  inflammatory bowel disease and, 117-118
  liver transplantation and, 125
  myringotomy and, 195-196
  pneumonia and, 33
  pyloric stenosis and, 129
  Reye's syndrome and, 93-94
  surgery and, 256
  total parenteral nutrition and, 295
  tracheoesophageal fistula and, 133-134
  tympanoplasty and, 198
Arnold-Chiari syndrome, 84
Arrhythmias, **40-42**
  assessment of, 40
  decreased cardiac output and, 40
  definition of, 40
  diversional activity deficit and, 41-42
  documentation checklist for, 42
  infection and, 41
  injury and, 40-41
  knowledge deficit and, 42
Arthritis, rheumatoid, **183-186**
  assessment of, 183
  body image disturbance and, 184-185
  definition of, 183
  documentation checklist for, 186
  ineffective family coping and, 185
  knowledge deficit and, 186
  pain and, 183-184
  self-care deficit and, 184

Aspiration, risk for, tracheostomy and, 299
Asthma, **2-7**. *See also* Bronchiolitis.
  altered nutrition and, 3, 6
  assessment of, 2
  definition of, 2
  diagnosis-related group information for, 4-5
  documentation checklist for, 7
  fatigue and, 3
  fluid volume deficit and, 6
  impaired gas exchange and, 2-3
  knowledge deficit and, 7
  noncompliance and, 6
Autism, **231-233**
  altered parenting and, 233
  assessment of, 231
  definition of, 231
  documentation checklist for, 233
  impaired communication and, 231-232
  violence and, 232

B

Biliary atresia, **104-106**
  altered growth and development and, 105
  assessment of, 104
  definition of, 104
  documentation checklist for, 106
  fluid volume deficit and, 104-105
  knowledge deficit and, 105-106
Blood pressure, normal, 305t
Body image disturbance
  anorexia nervosa and, 229
  colostomy and ileostomy and, 286
  Cushing's syndrome and, 218
  Hirschsprung's disease and, 116
  inflammatory bowel disease and, 119
  kidney transplantation and, 154
  liver transplantation and, 127
  rheumatoid arthritis and, 184-185
  spinal cord injury and, 100-101
Body temperature, normal, 305t
BPD. *See* Bronchopulmonary dysplasia.
Breathing pattern, ineffective
  anesthesia and, 255
  croup and, 18-19
  epiglottitis and, 26-27
  head injury and, 63-64
  liver transplantation and, 124

Boldface page numbers refer to major entries; i refers to an illustration; t refers to a table.

Index

Index

Boldface page numbers refer to major entries; i refers to an illustration; t refers to a table.